COMPREHENSIVE EXAM REVIEW

for the Pharmacy Technician

Second Edition

COMPREHENSIVE EXAM REVIEW

for the Pharmacy Technician

Second Edition

Jahangir Moini, MD, MPH, CPhT

Professor and Former Director Allied Health Sciences,
including the Pharmacy Technician Program
Everest University
Melbourne, Florida

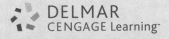
DELMAR
CENGAGE Learning™

Australia • Brazil • Japan • Korea • Mexico • Singapore • Spain • United Kingdom • United States

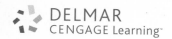
DELMAR
CENGAGE Learning

Comprehensive Exam Review for the Pharmacy Technician, 2nd Edition
Jahangir Moini

Vice President, Career and Professional Editorial: Dave Garza

Director of Learning Solutions: Matt Kane

Senior Acquisitions Editor: Tari Broderick

Managing Editor: Marah Bellegarde

Senior Product Manager: Juliet Steiner

Editorial Assistant: Ian Lewis

Vice President, Career and Professional Marketing: Jennifer Ann Baker

Marketing Director: Wendy Mapstone

Associate Marketing Manager: Jonathan Sheehan

Production Director: Carolyn Miller

Production Manager: Andrew Crouth

Senior Content Project Manager: Kenneth McGrath

Senior Art Director: Jack Pendleton

For product information and technology assistance, contact us at
Cengage Learning Customer & Sales Support, 1-800-354-9706

For permission to use material from this text or product,
submit all requests online at **www.cengage.com/permissions**.
Further permissions questions can be e-mailed to
permissionrequest@cengage.com

Library of Congress Control Number: 2010938581

ISBN-13: 978-1-111-12847-0

ISBN-10: 1-111-12847-2

Delmar
5 Maxwell Drive
Clifton Park, NY 12065-2919
USA

Cengage Learning is a leading provider of customized learning solutions with office locations around the globe, including Singapore, the United Kingdom, Australia, Mexico, Brazil, and Japan. Locate your local office at:
international.cengage.com/region

Cengage Learning products are represented in Canada by Nelson Education, Ltd.

To learn more about Delmar, visit **www.cengage.com/delmar**

Purchase any of our products at your local college store or at our preferred online store **www.cengagebrain.com**

Notice to the Reader

Printed in the United States of America
1 2 3 4 5 6 7 13 12 11 10

Dedication

This book is dedicated to my grand daughter, Laila Mabry.

Contents

SELF-EVALUATION

APPENDICES

Preface

During the past decade, the profession and the practice of pharmacy have been revolutionized. The reasons for this revolution include advanced technology and research, new diseases, new drugs, new treatments, and new health-care systems in the United States. Today, pharmacists and pharmacy technicians have greater responsibilities in the field of medicine. Because of changing health-care systems and the ever-increasing costs of patient care, management of insurance policies and operation of pharmacies have shifted into a new era of responsibility. This revolution has increased and changed the duties of both pharmacists and pharmacy technicians.

Pharmacy technicians must be more knowledgeable and skillful about preparing and dispensing medications in various types of pharmacy settings. Most states now require that pharmacy technicians become certified. To become a certified pharmacy technician, an individual must pass either the:

- Pharmacy Technician Certification Examination (PTCE) or
- Exam for the Certification of Pharmacy Technicians (ExCPT).

The Pharmacy Technician Certification Board (PTCB) administers the PTCE; the Institute for the Certification of Pharmacy Technicians (ICPT), the ExCPT.

SPECIAL FEATURES OF THE TEXT

This text provides a quick but thorough review of the main concepts covered on the two certification exams (PTCE and ExCPT). Each chapter begins with an outline and a glossary to support study and review. Photos, figures, and tables illustrate concepts covered in the review. Chapters end with "Exploring the Web," listing Web sites of interest to which students can link to find out more information, and "Review Questions," consisting of multiple-choice items related to the concepts covered in that chapter only (with answers provided at the back of the text). These items are similar to those found on each of the certification exams. This allows students to focus on topics covered in an individual chapter only, and they can use their performance scores on the chapter review questions to direct their study.

NEW TO THIS EDITION

This second edition of the text has been completely reorganized and has three sections and a total of 20 chapters. Completely revised and updated from the first edition, the three sections reflect the types of questions asked on the certification examinations:

- **Section I:** Introduction and General Knowledge
- **Section II:** Assisting the Pharmacist in Various Settings
- **Section III:** Administration and Management of Pharmacy Practice

At the end of the text are six self-examinations that offer additional questions for thorough practice. Each of these tests contains 100 questions, similar in set up to those on the certification examinations.

In addition, this text contains five appendices:

- **Appendix A: Pharmacy Technician Certification Examination.** Explaining the examination process and how the exams are formatted, Appendix A is designed to be an easy reference for students to ensure better understanding of what they will experience when taking the examination.

- **Appendix B: State Boards of Pharmacy.** Appendix B lists complete contact information for each state's board of pharmacy.

- **Appendix C: Professional Organizations.** Appendix C lists professional organizations and their contact information that relate to the practice of pharmacy.

- **Appendix D: Top 200 Prescription Drugs.** Appendix D lists the Brand and generic names of the top 200 drugs by prescription.

- **Appendix E: Vitamins.** In addition to discussing the benefits of vitamins, as well as vitamin deficiencies and toxicities, Appendix E lists the various fat-soluble and water-soluble vitamins.

The text also features a Glossary, Answer Keys, and an Index, all to support students' comprehension and to help them be successful on the certification examinations.

In addition to its overall reorganization, the text includes several new chapters:

- **Chapter 2: Pharmacy Law and Ethics for Technicians.** Chapter 2 provides updated law information, has an increased emphasis on scheduled drugs, provides detailed explanations of filing systems, and includes new information about hazardous waste disposal.

- **Chapter 4: Structures and Functions of Body Systems.** In the previous edition of the text, the structures and functions of body systems were incorporated into chapters about pharmacology and drug effects on various systems. The new Chapter 4 reorganizes the information so that the anatomy and physiology of the body is contained in just one chapter.

- **Chapter 5: Common Disorders and Conditions.** Chapter 5 uses the same approach as does Chapter 4—the common disorders and conditions are separated from the structures and functions for easier information access and are organized by body system.

- **Chapter 9: Pharmacology.** Following the format of Chapters 4 and 5, Chapter 9 now separates pharmacology information from structures/functions and disorders/conditions and also organizes the information by body system.

- **Chapter 15: Sterile and Nonsterile Compounding.** In the previous edition of the text, only nonsterile compounding was discussed. This expanded chapter now covers essential information about sterile compounding that pharmacy technicians must understand.

- **Chapter 20: Inventory Control and Management.** Chapter 20 includes recent information about inventory control systems, equipment, procedures, and drug formularies.

ANCILLARY MATERIALS

This text also contains a CD that offers a 600 multiple choice-item test bank, consisting of three topic areas similar to those on the certification examinations. These include:

- *Assisting the Pharmacist in Serving Patients* (66% of the questions),

- *Maintaining Medication and Inventory Control Systems* (22%), and

- *Participating in the Administration and Management of Pharmacy* (12%).

Timed and scored, these tests offer students as much practice in taking the same format of examination as they will encounter upon seeking to become certified. Because these exams are randomly generated to match the specifications of the exam, no two tries will be the same. Each quiz is unique, giving students the nearly unlimited opportunity for self-testing and review.

Student Resources

Flashcards for the Pharmacy Technician
ISBN-10: 1-439-05646-3
ISBN-13: 9798-1-4390-5646-2

The Author has also created 600 flash cards that may be purchased separately from this book. These flash cards are highly recommended by the Author for preparing to take the exams.

ACKNOWLEDGMENTS

The author would like to acknowledge the contributions of the following individuals:

Julia Waugaman
Maggie Carpenter, PharmD
Pharmacist Consultant
Melbourne, FL

Mahkameh Moini, DMD
Healthy Smile Dental
West Palm Beach, FL

Stephanie K. Mullen, RN, MSN, CPNP
Pediatric Nurse Practitioner
Cleveland, OH

Susan Neil, MBA, RNP, LMIF
Retired Nurse
Melbourne, FL

Norman Tomaka, CRPh, LHCRM
Pharmacist Consultant
Melbourne, FL

Vincent E. Trunzo, RPh, MSM
Former Director of Pharmacy, Health First Inc.
Holmes Regional Medical Center
Melbourne, FL

Greg Vadimsky, CPhT
Editorial Assistant
Melbourne, FL

From Delmar Cengage Learning: Tari Broderick, Darcy Scelsi, Juliet Steiner, Ian Lewis, Ken McGrath, Jack Pendleton, and Brian Davis.

Reviewers

Christy Bivins
Pharmacy Technology Program Director
North Georgia Tech College
Clarkesville, GA

Linda Calvert
Chair Allied Health/PHT Program Director
Front Range Community College
Westminster, CO

Michael Edwards, BS PharmD
Corporate Director of Pharmacy
Health First, Inc.
Melbourne, FL

Thomas Fridley
Instructor
Long Island University
Brookville, NY

Kathy Kundrat
Instructor
Community College Rhode Island
Warwick, RI

Paula Lambert, BS, MEd, CPhT
Pharmacy Technology Instructor
North Idaho College
Coeur d'Alene, ID

Elina Pierce, MSP, CPhT – ASHP, PTEC, NPA
Program Chair
Southeast Community College
Beatrice, NE

Ateequr Rahman
Associate Professor
Shenandoah University
Winchester, VA

Diana Rangaves, PharmD, Rph
Pharmacy Technician Program Coordinator
Santa Rosa Junior College
Santa Rosa, CA

Dawn Tesner, BS, CPhT
Program Director
Mid Michigan Community College
Harrison, MI

Shannon Trivett
Instructor
Edmonds Community College
Lynnwood, WA

Professor Uyen Thorstensen CPhT, BA, BS
UW Medical Center: Pharmacy Technician
North Seattle Community College
Seattle, WA

Stephanie Weiskind
Pharmacology Instructor
Cuyahoga Community College Eastern
Cleveland, OH

Kristen Zbikowski
Instructor
Hibbing Community College
Hibbing, MN

About the Author

For 9 years, Dr. Moini was assistant professor at Tehran University School of Medicine, where he taught medical and allied health students. A professor and former director (for 15 years) of allied health programs at Everest University (EU), Dr. Moini established several programs at EU's Melbourne campus. He established the Pharmacy Technician Associate Degree Program in 2000 and was the Director of the Pharmacy Technician Program for 5 years.

As a physician and instructor for the past 35 years, Dr. Moini understands the importance of pharmacy technicians in the modern health-care setting. He advocates the importance of pharmacy technicians becoming certified to assist pharmacists in a variety of functions in the pharmacy and to prevent medication errors.

Dr. Moini is actively involved in teaching and helping students prepare for service in various health professions. He worked with the Brevard County Health Department as an epidemiologist and health educator consultant for 18 years. Since 1999, he has been an internationally published author of various allied health books.

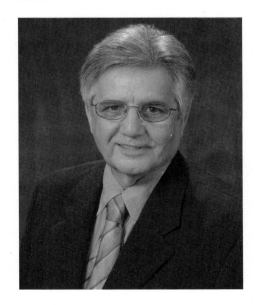

Pharmacy Technicians and Professional Organizations

OUTLINE

GLOSSARY

Drug control – a method of ensuring optimal safety in the distribution and use of medications by providing knowledge, procedures, controls, ethics, and other standards

Pharmaceutical care – the provision of drug therapy for the purpose of achieving the improvement of a patient's quality of life, which includes the prediction, detection, and resolution of drug therapy-related problems

Pharmacist – an individual who is educated and licensed to dispense drugs and to provide drug information to patients and other health-care providers

Pharmacy – the art and science of dispensing and preparing medication and providing drug-related information to the public

Pharmacy technician – an individual who helps licensed pharmacists provide medications and other health-care products to patients

Pharmacy Technician Certification Board – a national organization that provides certification to pharmacy technicians based on a national examination and on continuing education

PHARMACEUTICAL CARE

The current philosophy or approach to professional practice in pharmacy is referred to as pharmaceutical care. This concept holds that pharmacists have the important role of ensuring *the responsible provision of drug therapy for the purpose of achieving definite outcomes that improve a patient's quality of life.* It also includes the prediction, detection, and resolution of drug therapy-related problems. A pharmacist, then, is one who is educated and licensed to dispense drugs and to provide drug information to patients and other health-care providers. Experts in their field, pharmacists are the most accessible members of today's health-care team. Together with pharmacists' intensive knowledge of drugs and continual professional development, advances in medical progress, commerce, and technology have made pharmacy and pharmaceutical care even more important throughout the modern world.

The Profession of Pharmacy

The profession of pharmacy, as with other lawful occupations, involves positive benefits to society and a specialized body of knowledge. Practitioners perform highly useful social and health care-related functions. Working in the field of pharmacy is considered a socially useful profession, but social utility alone does not make an occupation a profession. Pharmacists are not professionals because they have good keying skills. Rather, their relevant professional knowledge about medications, patient care, and interactions of drugs sets pharmacists apart from other health-care professionals.

Pharmacists advise patients and prescribers concerning drug therapy, are alert for potential drug interactions, select appropriate product sources, and exercise professional judgment. The latter is an essential skill to the profession of pharmacy. In addition to these duties, pharmacists possess specific attitudes that also influence their professional behavior. Professionals are concerned with issues and practices that are vital to the health or well-being of their patients.

The Practice of Pharmacy

Pharmacy is the art and science of dispensing and preparing medications and providing drug-related information to the public. It involves interpreting prescription orders; compounding, labeling, and dispensing drugs and devices; selecting drug products and conducting drug utilization reviews; monitoring patients and intervening in their prescriptions of drugs as necessary; and providing cognitive services related to use of medications and devices. Today, pharmaceutical care is a necessary element of total health care. The doctorate of pharmacy (PharmD) degree curriculum usually requires six academic years to complete.

Pharmaceutical Testing, Analysis, and Control

Developing methods for standardizing and controlling medicines is vital. Control is a method used to eliminate or reduce the potential harm of the drug distributed. Drug control provides knowledge, understanding, judgments, procedures, skills, controls, and ethics that ensure optimal safety in the distribution and use of medications. In manufacturing laboratories, pharmacists often perform physical and chemical analyses either in the course of developing dosage forms of new products or in the control of standard products.

In small laboratories, pharmacy staff members may have the responsibility for performing analyses. However, even if pharmacists do not conduct analyses, they should at a minimum understand the basic principles involved in the standardization and control of the medicinal agents dispensed. The use of an analytical method is justified only after it has been proved to be valid, accurate, and selective. Drug control is the most important goal for medications that patients may take.

PHARMACY TECHNICIANS

To keep up with the increasing demand for pharmaceutical products and services, pharmacy technicians play a vital role in supporting pharmaceutical care.

A **pharmacy technician** helps licensed pharmacists provide medications and other health-care products to patients. Technicians usually perform routine tasks, such as counting tablets and labeling bottles, to help prepare prescribed medications for patients. Although technicians refer questions regarding prescriptions, drug information, or health issues to a pharmacist, they can, however, answer all questions that do not require professional judgment.

Two-thirds of all pharmacy technician jobs in the United States are in retail pharmacies; one-third, in hospitals. Pharmacy technicians who work in retail pharmacies have varying responsibilities, depending on the rules and regulations of the state in which they are working. If they work in hospitals, pharmacy technicians have additional responsibilities. In a hospital setting, they also read patient charts and prepare and deliver the medications to patients. Of course, the pharmacist must check the order before the technician can dispense the medication to the patient. Pharmacy technicians may also assemble a 24-hour supply of a medication for patients in an institutional setting.

National Certification Exams

Certification (via the two available national exams) is a valuable component for a pharmacy technician's career. The **Pharmacy Technician Certification Board (PTCB)** offers a standardized national exam that evaluates knowledge and competency in basic functions of and activities performed in the pharmacy. Skills are measured in three general areas:

1. Assisting the pharmacist in serving patients

2. Maintaining medication and inventory control systems

3. Participating in the administration and management of the pharmacy

The exam, which lasts for two hours, contains 90 multiple-choice questions. Ten of these questions, distributed randomly, are "pretest" questions used for statistical information for future exams and do not count toward the final score. The questions are not presented in distinct or separate sections relating to the three general areas being tested. Rather, they are presented randomly throughout the exam. A score of at least 650 (of a possible 300 to 900) is required to pass. The latest pricing information can be found at http://www.ptcb.org.

Another national exam for certification is the ExCPT exam, which the National Healthcareer Association (NHA) offers. Similar to the PTCB exam in content, the ExCPT exam contains 110 multiple-choice questions with ten of them being unscored and used for statistical information. The exam is given on computer and lasts for two hours. The latest pricing information can be found at http://www.nationaltechexam.org.

Assisting the Pharmacist in Serving Patients

Questions that address assisting pharmacists in serving patients make up more than 50% of the exam. This portion covers both retail and hospital settings. Technicians must prepare themselves for questions about interpretation of the prescription order; the structure and use of the patient profile; and the dispensing, labeling, storage, and delivery of medications. Questions related to this area also include drug calculations.

Maintaining Medication and Inventory Control Systems

Also on the exam are questions that address maintaining medications and inventory control systems. Accounting for nearly 25% of the exam, these include questions about storing medications in the pharmacy, the ordering and inventory process, prepackaging and unit dose distribution, labeling, and record keeping.

Participating in the Administration and Management of the Pharmacy

Making up the remainder of the exam are questions that test knowledge about participating in the administration and management of the pharmacy. These questions deal with topics such as safety, cleanliness, infection control, pharmacy law, communications, and computers.

Continuing Education

Pharmacy technicians must renew their certifications every two years. To become eligible for recertification, certified pharmacy technicians (CPhTs) must meet requirements of 20 contact hours of pharmacy-related continuing education. At least one contact hour must be in pharmacy law. Pharmacy technicians can accomplish this requirement through various means, such as educational meetings, seminars, workshops, and conventions. If employed under the direct supervision and instruction of a pharmacist, a pharmacy technician can earn up to 10 contact hours.

Continuing education is a lifelong process. The annual American Association of Pharmacy Technicians (AAPT) or National Pharmacy Technician Association (NPTA) convention provides an excellent forum for attaining knowledge through its educational offerings and for networking with other pharmacy technicians.

PROFESSIONAL ORGANIZATIONS

Similar to other professionals, people in the pharmaceutical care industry have created organizations or associations to advance the purposes of their professions. The better-known organizations in the pharmacy profession are discussed in the following sections. Many of these organizations have both state and local branches.

Accreditation Council for Pharmacy Education

The Accreditation Council for Pharmacy Education (ACPE), founded in 1932, is the national accrediting agency for pharmacy education programs recognized by the Secretary of Education.

American Association of Colleges of Pharmacy

As the national organization representing the interests of pharmaceutical education and educators, the American Association of Colleges of Pharmacy (AACP), established in 1900, represents all 112 pharmacy colleges and schools in the United States. The AACP publishes the *American Journal of Pharmaceutical Education*, a monthly newsletter, and other publications.

American Association of Pharmaceutical Scientists

Formerly an academy of the American Pharmacists Association, the American Association of Pharmaceutical Scientists (AAPS) represents pharmaceutical scientists employed in academia, industry, government, and other research institutions. Members can access the full article content of three journals: *Pharmaceutical Research*, *The AAPS Journal,* and *AAPS PharmSciTech*. The AAPS is also affiliated with (or sponsors) other journals.

American Association of Pharmacy Technicians

The AAPT, formerly called the APT, was founded in 1979. A national organization, AAPT has chapters in many states, represents pharmacy technicians, and promotes certification of technicians. The association has established a code of ethics for pharmacy technicians.

American College of Clinical Pharmacology

The American College of Clinical Pharmacology (ACCP) is a professional and scientific society that provides leadership, education, advocacy, and resources for clinical pharmacists.

American Pharmacists Association

The largest of the national pharmacy organizations, the American Pharmacists Association (APhA) consists of three academies: the Academy of Pharmacy Practice and Management (APhA-APPM), the Academy of Pharmaceutical Research and Science (APhA-APRS), and the Academy of Students of Pharmacy (APhA-APS). The APhA publishes the bimonthly *Journal of the American Pharmacists Association*, the monthly *Pharmacy Today Newsletter*, and the monthly *Journal of Pharmaceutical Sciences*.

The APhA also operates a political action committee, or PAC. According to the APhA, its mission is "to advocate the interests of pharmacists; influence the profession, government, and others in addressing essential pharmaceutical care issues; promote the highest professional and ethical standards; and foster science and research in support of the practice of pharmacy." (American Pharmacists Association (APhA) (n.d.). In *EMC/paradigm: College resource center: Health careers: Readings in subject area: Resources*. Retrieved March 30, 2010, from http://www.emcp.com).

American Society of Health-System Pharmacists

The American Society of Health-System Pharmacists (ASHP) represents pharmacists who practice in hospitals, health maintenance organizations (HMOs), long-term care facilities, home care agencies, and other institutions. A large national organization, the ASHP accredits pharmacy residency and pharmacy technician training programs. The ASHP publishes the *American Journal of Health-System Pharmacy*.

United States Drug Enforcement Administration

The U.S. Drug Enforcement Administration (DEA) enforces federal laws and regulations governing controlled substances.

United States Food and Drug Administration

The U.S. Food and Drug Administration (FDA) has the primary responsibility for creating regulations governing the safety of foods, drugs, and cosmetics.

The FDA enforces the Food, Drug, and Cosmetic Act of 1938 and its subsequent amendments, oversees new drug development, approves or disapproves applications to market new drugs, monitors reports of adverse reactions, and has the authority to recall drugs deemed dangerous.

Pharmacy Technician Certification Board

The Pharmacy Technician Certification Board (PTCB) administers the Pharmacy Technician Certification Examination (PTCE). Anyone who wishes to be a certified pharmacy technician in the United States voluntarily takes the PTCE. The PTCB also oversees a recertification program for technicians.

Pharmacy Technician Educators Council

The Pharmacy Technician Educators Council (PTEC) is an association of educators who prepare people for careers as pharmacy technicians. Its official publication is the *Journal of Pharmacy Technology*.

United States Pharmacopeia

A nonprofit organization, the U.S. Pharmacopeia (USP) sets standards for the identity, strength, quality, purity, packaging, and labeling of drug products. The USP also provides drug information online.

JOB OUTLOOK

For pharmacy technicians with formal training or previous experience, good job opportunities are expected for full-time and part-time work. As a result from the expansion of retail pharmacies and other employment settings and from the need to replace workers who leave the field, employment of pharmacy technicians is expected to increase by 25% from 2008 to 2018, which is much higher than the average for other occupations. This increase will result from the greater pharmaceutical needs of a larger and older population. The increased number of middle-aged and elderly people, who average more prescription drugs than do younger people, will spur demand for pharmacy technicians in all practice settings. In addition, the shortage of pharmacists will increase the demand for pharmacy technicians.

With advances in science, newer medications are becoming available to treat more health conditions. Cost-conscious insurers, pharmacies, and health systems will continue to emphasize the role of pharmacy technicians. As a result, pharmacy technicians will assume responsibility for more routine tasks that pharmacists previously performed. Pharmacy technicians also will need to learn and master new pharmacy technology as it surfaces. For example, robotic machines can dispense medications into containers, but pharmacy technicians must oversee the machines, stock the bins, and label the containers. Although it is increasingly incorporated into the job, automation will not necessarily reduce the need for pharmacy technicians.

EXPLORING THE WEB

Visit http://www.acpe-accredit.org for information about the Accreditation Council of Pharmacy Education.

Visit http://www.aacp.org to learn more about the American Association of Colleges of Pharmacy.

Visit http://www.aapspharmaceutica.com for more information on the American Association of Pharmaceutical Scientists.

Visit http://www.pharmacytechnician.com to learn about the American Association of Pharmacy Technicians.

Visit http://www.accp1.org for more information about the American College of Clinical Pharmacology.

Visit http://www.pharmacist.com to learn more about the American Pharmacists Association.

Visit http://www.ashp.org for more information on the American Society of Health-System Pharmacists.

Visit http://www.bls.gov/oco/ocos325.htm to learn more about the Bureau of Labor Statistics and about pharmacy technicians and aides.

Visit http://www.nationaltechexam.org/excptinfo.html for information on the exam for the Certification of Pharmacy Technicians.

Visit https://www.freece.com/freece/index.asp to learn about free online education for the healthcare profession.

Visit http://www.ptcb.org for more information about the Pharmacy Technician Certification Board.

Visit http://www.rxptec.org to learn about the Pharmacy Technician Educators Council.

Visit http://www.justice.gov/dea/index.htm for more information on the U.S. Drug Enforcement Administration.

Visit http://www.fda.gov to learn about the U.S. Food and Drug Administration.

Visit http://www.usp.org for more information about the U.S. Pharmacopeia.

REVIEW QUESTIONS

1. Which agency administers the national testing of pharmacy technicians?

   A. Illinois Council of Health-System Pharmacists
   B. American Society of Health-System Pharmacists
   C. Pharmacy Technician Certification Board
   D. National American Pharmacy Technicians

2. To be eligible for recertification, a pharmacy technician must complete:

   A. 10 contact hours every two years in pharmacy-related study
   B. 10 contact hours in pharmacy law
   C. 20 contact hours every two years in pharmacy-related study, including one contact hour in pharmacy law
   D. 40 contact hours that are not required for recertification

3. Pharmacists are those who are educated and licensed to:

   A. dispense drugs and provide drug information
   B. dispense information but not drugs
   C. dispense alternative remedies rather than the drugs prescribed
   D. test pharmacy technicians and provide their certification

4. The key traits of professionals in the pharmacy include all of the following except:

   A. using proper judgment
   B. having good keying skills
   C. having specific attitudes that influence professional behavior
   D. possessing relevant professional knowledge about drugs

5. Pharmacy is:

   A. the art of drug therapy
   B. only about drug product selection
   C. exclusively about interpreting prescriptions from doctors' handwriting
   D. the art and science of dispensing and preparing medication and providing drug-related information to the public

6. The most important goal for a patient's medication is:

   A. that it be inexpensive
   B. drug control
   C. that it be easy to open
   D. drug therapy

7. Pharmacy technicians perform routine tasks such as:

   A. prescribing medications
   B. counting tablets and labeling bottles
   C. referring questions to medical assistants
   D. counting patients and giving out free samples

8. On the national pharmacy technician certification exams, more than 50% of the questions concern:

   A. medication distribution and inventory control
   B. the Pharmacy Technician Certification Board
   C. pharmacy operations
   D. assisting the pharmacist in serving patients

9. *AAPT* stands for:

   A. American Association of Pharmaceutical Terminology
   B. Automatic Accreditation of Pharmacy Technicians
   C. American Association of Pharmacy Technicians
   D. American Association of Pharmaceutical Torts

10. Which government bureau enforces federal laws and regulations related to controlled substances?

   A. Drug Enforcement Administration
   B. Food and Drug Administration
   C. Drug Donors Administration
   D. Licensure Surety Division

CHAPTER 2

Pharmacy Law and Ethics for Technicians

OUTLINE

Regulatory Agencies

Bureau of Alcohol, Tobacco, Firearms and Explosives (ATF)

Centers for Disease Control and Prevention (CDC)

Centers for Medicare and Medicaid Services (CMS)

Drug Enforcement Agency (DEA)

Environmental Protection Agency (EPA)

Food and Drug Administration (FDA)

The Joint Commission (JCAHO)

National Association of the Boards of Pharmacy (NABP)

State Boards of Pharmacy (BOP)

United States Pharmacopeia (USP)

The Ethical Foundation of Pharmacy

GLOSSARY

Bioethics – a discipline dealing with the ethical and moral implications of biological research and applications

Ethics – the branch of philosophy that deals with the distinction between right and wrong and with the moral consequences of human actions

Law – a principle or rule that is advisable or obligatory to observe

National Drug Code (NDC) – a unique and permanent product code assigned to each new drug as it becomes available in the marketplace; identifying the manufacturer or distributor, the drug formulation, and the size and type of its packaging

National Formulary (NF) – a database of officially recognized drug names

Standards – established by authority, custom, or general consent as a model or example; something set up and established by authority as a rule for the measure of quantity, weight, extent, value, or quality

U.S. Pharmacopeia (USP) – a database of drugs and their preparation that serves as the standard for drugs used in the United States

LAW AND ETHICS IN PHARMACY

Laws, standards, and ethics exercise controls on pharmacy and drugs. A law is a rule or regulation that a governing body establishes and enacts both to protect society as a whole and to maintain order and standards of living. The study of values or principles, ethics govern personal relationships and determine whether actions are right or wrong. Based on morals, particular behaviors or rules of conduct, ethics are formed through the influences of family, culture, and society.

Professional organizations establish standards, or guidelines for practice. Professionals in a particular area of practice share a common philosophy (a basic viewpoint or shared beliefs, concepts, attitudes, and values) that dictates the etiquette, or standards of behavior, considered appropriate for that profession. The philosophy and etiquette established within a profession drive the standards that are established for the profession. Pharmacists and pharmacy technicians are responsible for upholding legal and ethical standards in their profession.

GOVERNING BODIES

Federal, state, and local governments create and uphold laws. In the United States, the federal government has three branches:

1. The legislative branch consists of the Congress (that is, the House of Representatives and the Senate) and is responsible for creating laws.

2. The executive branch enforces the laws and consists of the president, vice president, cabinets, and various smaller organizations.

3. The judicial branch interprets the laws and consists of the Supreme Court and lower federal courts.

The federal government creates, issues, and interprets laws for the general population. State and local governments are responsible for determining the specifics of certain laws within their jurisdictions. Regulatory agencies are government-based departments that create specific rules about what is and is not legal within a specific field or area of expertise. The regulatory agency for the field of pharmacy is the U.S. Food and Drug Administration (FDA), which is a branch of the Department of Health and Human Services. Among other services, the FDA regulates all drugs with the exception of illegal drugs. Once the FDA recognizes them, drugs are substances (or components of medications) that health-care professionals can use to diagnose, treat, or prevent disease.

Drugs differ from supplements, which the FDA considers as "foods." Supplements are dietary substances used to augment, enhance, or enrich a patient's nutritional status. Initiating, implementing, and enforcing all legislation pertaining to drug administration, the FDA is responsible for the approval of drugs, labeling of over-the-counter (OTC) and prescription drugs, and standards for drug manufacturing.

Pharmacy Laws, Regulations, and Agencies

Local, state, and federal governments enforce a series of rules, regulations, and laws that regulate pharmacy practice. In 1906, the U.S. Congress passed the first laws to regulate the development, compounding, distribution, storage, and dispensing of drugs.

Pure Food and Drug Act of 1906

The purpose of the Pure Food and Drug Act of 1906 was to forbid the interstate distribution or sale of adulterated and misbranded food and drugs. The act did not require that drugs be labeled, only that the label could not contain false information about the strength or purity of the drug. Therefore, after amendment, the act proved unenforceable, and new legislation was required. In 1937, the need for new legislation was tragically demonstrated when 107 people died after taking a sulfa drug product that contained diethylene glycol, used today as an antifreeze for automobile radiators.

Food, Drug, and Cosmetic Act of 1938

The Food, Drug, and Cosmetic Act (FD&C Act) of 1938 created the FDA and required pharmaceutical manufacturers to file a New Drug Application with the FDA. Under this act, manufacturers must maintain the purity, strength, effectiveness, safety, and packaging of drugs, foods, and cosmetics. The act empowers the FDA to approve or deny new drug applications, to conduct inspections to ensure compliance, to approve the investigational use of drugs on humans, and to ensure that all approved drugs are safe and effective. Any adverse reaction to a drug should be reported to the FDA. It is important to note that just because a drug is considered "safe" does not mean that it is without risks. When people use drugs as directed, the FDA emphasizes or upholds their safety.

Durham-Humphrey Amendment of 1951

The Durham-Humphrey Amendment of 1951 states that drug containers do not have to include "adequate directions for use," as long as they bear the legend "Caution: Federal law prohibits dispensing without a prescription." The pharmacist's dispensing of the drug with a label giving directions from the practitioner meets the law's requirements. Therefore, this amendment established the difference between legend (prescription) drugs and OTC (over-the-counter or nonprescription) drugs and authorized the acceptance of verbal prescriptions and the refilling of prescriptions.

Kefauver-Harris Amendment of 1962

The Kefauver-Harris Amendment of 1962 was passed in response to reports of severe birth defects in infants born to mothers who had taken the tranquilizer thalidomide. The act extended the FDA's requirement that drug products, both prescription and nonprescription, be shown to be effective and safe. At this time, provisions were added to the act concerning factory inspections and clinical studies, and the responsibility for regulating prescription drug advertising was shifted from the Federal Trade Commission (FTC) to the FDA.

Comprehensive Drug Abuse Prevention and Control Act of 1970

Known as the Controlled Substance Act (CSA), the Comprehensive Drug Abuse Prevention and Control Act of 1970 controls the manufacture, importation, sale, and distribution of drugs that have the potential for addiction and abuse. Drugs with a strong potential for abuse are identified, and their manufacture and distribution are monitored closely. Under this act, drugs are classified with potential for abuse into five types, or schedules (see Table 2–1).

The Drug Enforcement Administration (DEA), an arm of the Department of Justice, is primarily charged with enforcing laws and regulations related to the abuse of controlled substances, both legal and illegal. The DEA manages most of its funds and personnel toward preventing the illegal trafficking of Schedule I drugs. The agency also has responsibilities regarding the legal use of narcotics and other controlled substances. The DEA issues practitioners and pharmacies a license (number) that enables them to write prescriptions for scheduled drugs and, in the case of a pharmacy, order scheduled drugs from wholesalers. Pharmacists must use a special form— the DEA Form 222 (see Figure 2–1)—when ordering Schedule II narcotics.

DEA Registration for Controlled Substances

The DEA requires all nonexempt individuals who manufacture, dispense, or distribute any controlled substance to register. Pharmacy registrations with the DEA last for three years. The DEA assigns specific numbers to controlled substance distributors, manufacturers, wholesalers, and practitioners (who

TABLE 2–1 Drug Schedules

Schedule	Abuse Potential	Prescription Requirement	Examples
I	High abuse potential; no accepted medical use	No prescription permitted	Heroin, LSD, marijuana, mescaline, peyote, PCP, hashish, and amphetamine variants
II	High abuse potential; accepted medical use	Prescription required; no refills permitted without a new written prescription	Cocaine, codeine, amphetamine salts (Adderall), Desoxyn, methadone hydrochloride, morphine, opium, codeine, methylphenidate (Ritalin), meperidine (Demerol), and secobarbital (Seconal)
III	Moderate abuse potential; accepted medical use	Prescription required; 5 refills permitted in 6 months	Certain drugs compounded with small quantities of narcotics, other drugs with high potential for abuse (Tylenol or Empirin with codeine tablets), and certain barbiturates such as butabarbital (Butisol)
IV	Low abuse potential; accepted medical use	Prescription required; 5 refills permitted in 6 months	Barbital, chloral hydrate (Noctec), diazepam (Valium), chlordiazepoxide (Librium), pentazocine hydrochloride (Talwin), and propoxyphene (Darvon)
V	Low abuse potential; accepted medical use	No prescription required for individuals 18 or older	Cough syrups with codeine, diphenoxylate hydrochloride with atropine sulfate (Lomotil), and kaolin/pectin/opium (Parepectolin)

BLANK DEA FORM-222
U.S. OFFICIAL ORDER FORM—SCHEDULES I & II

See Reverse of PURCHASER'S Copy for Instructions	No order form may be issued for Schedules I and II substances unless a completed application form has been received, (21 CFR 1305.04).	OMB APPROVAL NO. 1117-0010

TO: *(Name of Supplier)* · STREET ADDRESS

CITY and STATE	DATE	TO BE FILLED IN BY SUPPLIER
		SUPPLIERS DEA REGISTRATION No.

LINE No.	No. of Packages	Size of Packages	Name of Item	National Drug Code	Packages Shipped	Date Shipped
	TO BE FILLED IN BY PURCHASER					
1						
2						
3						
4						
5						
6						
7						
8						
9						
10						

NO. OF LINES COMPLETED	SIGNATURE OF PURCHASER OR HIS ATTORNEY OR AGENT

Date Issued	DEA Registration No.	Name and Address of Registrant

Schedules
2, 2N, 3, 3N, 4, 5

Registered as a PHARMACY	No. of this Order Form

DEA Form-222   **U.S. OFFICIAL ORDER FORMS—SCHEDULES I & II**
DRUG ENFORCEMENT ADMINISTRATION
SUPPLIER'S COPY 1

Figure 2–1 DEA Form 222. (*Courtesy of DEA*)

may be dentists, physicians, scientists, veterinarians, hospitals, and pharmacies). All pharmacies must have a valid DEA registration, in accordance with state and federal laws. Registration requires the use of DEA Form 224 (see Figure 2–2). If a registrant is not the same person who either controls the pharmacy's operations or who orders the controlled substances, a Power of Attorney form may be used and must be kept on file for two years.

Regulation of Controlled Substances

Each state regulates the medical professionals who may prescribe controlled substances. If authorized, an individual may apply for a DEA number. In certain states, certified nurse practitioners and optometrists can prescribe controlled substances. Various CSA regulations govern record keeping, physician registration, pharmacy registration, and controlled substance inventories. Any ambulatory

Form-224

APPLICATION FOR REGISTRATION
Under the Controlled Substances Act

APPROVED OMB NO 1117-0014
FORM DEA-224 (10-06)
Previous editions are obsolete

INSTRUCTIONS

Save time - apply on-line at www.deadiversion.usdoj.gov

1. To apply by mail complete this application. Keep a copy for your records.
2. Print clearly, using black or blue ink, or use a typewriter.
3. Mail this form to the address provided in Section 7 or use enclosed envelope.
4. Include the correct payment amount. FEE IS NON-REFUNDABLE.
5. If you have any questions call 800-882-9539 prior to submitting your application.

IMPORTANT: DO NOT SEND THIS APPLICATION **AND** APPLY ON-LINE.

DEA OFFICIAL USE :

Do you have other DEA registration numbers?

☐ NO   ☐ YES

MAIL-TO ADDRESS

Please print mailing address changes to the right of the address in this box.

**FEE FOR THREE (3) YEARS IS $551
FEE IS NON-REFUNDABLE**

SECTION 1   APPLICANT IDENTIFICATION   ☐ **Individual Registration**   ☐ **Business Registration**

Name 1   (Last Name of individual -OR- Business or Facility Name)

Name 2   (First Name and Middle Name of individual - OR- Continuation of business name)

Street Address Line 1 (if applying for fee exemption, this must be address of the fee exempt institution)

Address Line 2

City   State   Zip Code

Business Phone Number   Point of Contact

Business Fax Number   Email Address

DEBT COLLECTION INFORMATION

Mandatory pursuant to Debt Collection Improvements Act

Social Security Number (*if registration is for individual*)   Tax Identification Number (*if registration is for business*)

Provide SSN or TIN.
See additional information note #3 on page 4.

FOR Practitioner or MLP ONLY:

Professional Degree : *select from list only*   Professional School :   Year of Graduation :

National Provider Identification: Date of Birth (*MM-DD-YYYY*):

M M - D D - Y Y Y Y

**SECTION 2
BUSINESS ACTIVITY**

Check one business activity box only

☐ Central Fill Pharmacy
☐ Retail Pharmacy
☐ Nursing Home
☐ Automated Dispensing System

☐ Practitioner (DDS, DMD, DO, DPM, DVM, MD or PHD)
☐ Practitioner Military (DDS, DMD, DO, DPM, DVM, MD or PHD)
☐ Mid-level Practitioner (MLP) (DOM, HMD, MP, ND, NP, OD, PA, or RPH)
☐ Euthanasia Technician

☐ Ambulance Service
☐ Animal Shelter
☐ Hospital/Clinic
☐ Teaching Institution

FOR Automated Dispensing System (ADS) ONLY: DEA Registration # of Retail Pharmacy for this ADS

An ADS is automatically fee-exempt.
Skip Section 6 and Section 7 on page 2.
You must attach a notorized affidavit.

**SECTION 3
DRUG SCHEDULES**

Check all that apply

☐ Schedule II Narcotic
☐ Schedule II Non-Narcotic

☐ Schedule III Narcotic
☐ Schedule III Non-Narcotic

☐ Schedule IV
☐ Schedule V

☐ Check this box if you require official order forms - for purchase or transfer of schedule 2 narcotic and/or schedule 2 non-narcotic controlled substances.

NEW - Page 1

Figure 2–2 DEA Form 224. (*Courtesy of DEA*)

SECTION 4

STATE LICENSE(S)

You MUST be currently authorized to prescribe, distribute, dispense, conduct research, or otherwise handle the controlled substances in the schedules for which you are applying under the laws of the **state** or jurisdiction in which you are operating or propose to operate.

Be sure to include both state license numbers if applicable

State License Number (required)

Expiration Date (required)   / / ____
MM - DD - YYYY

What state was this license issued in? _____

State Controlled Substance License Number (if required)

Expiration Date   / / ____
MM - DD - YYYY

What state was this license issued in? _____

SECTION 5

LIABILITY

IMPORTANT

All questions in this section must be answered.

1. Has the applicant ever been **convicted of a crime** in connection with controlled substance(s) under state or federal law, or is any such action pending?   YES ☐   NO ☐

Date(s) of incident MM-DD-YYYY: ☐☐-☐☐-☐☐☐☐

2. Has the applicant ever surrendered (for cause) or had a **federal** controlled substance registration revoked, suspended, restricted, or denied, or is any such action pending?   YES ☐   NO ☐

Date(s) of incident MM-DD-YYYY: ☐☐-☐☐-☐☐☐☐

3. Has the applicant ever surrendered (for cause) or had a **state** professional license or controlled substance registration revoked, suspended, denied, restricted, or placed on probation, or is any such action pending?   YES ☐   NO ☐

Date(s) of incident MM-DD-YYYY: ☐☐-☐☐-☐☐☐☐

4. If the applicant is a **corporation** (other than a corporation whose stock is owned and traded by the public), association, partnership, or pharmacy, has any officer, partner, stockholder, or proprietor been **convicted of a crime** in connection with controlled substance(s) under state or federal law, or ever surrendered, for cause, or had a **federal** controlled substance registration revoked, suspended, restricted, denied, or ever had a **state** professional license or controlled substance registration revoked, suspended, denied, restricted or placed on probation, or is any such action pending?   YES ☐   NO ☐

Date(s) of incident MM-DD-YYYY: ☐☐-☐☐-☐☐☐☐   *Note: If question 4 does not apply to you, be sure to mark 'NO'. It will slow down processing of your application if you leave it blank.*

EXPLANATION OF "YES" ANSWERS

Applicants who have answered "YES" to any of the four questions above **must provide a statement to explain each "YES" answer.**

Use this space or attach a separate sheet and return with application

Liability question # _____   Location(s) of incident: _____

Nature of incident:

Disposition of incident:

SECTION 6   EXEMPTION FROM APPLICATION FEE

☐ Check this box if the applicant is a federal, state, or local government official or institution. Does not apply to contractor-operated institutions.

Business or Facility Name of Fee Exempt Institution. **Be sure to enter the address of this exempt institution in Section 1.**

The undersigned hereby certifies that the applicant named hereon is a federal, state or local government official or institution, and is exempt from payment of the application fee.

FEE EXEMPT CERTIFIER

Provide the name and phone number of the certifying official

Signature of certifying official (**other than applicant**)   Date

Print or type name and title of certifying official   Telephone No. (required for verification)

SECTION 7

METHOD OF PAYMENT

Check one form of payment only

☐ Check   Make check payable to: **Drug Enforcement Administration**   See page 4 of instructions for important information.

☐ American Express ☐ Discover ☐ Master Card ☐ Visa

Credit Card Number   Expiration Date ☐☐-☐☐

Sign if paying by credit card

Signature of Card Holder

Printed Name of Card Holder

Mail this form with payment to:

U.S. Department of Justice
Drug Enforcement Administration
P.O. Box 28083
Washington, DC 20038-8083

FEE IS NON-REFUNDABLE

SECTION 8

APPLICANT'S SIGNATURE

Sign in ink

I certify that the foregoing information furnished on this application is true and correct.

Signature of applicant (sign in ink)   Date

Print or type name and title of applicant

WARNING: Section 843(a)(4)(A) of Title 21, United States Code states that any person who knowingly or intentionally furnishes false or fraudulent information in the application is subject to imprisonment for not more than four years, a fine of not more than $30,000, or both.

NEW - Page 2

Figure 2–2 DEA Form 224 (continued). (*Courtesy of DEA*)

care setting must keep complete, accurate records concerning the purchase, storage, management, and distribution of controlled substances. Also, pharmacy technicians and pharmacists must understand their state's legal requirements concerning controlled substances.

Ordering Controlled Substances

To order Schedule II controlled substances, pharmacists must use DEA Form 222. Anyone who orders controlled substances must have a DEA license. Orders for Schedule III, IV, or V substances do not require a Form 222 and can be ordered directly from manufacturers and other registrants. When filling out Form 222, pharmacists must include the following information: company name and address, order date, number of packages of each item, size of package of each item, name of each item, purchaser's signature or that of his or her attorney or agent, and the DEA registration number. Pharmacists may order a maximum of 10 items on one Form 222.

When they receive an order form, suppliers must add the following information: their DEA number, the National Drug Code (NDC) of each item, an indication of the packages being shipped, and the date of each shipment. Suppliers can only ship to the purchaser's address as it is listed on Form 222 and on the DEA certificate and cannot process an incorrectly completed form. If the Form 222 is incomplete, then the pharmacist must complete and submit a new form. For partial shipments, suppliers must ship the balance of these orders within 60 days of the original order date. The new "e222" form, an electronic version of Form 222, can reduce errors and paperwork. To access the e222, go to: http://www.deadiversion.usdoj.gov.

Prescriptions for Controlled Substances

Practitioners must issue controlled substance prescriptions for valid medical purposes only. Unless they have an emergency situation, practitioners cannot fax or call in Schedule II drug prescriptions. Although Schedule II prescriptions cannot be refilled, Schedule III or IV substances have restrictions concerning refills. "E-prescribing," the use of electronic prescribing technology, reduces errors and fraud and increases accuracy of controlled substance prescribing. When ordering these substances from a warehouse, pharmacists must always use DEA Form 222.

Filling Prescriptions for Controlled Substances

Schedule II prescriptions must be signed in ink. After seven days, practitioners must submit a new prescription if they prescribe additional quantities for their patients. Oral prescriptions are allowed only in emergencies. The prescriber must submit a written follow-up to an oral prescription to the pharmacy within 72 hours. Pharmacies must maintain controlled substance prescriptions in either a three-file, a two-file, or an alternate two-file system. These systems may be defined as follows:

- Three-file system: one file for all Schedule II prescriptions; one for all Schedule III, IV, and V prescriptions; and one for all other types of prescriptions.

- Two-file system: one file for Schedule II prescriptions and one for Schedule III, IV, and V prescriptions.

- Alternate two-file system: one file for all controlled drug prescriptions and one for prescription orders for all noncontrolled drugs that are dispensed.

Labeling of Controlled Substances

State and federal laws require controlled substance labels to contain the following information: the dispensing pharmacist's name and address, pharmacy name, drug serial number, the date the prescription was filled, the prescriber's name, the patient's name, directions for use, and any cautionary statements. Some states require the telephone number of the pharmacy and other information to be included also. Controlled substance containers must have a special manufacturer symbol printed on their stock bottles showing the schedule to which the medication belongs. These symbols include: CI or C-I, CII or C-II, CIII or C-III, CIV or C-IV, and CV or C-V. Schedule II,

III, and IV drugs must bear the legend: "Federal law prohibits the transfer of this drug to any person other than the patient for whom it is prescribed."

Distribution

Although the DEA requires separate registrations for the activities of manufacturing, distributing, dispensing, or research, a pharmacy that is registered to dispense controlled substances can distribute certain amounts of controlled substances to physicians, hospitals, nursing homes, or other pharmacies without separate registration as a distributor. In these cases, the following conditions apply:

- The pharmacy or practitioner receiving the controlled substances must be listed with the DEA.

- The pharmacy or pharmacist must use Form 222 to transfer Schedule I or II substances.

- The pharmacy or pharmacist must record the distribution, and the pharmacist or practitioner must record the receipt of the substances.

- The total number of dosage units cannot exceed 5% of all controlled substances that the pharmacy dispenses during the one-year period in which it is registered. Any more units than the 5% limit requires the pharmacy to secure a separate registration as a distributor.

Record Keeping

A pharmacy must maintain complete and accurate records of all its controlled substance dispensing and receiving activities for two to five years, depending on the state where the pharmacy is located. Schedule II records must be kept separately from all other records. DEA officials must be able to inspect all controlled substance records at any time. Record keeping includes inventory records, received drugs records, and dispersal records.

Returning Controlled Substances

Pharmacists must use DEA Form 222 when returning Schedule II substances, which can only be returned from one DEA registrant to another. To return the Schedule II substances, pharmacists must label each of them with the following information: product description, quantity, product name, size, strength, NDC number, and manufacturer name.

Handling Outdated Controlled Substances

To deal with outdated controlled substances, pharmacists must use DEA Form 41 (see Figure 2–3) and submit a cover letter with the form, explaining the situation and requesting permission to destroy the substances. Approval from the DEA is not needed if a representative from the state board of pharmacy witnesses the destruction of the drugs. Retail pharmacies may request DEA permission to destroy these substances once per year by sending the request two weeks prior to the intended destruction date. Two witnesses must witness the destruction. These witnesses may be physicians, pharmacists, mid-level practitioners, nurses, or law enforcement officers. If their pharmacies are part of a product-return system, pharmacists may also return outdated controlled substances for partial reimbursement.

Theft or Loss of Controlled Substances

If a controlled substance is stolen or lost, pharmacists must notify the nearest DEA office; and if it is a significant loss or theft, they must immediately make a report by phone. To report smaller amounts of drugs that are lost or stolen, pharmacists use DEA Form 106 (see Figure 2–4) to make the report. The form must include the company's name and address, DEA number, date of theft or loss, type of theft or loss, complete list of items stolen or lost, local police department information, and an explanation of the pharmacy's container-marking system with related costs. Pharmacists should send copies of the form to the DEA, board of pharmacy, and local police (depending on state requirements).

Refilling Prescriptions for Controlled Substances

According to Section 829, Title 21, of the CSA, pharmacists should not refill Schedule II controlled

OMB Approval No. 1117 - 0007	U. S. Department of Justice / Drug Enforcement Administration **REGISTRANTS INVENTORY OF DRUGS SURRENDERED**	PACKAGE NO.

The following schedule is an inventory of controlled substances which is hereby surrendered to you for proper disposition.

FROM: *(Include Name, Street, City, State and ZIP Code in space provided below.)*

Signature of applicant or authorized agent

Registrant's DEA Number

Registrant's Telephone Number

NOTE: CERTIFIED MAIL (Return Receipt Requested) IS REQUIRED FOR SHIPMENTS OF DRUGS VIA U.S. POSTAL SERVICE. See instructions on reverse (page 2) of form.

NAME OF DRUG OR PREPARATION Registrants will fill in Columns 1,2,3, and 4 ONLY. 1	Number of Containers 2	CONTENTS (Number of grams, tablets, ounces or other units per container) 3	Controlled Substance Content, (Each Unit) 4	**FOR DEA USE ONLY** DISPOSITION 5	QUANTITY GMS. 6	MGS. 7
1						
2						
3						
4						
5						
6						
7						
8						
9						
10						
11						
12						
13						
14						
15						
16						

FORM DEA-41 (9-01)   Previous edition dated **6-86** is usable.   *See instructions on reverse (page 2) of form.*

Figure 2–3 DEA Form 41. (*Courtesy of DEA*)

DEA-41 (6/1986) Pg. 2

NAME OF DRUG OR PREPARATION	Number of Containers	CONTENTS (Number of grams, tablets, ounces or other units per container)	Controlled Substance Content, (Each Unit)	FOR DEA USE ONLY		
				DISPOSITION	QUANTITY	
					GMS.	MGS.
Registrants will fill in Columns 1,2,3, and 4 ONLY. 1	2	3	4	5	6	7
17						
18						
19						
20						
21						
22						
23						
24						

The controlled substances surrendered in accordance with Title 21 of the Code of Federal Regulations, Section 1307.21, have been received in _____ packages purporting to contain the drugs listed on this inventory and have been: ** (1) Forwarded tape-sealed without opening; (2) Destroyed as indicated and the remainder forwarded tape-sealed after verifying contents; (3) Forwarded tape-sealed after verifying contents.

DATE _____   DESTROYED BY: _____

** *Strike out lines not applicable.*

WITNESSED BY: _____

INSTRUCTIONS

1. List the name of the drug in column 1, the number of containers in column 2, the size of each container in column 3, and in column 4 the controlled substance content of each unit described in column 3; e.g., morphine sulfate tabs., 3 pkgs., 100 tabs., 1/4 gr. (16 mg.) or morphine sulfate tabs., 1 pkg., 83 tabs., 1/2 gr. (32mg.), etc.

2. All packages included on a single line should be identical in name, content and controlled substance strength.

3. Prepare this form in quadruplicate. Mail two (2) copies of this form to the Special Agent in Charge, under separate cover. Enclose one additional copy in the shipment with the drugs. Retain one copy for your records. One copy will be returned to you as a receipt. No further receipt will be furnished to you unless specifically requested. Any further inquiries concerning these drugs should be addressed to the DEA District Office which serves your area.

4. There is no provision for payment for drugs surrendered. This is merely a service rendered to registrants enabling them to clear their stocks and records of unwanted items.

5. Drugs should be shipped tape-sealed via prepaid express or certified mail (**return receipt requested**) to Special Agent in Charge, Drug Enforcement Administration, of the DEA District Office which serves your area.

PRIVACY ACT INFORMATION

AUTHORITY: Section 307 of the Controlled Substances Act of 1970 (PL 91-513).
PURPOSE: To document the surrender of controlled substances which have been forwarded by registrants to DEA for disposal.
ROUTINE USES: This form is required by Federal Regulations for the surrender of unwanted Controlled Substances. Disclosures of information from this system are made to the following categories of users for the purposes stated.
    A. Other Federal law enforcement and regulatory agencies for law enforcement and regulatory purposes.
    B. State and local law enforcement and regulatory agencies for law enforcement and regulatory purposes.
EFFECT: Failure to document the surrender of unwanted Controlled Substances may result in prosecution for violation of the Controlled Substances Act.

Under the Paperwork Reduction Act, a person is not required to respond to a collection of information unless it displays a currently valid OMB control number. Public reporting burden for this collection of information is estimated to average 30 minutes per response, including the time for reviewing instructions, searching existing data sources, gathering and maintaining the data needed, and completing and reviewing the collection of information. Send comments regarding this burden estimate or any other aspect of this collection of information, including suggestions for reducing this burden, to the Drug Enforcement Administration, FOI and Records Management Section, Washington, D.C. 20537; and to the Office of Management and Budget, Paperwork Reduction Project no. 1117-0007, Washington, D.C. 20503.

Figure 2–3 DEA Form 41 (continued). (*Courtesy of DEA*)

REPORT OF THEFT OR LOSS OF CONTROLLED SUBSTANCES

Federal Regulations require registrants to submit a detailed report of any theft or loss of Controlled Substances to the Drug Enforcement Administration.

Complete the front and back of this form in triplicate. Forward the original and duplicate copies to the nearest DEA Office. Retain the triplicate copy for your records. Some states may also require a copy of this report.

OMB APPROVAL
No. 1117-0001

1. Name and Address of Registrant (include ZIP Code)

ZIP CODE

2. Phone No. (Include Area Code)

3. DEA Registration Number
2 ltr. prefix   7 digit suffix

4. Date of Theft or Loss

5. Principal Business of Registrant (Check one)
1 ☐ Pharmacy   5 ☐ Distributor
2 ☐ Practitioner   6 ☐ Methadone Program
3 ☐ Manufacturer   7 ☐ Other (Specify)
4 ☐ Hospital/Clinic

6. County in which Registrant is located

7. Was Theft reported to Police?
☐ Yes   ☐ No

8. Name and Telephone Number of Police Department (Include Area Code)

9. Number of Thefts or Losses Registrant has experienced in the past 24 months

10. Type of Theft or Loss (Check one and complete items below as appropriate)
1 ☐ Night break-in   3 ☐ Employee pilferage   5 ☐ Other (Explain)
2 ☐ Armed robbery   4 ☐ Customer theft   6 ☐ Lost in transit (Complete Item 14)

11. If Armed Robbery, was anyone:
Killed? ☐ No ☐ Yes (How many) _____
Injured? ☐ No ☐ Yes (How many) _____

12. Purchase value to registrant of Controlled Substances taken?
$

13. Were any pharmaceuticals or merchandise taken?
☐ No   ☐ Yes (Est. Value)
$

14. IF LOST IN TRANSIT, COMPLETE THE FOLLOWING:

A. Name of Common Carrier

B. Name of Consignee

C. Consignee's DEA Registration Number

D. Was the carton received by the customer?
☐ Yes   ☐ No

E. If received, did it appear to be tampered with?
☐ Yes   ☐ No

F. Have you experienced losses in transit from this same carrier in the past?
☐ No   ☐ Yes (How Many) _____

15. What identifying marks, symbols, or price codes were on the labels of these containers that would assist in identifying the products?

16. If Official Controlled Substance Order Forms (DEA-222) were stolen, give numbers.

17. What security measures have been taken to prevent future thefts or losses?

FORM DEA - 106 (11-00) *Previous editions obsolete*

CONTINUE ON REVERSE

Figure 2–4 DEA Form 106. *(Courtesy of DEA)*

FORM DEA-106 (Nov. 2000) Pg. 2

LIST OF CONTROLLED SUBSTANCES LOST

Trade Name of Substance or Preparation	Name of Controlled Substance in Preparation	Dosage Strength and Form	Quantity
Examples: Desoxyn	Methamphetamine Hydrochloride	5 mg Tablets	3 x 100
Demerol	Meperidine Hydrochloride	50 mg/ml Vial	5 x 30 ml
Robitussin A-C	Codeine Phosphate	2 mg/cc Liquid	12 Pints
1.			
2.			
3.			
4.			
5.			
6.			
7.			
8.			
9.			
10.			
11.			
12.			
13.			
14.			
15.			
16.			
17.			
18.			
19.			
20.			
21.			
22.			
23.			
24.			
25.			
26.			
27.			
28.			
29.			
30.			
31.			
32.			
33.			
34.			
35.			
36.			
37.			
38.			
39.			
40.			
41.			
42.			
43.			
44.			
45.			
46.			
47.			
48.			
49.			
50.			

I certify that the foregoing information is correct to the best of my knowledge and belief.

_____   _____   _____
Signature   Title   Date

Figure 2–4 DEA Form 106 (continued). (*Courtesy of DEA*)

substance prescriptions and may refill Schedule III and IV controlled substance prescriptions if the prescriber authorizes the refills. The total quantity that pharmacists dispense in a partial filling cannot exceed the total prescribed quantity. No dispensing can occur after six months past the date of issue. Certain states allow partial refills of Schedule II drugs to ambulatory patients within 72 hours of the original prescription.

Facsimile Prescriptions

The DEA allows faxed copies of Schedule II through V prescriptions, as long as they are sent directly from a practitioner to a pharmacy. Except in limited circumstances, pharmacists must review the original, signed prescriptions for all Schedule II substances. DEA regulations do not authorize practitioners to prescribe, or pharmacists to dispense, controlled substances via faxed prescriptions unless approved by state law.

Storage and Security Requirements

Pharmacies must store Schedule II substances in securely constructed, locked cabinets. Schedule III through V substances should be similarly stored, although they may be dispersed throughout as non-controlled substances in order to obstruct theft or diversion. To protect themselves from theft or diversion of controlled substances, pharmacies should undertake the following security measures:

- Controlled accessibility
- Electronic alarm systems
- Key control systems
- Perimeter security
- Self-locking and self-closing doors

DEA Inspections

The CSA requires administrative search warrants for most nonconsensual DEA inspections. Agents must enter DEA-registered premises by stating the purpose of their inspection and presenting appropriate identification. If an administrative inspection warrant has not been issued, the agent must secure informed consent from the registrant, unless the inspection is of a special state statute category. Inspection warrants are not required for initial registration inspections, mobile vehicle inspections, emergencies, or in dangerous health situations. Pharmacy technicians must immediately refer any DEA agent to the pharmacist in charge.

Poison Prevention Packaging Act of 1970

The Poison Prevention Packaging Act of 1970 required that the majority of OTC and prescription drugs be packaged in child-resistant containers. Eighty percent of children younger than age 5 cannot open these containers, whereas 90% of adults can open them. The Consumer Product Safety Commission enforces this act. However, this law allows certain medications, such as nitroglycerin medications and nasal inhalers, to be dispensed without a child-resistant container.

Occupational Safety and Health Act of 1970

Because of increasing workplace diseases and injuries, Congress passed the Occupational Safety and Health Act (OSHA) in 1970. Having a general purpose of requiring all employers to ensure employee safety and health, OSHA regulates actual workplaces, first aid, job-related materials, equipment, and machinery. Workplaces must be free of recognized hazards such as dangerous machinery, excessive noise, extreme temperatures, toxic chemicals, and unsanitary conditions. The act also established the Occupational Safety and Health Administration (also abbreviated OSHA). OSHA oversees workplace health and safety for governmental, as well as private sector, workers. The Occupational Safety and Health Review Commission enforces OSHA standards.

Drug Listing Act of 1972

Under the Drug Listing Act of 1972, each new drug is assigned a unique and permanent product code, known as a *National Drug Code (NDC)* that identifies the manufacturer or distributor, the drug formulation, and the size and type of its packaging. Using this code, the FDA maintains a database of drugs by use, manufacturer, and active ingredients and of newly marketed, discontinued, and remarketed drugs. The NDC for one product may not be used for another. If any changes occur in a product's characteristic, a new NDC number must be assigned to the new product version.

Medical Device Amendments of 1976

Previous to these amendments, medical devices were controlled only under the Food, Drug, and Cosmetic Act. As a result of rapidly growing developments in scientific and medical technology, the Medical Device Amendments of 1976 classified medical devices into three different regulatory classes. These classes depended upon how each device actually functioned. Class III devices, such as those used for life-sustaining and life-supporting measures, were required to have premarket approval from the FDA. Problems and failures with intrauterine devices (IUDs) and pacemakers promoted the passing of these amendments. Examples of other medical devices covered by these amendments include tablet-counting devices, scales, crutches, and wheelchairs. Class I and II devices do not require premarket approval by the FDA.

Resource Conservation and Recovery Act of 1976

Also known as the Solid Waste Disposal Act, the Resource Conservation and Recovery Act (RCRA) of 1976 regulates how solid wastes are handled and authorizes environmental agencies for the proper cleanup of contaminated sites. As a result of many problems with inadequate disposal of environmental wastes, the act was established to regulate solid waste landfills and to set guidelines for pollution reduction and elimination. Drugs that are cytotoxic or radioactive, for example, must be disposed of by using methods established under this act. Therefore, pharmacy employees will handle some substances that fall under the regulations the RCRA establishes.

Pharmaceutical waste may include any of the following medications: expired drugs, medications that patients discard, waste materials containing chemotherapy drug residues, and drugs that healthcare practitioners discard. Pharmaceutical waste also includes used containers (syringes, IV bags, tubing, vials, etc.), open containers of drugs that cannot be used, containers that previously held acute hazardous waste (*P-listed drugs*), contaminated garments, absorbents, and spill cleanup materials.

Drug Regulation Reform Act of 1978

Enacted to permit a shorter period for the investigation of new drugs, the Drug Regulation Reform Act of 1978 was in response to public pressure to allow quicker consumer access.

Orphan Drug Act of 1983

The Orphan Drug Act of 1983 offers federal financial incentives to commercial and nonprofit organizations to develop and market drugs previously unavailable in the United States. The orphan drug can be used to treat a rare disease that affects fewer than 200,000 people in the United States. The law offers tax breaks and a seven-year monopoly on drug sales to encourage companies to undertake the development and manufacture of such drugs. Since the 1983 act went into effect, more than 200 orphan drugs have been approved, including those for the treatment of such conditions as acquired immunodeficiency syndrome (AIDS), cystic fibrosis, blepharospasm (uncontrolled rapid blinking), and snake bites.

Drug Price Competition and Patent Term Restoration Act of 1984

The Drug Price Competition and Patent Term Restoration Act of 1984 encouraged the creation of both generic drugs (those not protected by trademark) and innovative new drugs. The act streamlined the process for generic drug approval and extended patent license as a function of the time required for the drug application approval process.

Prescription Drug Marketing Act of 1987

The Prescription Drug Marketing Act of 1987 deals with safety and competition issues that secondary markets raised for drugs and prohibits the re-importation of a drug into the United States by anyone except the manufacturer. The act also prohibits the sale or trading of drug samples, the distribution of samples to persons other than those licensed to prescribe them, and the distribution of samples except by mail or by common carrier.

Omnibus Budget Reconciliation Act of 1990

The Omnibus Budget Reconciliation Act of 1990 (OBRA-90) requires pharmacists to offer to discuss information about new and refill prescriptions with each patient. In counseling patients, pharmacists should give them the following information:

- Name and description of medication
- Dosage form, dosage, route of administration, and duration of drug therapy
- Common severe side effects or adverse effects
- Interactions (with other drugs or food) and therapeutic contraindications
- Self-monitoring of the medication therapy
- Proper storage
- Action in the event of a missed dose
- Special directions and precautions that the patient should take

FDA Safe Medical Devices Act of 1990

The Safe Medical Devices Act (SMDA) of 1990 increases the FDA's ability to regulate medical devices and products used in medical diagnostic procedures. Medical device reports regarding patient harm or death must be filed on a timely basis, and devices must go through a specific approval procedure before being marketed. Anyone violating the FD&C Act's medical devices policy faces increased civil penalties.

Previous to this act, patients harmed or killed by medical devices had little likelihood of receiving federal support. In addition, manufacturers must maintain better quality control and tracking of the devices they market.

Anabolic Steroid Control Act of 1990

Increasing the CSA's powers to regulate anabolic steroids, hormonal substances that promote muscle growth, the Anabolic Steroid Control Act of 1990 was in response to reports of athletes abusing anabolic steroids to increase their physical performance. "Performance-enhancing" steroids have caused serious harm, even death, to many athletes who used them illegally; and the Anabolic Steroid Control Act increased penalties for misuse and abuse of these drugs, including illegal distribution. Under the terms of this act, anabolic steroids are now listed in Schedule III of the CSA. Human growth hormone is also regulated through this act.

Americans with Disabilities Act of 1990

In areas focusing on employment, public services and transportation, telecommunications, public accommodations, commercial facilities, and more, the Americans with Disabilities Act (ADA) of 1990 prohibits discrimination against people with disabilities. Not only does the ADA oversee accommodations and devices for people with disabilities that help them to live as normally as possible, but it also prohibits employers from requiring medical examinations prior to employment for people with disabilities if employers do not require the same for prospective employees who have no apparent disabilities. The act was in response to some employers denying employment to individuals with physical or mental disabilities.

Dietary Supplement Health and Education Act of 1994

The Dietary Supplement Health and Education Act (DSHEA) of 1994 amended the FD&C Act to increase regulations on dietary supplements and how they are labeled. Dietary supplements are foods, not drugs, and manufacturers are responsible for ensuring that their supplements are safe to use. These supplements include amino acids, botanicals, herbs, certain hormones, minerals, vitamins, and others. DSHEA controls the display of, recommendation of, and stocking of dietary supplements. For example, pharmacy technicians cannot attach extraneous labeling or stickers to dietary supplement packages. Prior to DSHEA, dietary supplements had little regulation; and some patients who took dietary supplements had life-threatening interactions with prescription and OTC drugs.

Health Insurance Portability and Accountability Act of 1996

The Health Insurance Portability and Accountability Act (HIPAA) of 1996 was signed into law on August 21, 1996, and required all health-care providers to be in compliance by April 14, 2003. HIPAA was designed with many goals in mind; limiting administrative costs of health care and privacy issues and preventing fraud and abuse were of primary importance.

Although using electronic transmissions was thought to lower the administrative costs of providing health care, it has led to problems related to privacy of health information. Therefore, the law also had to provide security and confidentiality guarantees for each individual patient. Extensive privacy rules, including the use of unique identifiers, have shaped the law.

The final regulations regarding the privacy legislation sections of HIPAA were published in December 2000, after the Centers for Medicare and Medicaid Services (CMS) reviewed more than 50,000 comments and concerns on this important subject. All health-care organizations that transmit any health information electronically must comply with HIPAA; those who do not comply can be fined and imprisoned.

FDA Modernization Act of 1997

Reforming regulation of cosmetics, foods, and medical products, the FDA Modernization Act (FDAMA) of 1997 affected user fees, compounding in the pharmacy, safety, and medical device regulation. The FDAMA

also gave manufacturers six-month extensions on new pediatric drugs that had undergone drug trials and required risk assessment reviews of all drugs and foods containing mercury. Manufacturers were required to label all prescription drugs with the symbol "Rx." Also, as part of the FDAMA, Medicare Part D established prescription drug costs for Medicare beneficiaries, covering drugs approved by the FDA, with certain exclusions. The act was designed to speed up the drug approval process and to improve FDA regulation of drugs, biologics, foods, and medical devices.

Medicare Prescription Drug, Improvement, and Modernization Act of 2003

Extensively overhauling Medicare, the Medicare Prescription Drug, Improvement, and Modernization Act (MMA) of 2003 introduced prescription drug tax breaks and subsidies. MMA also offered new Medicare "Advantage" plans with increased choices about care, providers, coverages, and federal reimbursements. It partially privatized the Medicare system, offering pretax medical savings accounts. Established to help many senior citizens afford new drugs, the MMA also gave employers the ability to offer their employees drug benefits via the drug subsidies it created.

Isotretinoin (Accutane®) Safety and Risk Management Act (Proposal only) of 2004

Although this act was not passed, it proposed the restriction of drugs containing isotretinoin as a result of severe, adverse effects. Used for the treatment of acne, isotretinoin was shown to cause severe birth defects in the fetuses of patients who took the drug during pregnancy. It is also linked to spontaneous abortions of fetuses, depression, psychosis, and suicide. As a result of the failure of this act to pass, the FDA instituted the System to Manage Accutane-Related Teratogenicity (SMART). As of this date, the SMART program has, unfortunately, not significantly reduced cases of isotretinoin (Accutane®) adverse effects.

Combat Methamphetamine Epidemic Act of 2005

An extension of the Patriot Act, or the USA Patriot Improvements and Reauthorization Act, the Combat Methamphetamine Epidemic Act of 2005 focused on the methamphetamine provisions with more intensity to stop illegal methamphetamine use, especially as it related to the funding of terrorist activities. The government can confiscate the property of anyone involved in methamphetamine-financed terrorism. The act also controls other drugs such as crack cocaine when involved in funding terrorism.

Drugs used for the manufacture of methamphetamine, including pure ephedrine and pseudoephedrine, must be behind counters or in locked cases. Patients or customers can buy a maximum of 9 grams per month per person and must show identification, as well as sign a sales log. Pharmacy technicians can help pharmacists by keeping these drug products out of reach of customers and by accurately maintaining the sales log for these products. Selling these drug products requires registration with the U.S. Attorney General's office and specific training.

Medical Tamper-Resistant Prescription Act of 2008

The Medical Tamper-Resistant Prescription Act of 2008 requires written prescriptions for Medicaid-covered outpatient drugs to be executed on a tamper-resistant prescription. The second phase of this act applies only to written prescriptions for covered outpatient drugs, not those that are verbal, faxed, or sent electronically. To be considered tamper-resistant, a prescription must have the following three characteristics:

1. One or more industry-recognized features designed to prevent unauthorized copying of a completed or blank prescription form

2. One or more industry-recognized features designed to prevent the erasure or modification of information written on the prescription pad by the prescriber

3. One or more industry-recognized features designed to prevent the use of counterfeit prescription forms

Each state Medicaid agency has issued its own guidance on the provisions of this act.

DRUG RECALLS

When a manufacturer determines that one of its drug products is harmful, it may issue a drug recall and inform the FDA of the situation. The FDA can recommend that a manufacturer issue a drug recall and can also obtain a warrant to seize defective products. To avoid governmental legal action, manufacturers usually voluntarily announce drug recalls. Some of the drugs recalled or withdrawn from the market in recent years include: Avandia, Ortho Evra birth control patch, Vioxx, and Ceclor suspension.

DRUG STANDARDS

Drug standards are the sets or sections of requirements for the formulation of drug substances, ingredients, and dosage forms. Drugs stocked in the pharmacy must be compendia drugs, and the pharmacy must maintain a drug formulary, or list of drugs it stocks. The pharmaceutical services must be under the general supervision of a licensed pharmacist, who must schedule regular visits to the facility to supervise the drug handling and administration procedures. At least monthly, the pharmacist must review the drug regimen of each patient and report any discrepancies or irregularities to the administrator and the medical director. This is a significant requirement in terms of patient safety and professional integrity. Drug standards are contained in the **U.S. Pharmacopeia (USP)** and the **National Formulary (NF)**, published by the U.S. Pharmacopeia.

REGULATORY AGENCIES

Many regulatory agencies of the federal and state governments in the United States influence the practice of pharmacy. All pharmacy technicians must be familiar with the policies of these regulatory agencies, which are listed below.

Bureau of Alcohol, Tobacco, Firearms and Explosives

As its title implies, the Bureau of Alcohol, Tobacco, Firearms and Expolsives (ATF) regulates alcohol, tobacco, firearms, and explosives. It also investigates acts of arson and is dedicated toward the prevention of terrorism, the reduction of violent crime, and the general protection of the United States.

Centers for Disease Control and Prevention

The Centers for Disease Control and Prevention (CDC) is a federal agency that provides facilities and services for the investigation, identification, prevention, and control of disease, injury, and disability. It provides statistics and information to health professionals about the treatment of common and rare diseases worldwide. Its primary function is to issue regulations for infection control. It was established in 1946 as the Communicable Disease Center and became the Center for Disease Control in 1970; "and Prevention" was added in 1992, but Congress requested that "CDC" remain the agency's acronym. This agency has also been deeply involved in the war against human immunodeficiency virus (HIV) infection and AIDS.

Centers for Medicare and Medicaid Services

The Centers for Medicare and Medicaid Services (CMS) strives to modernize the health-care system, promoting effective and up-to-date health-care coverage. It also promotes quality health care for beneficiaries.

Drug Enforcement Agency

The Drug Enforcement Agency (DEA) enforces controlled substances legislation, promotes reduction of illegal substances, and brings offenders to justice. To do this, the DEA cooperates with local, regional, national, and international agencies. The agency investigates and prosecutes major violators, focusing heavily on individuals, groups, and gangs who use violence to promote their activities. The DEA manages a national drug intelligence program, which has ties into many other countries. As part of its enforcement activities, the DEA often seizes the assets of those involved in illegal drug activities.

Environmental Protection Agency

Focusing on protection of the environment and the health of human beings, The Environmental Protection Agency (EPA) develops and enforces environmental legislation. The EPA also offers state environmental program grants, publishes educational information, and continually establishes voluntary environmental programs and partnerships.

Food and Drug Administration

The Food and Drug Administration (FDA) promotes public health by controlling the safety and effectiveness of foods, drugs, biological products, medical devices, cosmetics, and radioactive substances. Whenever adverse reactions, quality problems, or product-use errors occur, individuals and organizations are encouraged to report them to the FDA by using its MedWatch system. Information on MedWatch can be found at http://www.fda.gov.

The Joint Commission

The Joint Commission, formerly the Joint Commission on Accreditation of Health-care Organizations (JCAHO), is a not-for-profit, independent organization that accredits and certifies health-care organizations in the United States. It strives for continual quality improvement so that accredited organizations offer increased patient safety.

National Association of the Boards of Pharmacy

By developing uniform standards, the National Association of the Boards of Pharmacy (NABP) promotes public health. NABP implements these standards to reduce potential public harm that can result because of the increasing complexity of medications and medication delivery systems.

State Boards of Pharmacy

Each state's board of pharmacy (BOP) regulates and controls the practice of pharmacy in that state. State board of pharmacy laws affect pharmacy practice directly to protect the public's health. Each state's board of pharmacy is part of the state Department of Health (DOH).

United States Pharmacopeia

As the official authority that sets standards for all prescription and OTC medications, the USP also standardizes dietary supplements and other healthcare products made and sold in the United States.

THE ETHICAL FOUNDATION OF PHARMACY

Ethics concern the thoughts, judgments, and actions on issues that have the greater implications of moral right and wrong. Physicians, pharmacists, and nurses have the ethical responsibility to provide information about the risks and side effects of drug regimens. Providing that information is grounded in the principle of respect for the distinctive capacity of humans to make their own choices about their own lives. Patients must be aware of the benefits and risks of drugs that they may take.

Bioethics, relating to the sciences that underlie medicine, is a discipline dealing with the ethical and moral implications of biological research and applications, especially as they relate to life and death. These include pharmacology, anatomy, physiology, microbiology, pathology, and biochemistry. The field of bioethics is a new area of ethics resulting from genetic research in the current era.

EXPLORING THE WEB

Visit http://www.aspl.org for information about the American Society for Pharmacy Law.

Visit http://www.cdc.gov to learn about the Centers for Disease Control and Prevention.

Visit http://www.presidency.ucsb.edu to learn about the Comprehensive Drug Abuse Prevention and Control Act. From this link, search for Comprehensive Drug Abuse Prevention and Control Act; 10/27/1970.

Visit http://www.drugrecalls.com for listings of current drug recalls.

Visit http://www.fdareview.org to review the history of the Food and Drug Administration.

Visit http://www.osha.gov to learn more about the Occupational Safety and Health Association.

Visit http://www.usdoj.gov/dea for information about the Drug Enforcement Administration.

Visit http://www.hhs.gov to learn more about the many services of the Department of Health and Human Services.

Visit http://www.fda.gov for information on the Food and Drug Administration.

Visit http://www.usp.org to learn more about the U.S. Pharmacopeia.

REVIEW QUESTIONS

1. Which act requires pharmaceutical manufacturers to file a New Drug Application with the FDA?

   A. Pure Food and Drug Act of 1906
   B. Comprehensive Drug Abuse Prevention and Control Act of 1970
   C. Drug Listing Act of 1972
   D. Food, Drug, and Cosmetic Act of 1938

2. Which form must pharmacists use to order Schedule II narcotics?

   A. Form 224
   B. Form 222
   C. Form 41
   D. Form 106

3. Which of these laws permits a shorter period for the investigation of new drugs?

   A. Orphan Drug Act of 1983
   B. Drug Regulation Reform Act of 1978
   C. Prescription Drug Marketing Act of 1987
   D. Food, Drug, and Cosmetic Act of 1938

4. Of which agency is the Drug Enforcement Administration a branch?

   A. Department of Health and Human Services
   B. Department of Justice
   C. Department of Labor
   D. Centers for Disease Control and Prevention

5. Which agency has been deeply involved in the war against HIV and AIDS?

   A. Department of Labor
   B. American Red Cross
   C. Department of Health and Human Services
   D. Centers for Disease Control and Prevention

6. Which activity is governed by the FD&C Act of 1938?

   A. Applying labels bearing the legend "Caution: Federal law prohibits dispensing without a prescription"
   B. Classifying drugs into types or schedules
   C. Issuing pharmacies and practitioners a license
   D. Approving or denying new drug applications

7. The Durham-Humphrey Amendment of 1951 established the difference between:

   A. the pharmacist and technician
   B. prescription and nonprescription drugs
   C. legend and OTC drugs
   D. B and C

8. Which federal law was enacted in 1970 to regulate the use and distribution of substances with high abuse potential?

   A. Food and Drug Act
   B. Drug Enforcement Act
   C. Environmental Protection Act
   D. Controlled Substances Act

9. Which of the following is OSHA's general purpose?

   A. To ensure safe and effective drug therapy
   B. To ensure a safe and healthful workplace
   C. To ensure that all drugs are labeled
   D. To control outdated drugs

10. To which agency does one send a report of adverse reaction to drugs?

    A. Food and Drug Administration
    B. Drug Enforcement Agency
    C. Farmers' Advocacy Agency
    D. Controlled Substances Agency

Pharmaceutical Terminology and Abbreviations

OUTLINE

GLOSSARY

Abbreviations – shortened forms of words

Root – the main part of a word that gives the word its central meaning

Prefix – a part of a word structure that occurs before or in front of the word and modifies the meaning of the root

Suffix – a word ending that modifies the meaning of the root

WORD BUILDING

To communicate precisely with other health-care professionals, pharmacy technicians must have appropriate knowledge and understanding of specialized words, phrases, abbreviations, and symbols used in pharmacy and medicine. They must learn and use terminology, words, and phrases to explain the particular elements of their field. Medical terminology is derived from word parts placed together to form specific words and phrases in the medical fields, a process called *word building*. Word building is accomplished through the use of roots, prefixes, and suffixes.

Roots

The main part of a word that gives the word its central meaning is its root. Word parts can be added to the root to offer more specific meanings to words. For example, *brady-* is a prefix meaning "slow" and *cardi-* is a root meaning "heart." If the two word parts are placed together to form the word *bradycardia*, the meaning is "slowness of the heart." This can be further defined as a slow heartbeat marked by a pulse rate below 60 beats per minute in an adult. Some examples of roots are shown in Table 3–1.

Prefixes

A structure at the beginning of a word that modifies the meaning of the root is a prefix. For example, the word *lateral* means "side." Adding the prefix *bi-*, meaning "two," forms the new word *bilateral*, which means "both sides." Another example begins with the word *venous*, which means "of the veins." Adding the prefix *intra-*, meaning "within or inside," forms the new word *intravenous*, which means "within or inside the veins." Not all medical words

TABLE 3–1 Commonly Used General Roots

Root	Meaning	Example
acu	abrupt, sudden, sharp	Acute
adeno	gland	Adenoid
adipo	fat	Adipose
aero	air	Aerosol
alb	white	Albumin
ambulo	walk	ambulatory
andro	male	androgen
angio	vessel	angiogram
arthr	joint	arthritis
bucc/a	inside of cheek	buccal
carcin/o	crab, cancer	carcinogen
cardi	heart	cardiology
cereb	brain	cerebrum
chemo	chemistry, chemical	chemotherapy
chol	bile	cholangiogram
cyst	urinary bladder	cystoscopy
cyt	cell	cytology
dactyl	finger	syndactylism
dermat	skin	dermatology
encephal	brain	electroencephalogram
erythro	red	erythrocyte
gastr	stomach	gastric acid
gluco	sugar	glucose
hemo	blood	hematoma
hepat	liver	hepatoma
hydro	water	hydrocephalus
lachry	tear	lachrymal fluid
lacto	milk	lactose
lapar	abdomen	laparoscope
laryng	larynx (voice box)	laryngitis
leuko	white	leukemia
lingua/o	tongue	sublingual
mal	bad	malpractice
mast, mamm	breast	mastectomy
melano	black	melanoma

Root	Meaning	Example
meter	measure	thermometer
my	muscle	myalgia
nas	nose	nasal
necro	dead	necrosis
nephr	kidney	nephrosis
ocul/o	eye	ocular
odont	shaped like a tooth	orthodontist
onc/o	tumor	oncology
ophthalm	eye	ophthalmoscope
optic/o	eye	optician
oste	bone	osteoarthritis
ot	ear	otalgia
patho	disease	pathology
phleb/o, ven/o	vein	phlebotomy, venipuncture
procto	rectum	proctologist
psych	mind	psychology
ren	kidney	renal
rhino	nose	rhinovirus
spir	breathing	spirometer
thrombo	blood clot	thrombolysis
tom/e	cut	phlebotomy
tox/o	poisonous	toxic, toxicology
uro	urine	urology
uter/o, hyster/o	uterus	intrauterine, hysterectomy
vaso	blood vessel	vasoconstriction
xanth/o	yellow	xanthin
xero	dry	xeroderma
zyme	ferment	enzyme

have a prefix, but every medical word has a root and ending, which is either a suffix or another root, which is itself a word. *Hyperglycemia* is an example of a word containing a prefix. *Hyper-* is the prefix, *glyc* is the root, and *-emia* is the suffix. For a list of common prefixes, see Table 3–2. Prefixes in this text will be followed by a hyphen to show that other word parts will be added to each prefix to form a new word.

TABLE 3–2   Commonly Used General Prefixes

Prefix	Meaning	Example
a-	without	aphonia
ab-	from, away from	abduct
ad-	toward	adduct
ambi-	both	ambidextrous
ana-	up, against, back	anaphylactic
ante-	before	antecubital
auto-	self	autoimmune
bi-	two, double	biceps, bilateral
bio-	life	biopsy, biology
brady-	slow	bradycardia
cata-	down	cataleptic
circum-	around	circumcision
con-	together	congestion
contra-	against	contraceptive
de-	from, away from, down	decalcify
deca-	ten	dekaliter
dia-	through, complete	diagnosis
dis-	separate, apart	dislocation
dys-	bad, abnormal, painful	dyspepsia, dysuria
ec-	out, away	ectopic
ecto-	outside	ectoplasm
em-	in	embolism
en-	in	endemic
endo-	into, within	endoscope, endometriosis
epi-	upon, high	epidermis
eu-	well, good	eupnea
intra-	within, inside	intravenous
iso-	equal	isometric
juxta-	near, beside	juxtaarticular
macro-	large, long	macrocytic
mal-	bad, poor	malnutrition
mega-	large	megacephaly
meso-	middle	mesoderm
meta-	change, after	metastasis

Prefix	Meaning	Example
micro-	small	microscope
milli-	one-thousandth	milliliter
neo-	new	neonatal
non-	not	noninvasive
para-	near, beside, beyond	paramedic
per-	through	percutaneous
peri-	around	perianal
poly-	many	polyarthritis
post-	behind, after	postpartum
pre-	before	premature
re-	again, back	reactivate
retro-	backward, behind	retrograde
semi-	half	semiconscious
sub-	under, beneath, below	sublingual
super-	above, over	superficial
supra-	above, excessive	suprarenal
syn-	together, with	synthetic
tri-	three	triceps
uni-	one	unicellular
ultra-	beyond, excessive	ultrasound

Suffixes

A word ending that modifies the meaning of the root is called a suffix. The root to which a suffix is attached may or may not need a combining vowel. Not all words have a suffix. An example of a word with a suffix is *pharmacology*. *Pharmaco* is the root and *-logy* is the suffix. For a list of common suffixes, see Table 3–3.

ABBREVIATIONS

Abbreviations are shortened forms of words. Pharmacy technicians are required to know many abbreviations. The most common abbreviations associated with measurements are shown in Table 3–4, and

TABLE 3-3 Commonly Used General Suffixes

Suffix	Meaning	Example
-ar	pertaining to	lumbar
-clasis	break	osteoclasis
-desis	binding	arthrodesis
-dipsia	thirst	polydipsia
-ectomy	cut out, remove	appendectomy
-emesis	vomit	hematemesis
-form	resembling, like	vermiform
-genic	originating, producing	toxigenic
-gram	record	electrocardiogram
-graph	device for recording	electrocardiograph
-iasis	condition	nephrolithiasis
-iatry	treatment	podiatry
-ic	pertaining to	thoracic
-ical	pertaining to	neurological
-ism	condition	alcoholism
-ist	specialist	cardiologist
-itis	inflammation	nephritis
-logist	specialist in the study of	microbiologist
-logy	study of	etiology
-lysis	breaking down	hemolysis
-megaly	enlargement	hepatomegaly
-ol	alcohol	ethanol
-oma	tumor	melanoma
-opia	vision	hyperopia
-ose	carbohydrate	glucose
-pathy	disease	homeopathy
-penia	abnormal reduction	leukocytopenia
-pepsia	digestion	dyspepsia
-philia	attraction	hydrophilia
-phobia	abnormal fear	photophobia
-plasty	surgical repair	rhinoplasty
-rrhea	discharge, flow	diarrhea
-sis	process	diagnosis
-stasis	control, stoppage	hemostasis
-stomy	surgical opening	colostomy
-tomy	cut, incision	nephrotomy
-tropia	turning	hypertropia

TABLE 3-4 Abbreviations Commonly Used for Measurements

Abbreviation	Meaning
C or °C	Celsius
cc	cubic centimeter (1cc = 1 ml)
cm	centimeter (2.54 cm = 1 inch)
°F	Fahrenheit
g or gm	gram
gr	grain
gtt	drop(s)
ht.	height
L or l	Liter = 100 mL (1 gallon = 4 quarts = 8 pints)
lb	pound
kg	kilogram (kg = 1000 gm = 2.2 pounds)
m^2	square meter
mcg	microgram
mEq	milliequivalent
mg	milligram
mg/kg	milligram of drug per kilogram of body weight
ml, mL	milliliter
mm	millimeter
no or NO	number
ss	one-half
Tbsp or T	tablespoon
Tsp	teaspoon
U	unit
wt.	weight
w/v.	weight-to-volume ratio

the abbreviations used for writing prescriptions are listed in Table 3–5.

Although they may be convenient to use, abbreviations can be confusing. In the medical and pharmaceutical fields, confusion can lead to medication errors

TABLE 3–5 Abbreviations Commonly Used in Prescriptions

Abbreviation	Meaning
ā	before
āā, aa	of each
a.c.	before meals
ad	to, up to
ad lib.	as desired
AM, a.m.	morning
amt.	amount
aq., AQ	water
b.i.d.	twice a day
BSA	body surface area
buc.	buccal
c̄	with
cap.	capsule
comp.	compound
d	day
dil	dilute
disp.	dispense
el., elix.	elixir
fl, fld	fluid
h, hr	hour
IM	intramuscular
IV	intravenous
liq	liquid
m.	mix
mixt., mist.	a mixture
no.	number
noc.	night
Non. Rep., n.r.	do not repeat, no refills
NPO	nothing by mouth
oint., ung.	ointment
P	after
p.c.	after meals
per.	by, through

Abbreviation	Meaning
PM, p.m.	after noon
PO, p.o.	by mouth, orally
PR, p.r.	through the rectum
PRN, p.r.n.	as needed
PV, vag.	through the vagina
pulv.	a powder
q	every
q AM	every morning
q h	every hour
q2h	every two hours
q.i.d.	four times a day
q.v.	as much as you wish
®	registered trademark
Rχ	prescription, take
s̄	without
sat.	saturated
sig.	instruction to patient
SL, sl	sublingual
sol., Soln.	solution
SP	spirits
S.O.S.	there is a need
stat	immediately
supp., suppos.	suppository
syr.	syrup
T	temperature
tab	tablet
t.i.d., TID	three times a day
tr., tinct.	tincture
w.a.	while awake
WK, wk	week
X	times, for

and harm to patients. Therefore, some abbreviations should be avoided because of their potential to cause confusion. These abbreviations are listed in Table 3–6.

TABLE 3–6 Abbreviations That Should Be Avoided

Abbreviation	Meaning	Reason to Avoid	Use Instead
AD, AS, AU	right ear, left ear, both ears	May be mistaken as "OD", "OS", "OU" (right eye, left eye, both eyes)	Use "right ear," "left ear," "both ears."
BT	bedtime	May be mistaken as "BID" (twice daily)	Use "bedtime."
D/C	discharge or discontinue	May be confused for intended meaning	Use "discharge" or "discontinue."
HS or hs	half-strength	May be mistaken as "hour of sleep" or "bedtime"	Use "half-strength."
i/d	one daily	May be mistaken as "tid" (three times daily)	Use "one daily."
IJ	injection	May be mistaken as "IV" or "intrajugular"	Use "injection."
IN	intranasal	May be mistaken as "IM" or "IV"	Use "intranasal" or "NAS."
OJ	orange juice	May be mistaken as "OD" or "OS"	Use "orange juice."
o.d. or OD	once daily	May be mistaken as "OD" (right eye)	Use "once daily."
OD, OS, OU	right eye, left eye, both eyes	May be mistaken as "AD", "AS", or "AU" (right ear, left ear, both ears)	Use "right eye," "left eye," or "both eyes."
per os	by mouth, or orally	"os" may be mistaken for "OS" (left eye)	Use "PO," "by mouth," or "orally."
q.d. or QD	every day	May be mistaken as "q.i.d." (four times a day)	Use "every day" or "daily."
qhs or qn	nightly at bedtime	May be mistaken as "qhr" (every hour)	Use "nightly at bedtime" or "nightly."
q.o.d. or QOD	every other day	May be mistaken as "q.d." (every day) or "q.i.d." (four times a day)	Use "every other day."
q1d	daily	May be mistaken as "four times a day"	Use "daily."
q6PM (or any other number in this type of abbreviation)	every evening at 6 pm	May be mistaken as "every 6 hours"	Use "6 PM nightly" or "6 PM daily."
SC, SQ, sub q	subcutaneous	May be mistaken as "SL" (sublingual), "5 every", "substitute every"	Use "subcutaneously."
$\bar{s}\bar{s}$	sliding scale or one-half	May be confused or may be mistaken for "55"	Use "sliding scale." "one-half," or "1/2."
SSI	sliding scale insulin	May be mistaken as "Strong Solution of Iodine" (Lugol's)	Use "sliding scale insulin."
SSRI	sliding scale regular insulin or selective serotonin reuptake inhibitor	May be confused	Use "sliding scale regular insulin" or "selective serotonin reuptake inhibitor."
TIW or tiw	3 times a week	May be mistaken as "3 times a day" or "twice in a week"	Use "3 times a week."

BRAND OR TRADE NAMES AND GENERIC NAMES

Pharmacy technicians must know all names for a given drug. Pharmaceutical literature usually has three different names listed for each medication:

1. Generic name
2. Trade name or brand name
3. Chemical name

A drug's generic name is also referred to as its *nonproprietary* or *nonbrand* name. Usually derived from the drug's longer chemical name, generic names are standardized and approved by the Food and Drug Administration for the sake of uniformity. For example, *acetaminophen* is the generic name of the trademarked product known as *Tylenol*®, as well as for hundreds of other products using acetaminophen as their primary ingredient.

The trade name is a specific, trademarked designation given to one company's product. Each trade name is capitalized and followed by the symbol®, which indicates that the name is registered to a specific manufacturer or owner and no one else can use it. Derived from the chemical composition of the drug, the chemical name is usually hyphenated and may be long. Table 3–7 shows the brand names (or trade names) and the corresponding generic names of some commonly used medications.

TABLE 3–7   Brand/Trade Names and Generic Names of Commonly Used Drugs

Brand/Trade	Generic
Achromycin	tetracycline
Activase	alteplase, recombinant
Adalat	nifedipine
Advil	ibuprofen
Airet	albuterol sulfate
Aldomet	methyldopa
Amerge	naratriptan

Brand/Trade	Generic
Amoxil	amoxicillin
Amphojel	aluminum hydroxide
Ancef	cefazolin
Anzemet	dolasetron
Apresoline	hydralazine
Atarax	hydroxyzine
Ativan	lorazepam
Axid	nizatidine
Bactrim	trimethoprim/sulfamethoxazole
Benadryl	diphenhydramine
Bentyl	dicyclomine
Brethine	terbutaline
Biaxin	clarithromycin
Biomox	amoxicillin trihydrate
Bufferin	aspirin
BuSpar	buspirone
Capoten	captopril
Carafate	sucralfate
Cardizem	diltiazem
Catapres	clonidine
Ceclor	cefaclor
Celexa	citalopram
Cipro	ciprofloxacin
Claritin	loratadine
Cleocin	clindamycin
Compazine	prochlorperazine
Corgard	nadolol
Corlopam	fenoldopam
Coumadin	warfarin
Crystodigin	digitoxin
Cytotec	misoprostol
Decadron	dexamethasone
Deltasone	prednisone
Demerol	meperidine
Depakene	valproic acid
DiaBeta	glyburide
Diabinese	chlorpropamide

(continued)

TABLE 3–7 (continued)

Brand/Trade	Generic
Diamox	acetazolamide
Dilantin	phenytoin
Dramamine	dimenhydrinate
Dulcolax	bisacodyl
Dyazide	hydrochlorothiazide/triamterene
Effexor	venlafaxine
Elavil	amitriptyline
Ery-Tab	erythromycin base
Flagyl	metronidazole
Floxin	ofloxacin
Folvite	folic acid
Fungizone	amphotericin B
Garamycin	gentamicin
Genprin	aspirin
Glucotrol	glipizide
Haldol	haloperidol
Hexadrol	dexamethasone
Hycort	hydrocortisone, topical
Hytrin	terazosin
Ilosone	erythromycin estolate
Ilotycin	erythromycin base
Impril	imipramine HCl
Inderal	propranolol
Indocin	indomethacin
Integrilin	eptifibatide
Isoptin	verapamil
Kantrex	kanamycin sulfate
Keflex	cephalexin
Kefzol	cefazolin
Kenalog	triamcinolone
Klonopin	clonazepam
Lanoxin	digoxin
Lasix	furosemide
Levate	amitriptyline HCl
Lipitor	atorvastatin
Lopid	gemfibrozil

Brand/Trade	Generic
Lopressor	metoprolol
Maxalt	rizatriptan
Mefoxin	cefoxitin
Mellaril	thioridazine
Micronase	glyburide
Minipress	prazosin
Motrin	ibuprofen
Mycostatin	nystatin
Mylicon	simethicone
Naprosyn	naproxen
Nebcin	tobramycin
Nizoral	ketoconazole
Nolvadex	tamoxifen citrate
Oretic	hydrochlorothiazide
Pepcid	famotidine
Phenergan	promethazine
Prilosec	omeprazole
Prinivil	lisinopril
Procardia	nifedipine
Pronestyl	procainamide
Prozac	fluoxetine
Proventil	albuterol
Retrovir	zidovudine
Robitussin	guaifenesin
Rocephin	ceftriaxone
Rufen	ibuprofen
Septra	trimethoprim/sulfamethoxazole
Stadol	butorphanol
Synthroid	levothyroxine
Tagamet HB	cimetidine
Talwin	pentazocine
Tapazole	methimazole
Tavist	clemastine fumarate
Teargen	artificial tears solution
Tebamide	trimethobenzamide HCl
Tebrazid	pyrazinamide
Tega-cort	hydrocortisone, topical

TABLE 3–7 (continued)

Brand/Trade	Generic
Tegopen	cloxacillin sodium
Tegretol	carbamazepine
Terramycin	oxytetracycline HCl
Tobrex	tobramycin
Tofranil	imipramine
Totacillin	ampicillin, oral
Trilafon	perphenazine
Tums	calcium carbonate
Tylenol	acetaminophen
Tyzine	tetrahydrozoline HCl, nasal
Ultiva	remifentanil HCl
Ultram	tramadol
Urobak	sulfamethoxazole
Vasotec	enalapril
Valisone	betamethasone valerate
Valium	diazepam
V-Cillin K	penicillin V potassium
Ventolin	albuterol
Vibramycin	doxycycline
Virilon	methyltestosterone
Vivarin	caffeine
Vivol	diazepam
Volmax	albuterol sulfate
Wellferon	interferon alfa-N1
Wycillin	penicillin G procaine
Xalatan	latanoprost
Xanax	alprazolam
Xylocaine	lidocaine HCl, local
YF-Vax	yellow fever vaccine
Yocon	yohimbine HCl
Zantac	ranitidine
Zestril	lisinopril
Zetar	coal tar
Zincate	zinc sulfate
Zithromax	azithromycin
Zocor	simvastatin

Brand/Trade	Generic
Zonalon	doxepin, topical
Zovirax	acyclovir
Zyloprim	allopurinol
Zyrtec	cetirizine HCl

COMMONLY USED APOTHECARY SYMBOLS

The definitions of all apothecary symbols are not absolute; that is, many of them have more than one meaning when used in different contexts. The symbols used most commonly in medicine are shown in Table 3–8.

TABLE 3–8 Symbols Commonly Used in Medicine

Symbol	Meaning
>	greater than
<	less than
=	equal to
↑	increase
↓	decrease
Ø	none
Δ	change
'	minutes
"	seconds
°	hours
1°	primary
2°	secondary
℥	ounce
ℳ	minim
#	pound
X	times (as in two times a week)
♀	female
♂	male

EXPLORING THE WEB

Visit http://www.latinrootsofenglish.com to discover how many medical terms have Latin roots.

Visit http://www.lib.umich.edu/tcp/docs/dox/medical.html to see several apothecary symbols.

Visit http://www.macroevolution.net/medical-suffixes.html for an online dictionary of biological and medical suffixes and prefixes.

Visit http://www.medilexicon.com/medicalabbreviations.php to search an online database of over 200,000 medical, biotech, pharmaceutical, and health-care acronym abbreviations.

Visit http://www.medword.com/prefixes.html for an online source of medical terms, especially the basics—suffixes, prefixes, terms.

Visit http://www.merck.com/mmhe/appendixes/ap3/ap3a.html for an online source of generic and trade names of many drugs.

Visit http://www.pharmaceutical-drug-manufacturers.com/pharmaceutical-glossary/pharmaceutical-abbreviations.html for an online source of pharmaceutical drug manufacturers and for a quick reference on abbreviations, weights and measures, and conversions.

REVIEW QUESTIONS

1. Which abbreviation means "centimeter"?

   A. ct   **C.** cn
   B. cr   **D.** cm

2. Which abbreviation means "four times a day"?

   A. q 4h   **C.** q id
   B. q.o.d.   **D.** b.i.d.

3. The suffix *-itis* means:

   A. pain   **C.** softening
   B. swelling   **D.** inflammation

4. Which prefix means "surrounding tissue"?

   A. *pre-*   **C.** *post-*
   B. *peri-*   **D.** *para-*

5. The abbreviation that means "right eye" is:

   A. OC   **C.** OS
   B. OD   **D.** OU

6. Which prefix means "around"?

   A. *dys-*   **C.** *endo-*
   B. *ecto-*   **D.** *circum-*

7. The abbreviation that means "every other day" is:

   A. q.i.d.   **C.** q.o.h.
   B. q.o.d.   **D.** q.d.

8. Which term means "death of tissue"?

   A. *necrosis*   **C.** *ntenesis*
   B. *nephrosis*   **D.** *sclerosis*

9. The abbreviation that means "drops" is:

   A. g   **C.** gt
   B. gr   **D.** gtt

10. Which abbreviation means "before meals"?

    A. ā   **C.** a.c.
    B. āā   **D.** ad

CHAPTER 4

Structures and Functions of Body Systems

OUTLINE

GLOSSARY

Acetylcholine (ACh) – a neurotransmitter

Agranulocyte – a type of white blood cell, including monocytes and lymphocytes, that is characterized by an absence of granules in its cytoplasm (cellular fluid)

Alveolar sacs (alveoli) – the cluster-like air sacs located at the end of each alveolar duct in the lungs

Anatomy – the branch of science that deals with the structure of body parts, their forms, and their organization

Bowman's glomerular capsule – a sac that collects fluids from the blood in the glomerulus of the kidney and, through a process called *ultrafiltration*, processes the fluids to form urine

Corpus callosum – a structure in the longitudinal fissure of the brain that connects the left and right cerebral hemispheres

Diaphragm – a sheet of muscle, important in the process of respiration, that extends across the bottom part of the rib cage

Distal convoluted tubule – a portion of the nephron of the kidney, located between the loop of Henle and the collecting ducts, that is partly responsible for regulating potassium, sodium, calcium, and pH

Endorphins – naturally occurring substances that, as part of the body's pain control system, mimic many of the effects of narcotics

Glomerulus – a knot of capillaries, surrounded by the Bowman's glomerular capsule, that receives blood from the renal circulation; each glomerulus and its surrounding capsule make up a renal corpuscle

Glucagon – an important hormone, antagonistic to insulin, involved in carbohydrate metabolism

Granulocyte – a type of white blood cell, having granules in its cytoplasm, that includes neutrophils, eosinophils, and basophils

Hormones – regulating and controlling organ and tissue activity, natural chemical substances secreted into the bloodstream from the endocrine glands

Insulin – a hormone, secreted when the blood glucose level rises, that extensively affects metabolism and many other body systems

Liver – one of the largest organs in the digestive system; among its many functions are manufacture of plasma proteins, storage of starch and vitamins, and the production of bile salts

Loop of Henle – a U-shaped structure, whose function is to reabsorb water and ions from the urine, that is located in the proximal convoluted tubule of the kidney

Mechanical digestion – the breakdown of large food particles into smaller pieces by chewing and the mashing actions of muscles in the digestive tract

Mediastinum – the central compartment of the thoracic cavity within the chest

Melanin – a dark pigment that provides skin color and absorbs ultraviolet radiation in sunlight

Neurohormones – hormones produced and released by neurons

Neurohypophysis – posterior lobe of the pituitary gland

Neuron – the basic cell of the nervous system

Phagocytize – to engulf solid particles within a cell membrane to form an internal food vacuole (membrane-bound compartment)

Physiology – the branch of science that deals with how body parts work and what they accomplish

Renal corpuscle – a filtration unit in the kidney that consists of a knot of capillaries (the glomerulus) surrounded by the Bowman's glomerular capsule

Renal tubule – the portion of the nephron in the kidney that contains the tubular fluid filtered through the glomerulus

Sebaceous – skin glands that secrete an oily substance called "sebum"

Venae cavae – the collective name for the superior and inferior *vena cava*, which are the veins that return deoxygenated blood from the body into the right atrium of the heart

OVERVIEW

Anatomy is the branch of science that deals with the structure of body parts, their forms, and their organization. How these body parts work and what they accomplish is the science of **physiology**. To comprehend the effects of different drugs, pharmacy technicians must understand the body's normal functions and structures. This chapter gives a brief overview of anatomy and physiology.

CARDIOVASCULAR SYSTEM

The cardiovascular system consists of the heart and blood vessels.

Heart

A hollow muscular organ, the heart is located within the **mediastinum**, resting on the **diaphragm**. The wall of the heart has three layers (the epicardium, myocardium, and endocardium) as shown in Figure 4–1.

The heart is divided into two atria and two ventricles. Receiving blood from the venae cavae, the right atrium is separated from the right ventricle by a *tricuspid valve*. Pulmonary arteries transfer low-oxygen blood away from the heart to the lungs. Receiving blood from the pulmonary veins, the left atrium is separated from the left ventricle by the *mitral valve*. The coronary arteries supply blood to the myocardium. Blood returns to the right atrium through the cardiac veins and the coronary sinus (see Figure 4–2).

The blood vessels include the arteries, capillaries, and veins. The heart's pumping forces blood through the arteries, which connect to the smaller-diameter vessels. The tiniest tubes, the capillaries, are the sites of nutrient, electrolyte, gas, and waste exchange. Capillaries converge into venules, which in turn converge into veins that return blood to the heart, completing the closed system of blood circulation. In addition to removing wastes, the cardiovascular system brings oxygen and nutrients to all body cells.

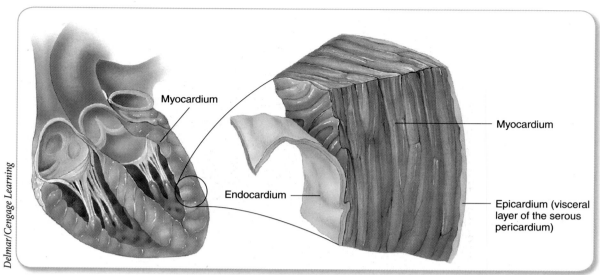

Figure 4–1 The walls of the heart.

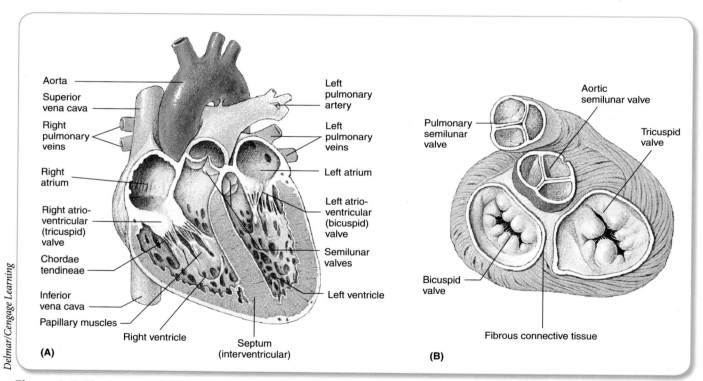

Figure 4–2 The interior of the heart. A. Cross section of the heart showing the chambers, valves, septum, chordae tendineae, and vessels. B. Superior view of valves.

Blood

Blood consists of red blood cells, white blood cells, and platelets suspended in a liquid known as *plasma*. Blood consists mostly of red blood cells, and its plasma includes water, gases, hormones, plasma proteins, nutrients, electrolytes, and cellular wastes. Red blood cells contain hemoglobin, which combines with oxygen. Mature red blood cells do not have nuclei. White blood cells are either granulocytes (neutrophils, eosinophils, and basophils) or agranulocytes (which include monocytes and lymphocytes) as shown in Figure 4–3.

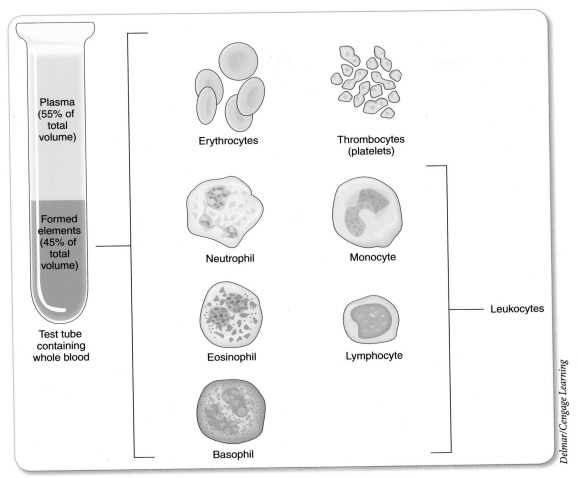

Plasma (55% of total volume)

Formed elements (45% of total volume)

Test tube containing whole blood

Erythrocytes

Neutrophil

Eosinophil

Basophil

Thrombocytes (platelets)

Monocyte

Lymphocyte

Leukocytes

Delmar/Cengage Learning

Figure 4–3 The major components of blood.

Neutrophils and monocytes phagocytize (engulf) foreign particles. Eosinophils are capable of destroying bacteria and increase in number during allergic reactions. Basophils release heparin, which inhibits blood clotting, and histamine, which increases blood flow to injured tissues. Lymphocytes produce antibodies that attack specific foreign substances, and platelets help to close breaks in blood vessels. An antibody is also called an *immunoglobulin* or *gamma globulin*.

NERVOUS SYSTEM

Composed of the brain, spinal cord, and nerves (see Figure 4–4), the nervous system is divided into two sections: the central nervous system (CNS) and the peripheral nervous system (PNS). The nervous system controls sensory functions, integrative functions, and motor functions. Subdivision of these two systems is summarized in Figure 4–5.

The brain is subdivided into the cerebrum, diencephalon, brainstem, and cerebellum. The cerebrum consists of two cerebral hemispheres, connected by the corpus callosum. The diencephalon contains the thalamus (which relays incoming sensory impulses) and the hypothalamus (which maintains homeostasis). The brainstem consists of the midbrain, pons, and medulla oblongata. The cerebellum consists of two hemispheres, coordinating skeletal muscle movements and maintaining equilibrium (see Figure 4–6).

Subdivided into the somatic and autonomic nervous systems, the PNS consists of cranial and spinal nerves, which branch from the brain and spinal cord to all body parts. Twelve pairs of cranial nerves connect the brain to various structures in the head, neck,

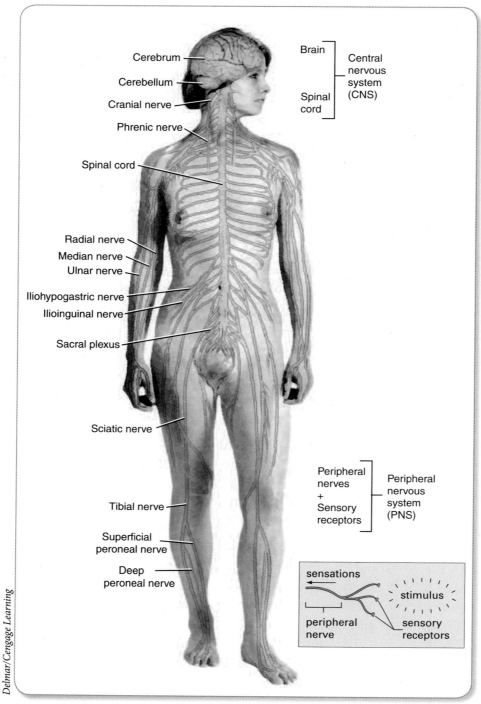

Cerebrum

Cerebellum

Cranial nerve

Phrenic nerve

Spinal cord

Radial nerve
Median nerve
Ulnar nerve

Iliohypogastric nerve

Ilioinguinal nerve

Sacral plexus

Sciatic nerve

Tibial nerve

Superficial
peroneal nerve

Deep
peroneal nerve

Brain

Spinal
cord

Central
nervous
system
(CNS)

Peripheral
nerves
+
Sensory
receptors

Peripheral
nervous
system
(PNS)

sensations

stimulus

peripheral
nerve

sensory
receptors

Delmar/Cengage Learning

Figure 4–4 The nervous system.

and trunk (see Figure 4–7). Thirty-one pairs of spinal nerves originate from the spinal cord.

Regulating the visceral activities that maintain homeostasis, the ANS functions without any conscious effort. The ANS is subdivided into the sympathetic and parasympathetic nervous systems (see Figure 4–8).

The sympathetic nervous system responds to stress and emergency situations. The parasympathetic nervous system is most active under ordinary conditions.

Carrying nerve impulses from one part of the body to another, the **neuron** is the basic cell of the nervous system. It consists of three parts: dendrites,

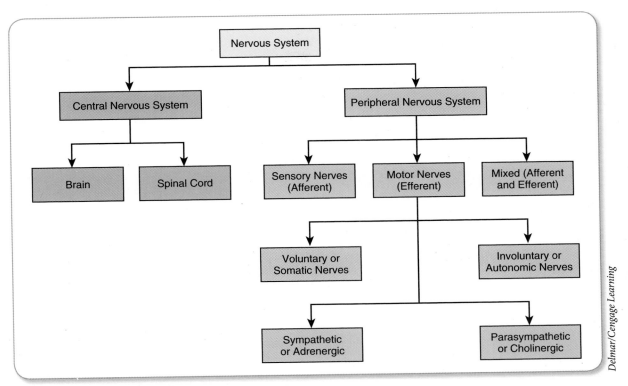

Figure 4–5 Organization of the nervous system.

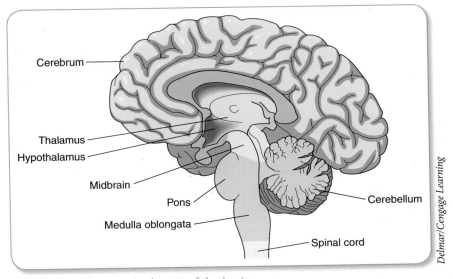

Figure 4–6 The principal parts of the brain.

cell body, and axons (see Figure 4–9). Dendrites are the receptors that carry information to the nerve cell body, whereas axons carry nerve information away from the nerve cell body. The junction between two neurons is called a *synapse*. At the junction of neurons, the continuation of messages is performed by neurotransmitters, such as acetylcholine (ACh), which stimulate the nerve endings. ACh is broken

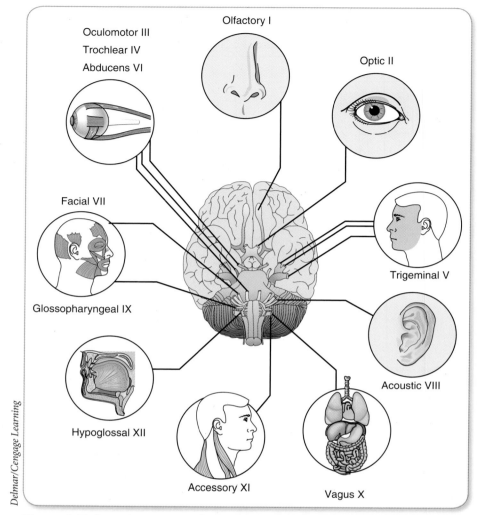

Figure 4–7 Cranial nerves are identified with Roman numerals and are named for the area, or function, they serve.

Delmar/Cengage Learning

down by the enzyme known as *cholinesterase*. Other neurotransmitters, or **neurohormones**, include the catecholamines (norepinephrine, epinephrine, and dopamine), serotonin, and **endorphins**.

ENDOCRINE SYSTEM

The endocrine system consists of specialized cell clusters, glands, hormones, and target tissues. The glands and cell clusters secrete hormones and chemical transmitters in response to stimulation from the nervous system and other sites. Together with the nervous system, the endocrine system regulates and integrates the body's metabolic activities and maintains internal homeostasis.

The endocrine system is composed of endocrine glands that are distributed throughout the body. Endocrine glands secrete hormones, or chemical messengers, directly into the bloodstream. The major organs of the endocrine system are the hypothalamus, pituitary gland, thyroid gland, parathyroid glands, adrenal glands, pancreas, testes, and ovaries (see Figure 4–10).

Sometimes called the *master gland*, the pituitary gland controls most glandular activity. The pituitary itself is controlled by the hypothalamus. Being

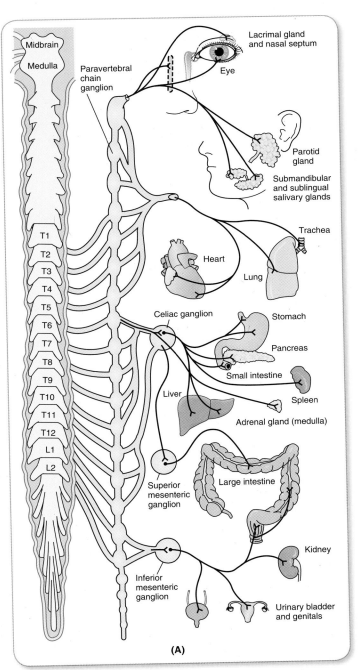
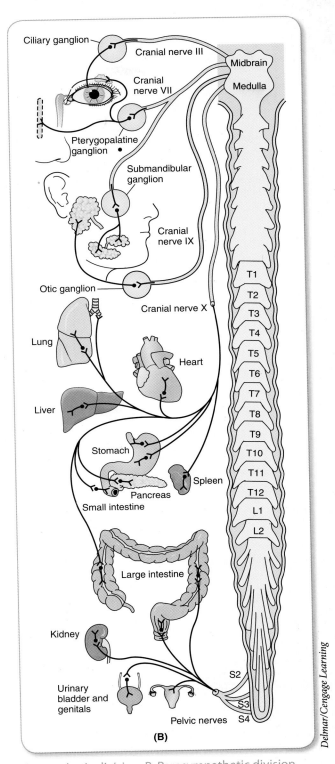

Figure 4–8 The nerve pathways of the autonomic nervous system. A. Sympathetic division. B. Parasympathetic division.

Delmar/Cengage Learning

conservative, the body secretes hormones only as needed. For example, insulin is secreted when the blood glucose level rises. Another hormone, glucagon, works antagonistically to insulin and is released when the blood glucose level falls below normal. Hormones are potent chemicals; hence, their circulating levels must be carefully controlled. When its level is adequate, a hormone stops releasing.

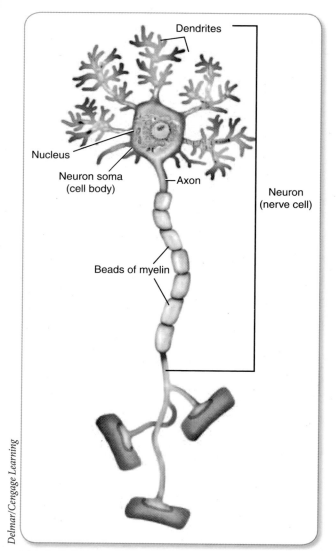

Delmar/Cengage Learning

Figure 4–9 The neuron.

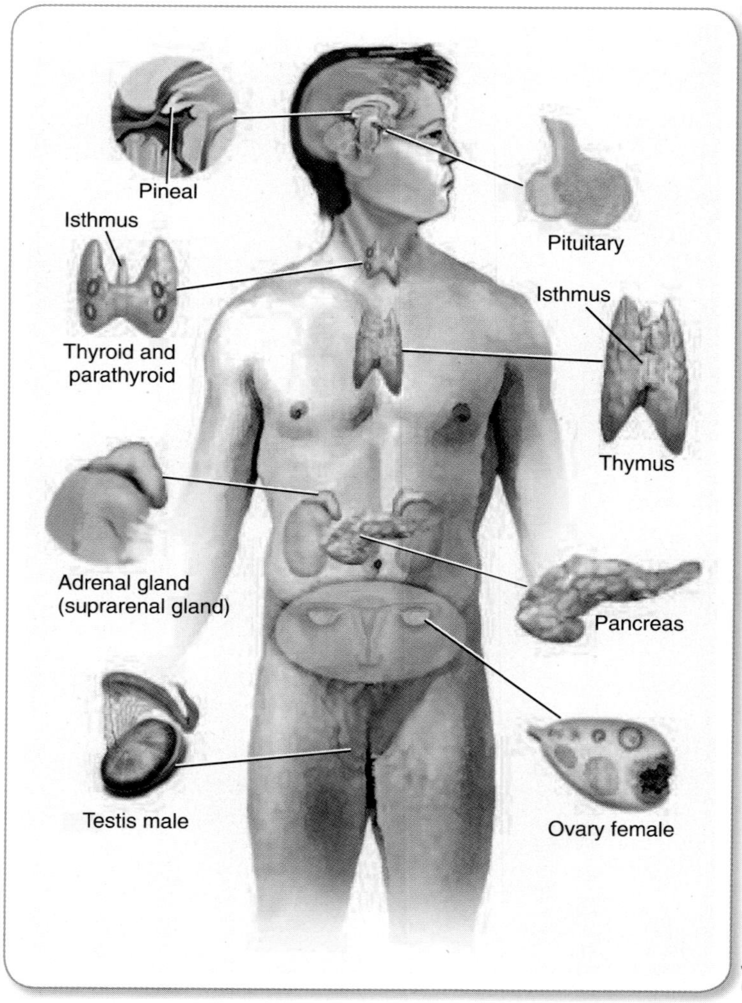

Figure 4–10 The endocrine system.

Delmar/Cengage Learning

Hormonal Regulation

The hypothalamus is the main integrative center for the endocrine and autonomic nervous systems. By neural and hormonal pathways, the hypothalamus helps control some endocrine glands. Neural pathways connect the hypothalamus to the posterior pituitary gland. Neural stimulation of the posterior pituitary causes the secretion of two effector hormones: antidiuretic hormone (also known as vasopressin) and oxytocin.

By releasing and inhibiting hormones and factors, which arrive by a portal system, the hypothalamus also exerts hormonal control at the anterior pituitary gland. Hypothalamic hormones stimulate the pituitary glands to synthesize and release trophic hormones. These hormones include corticotropin (also called *adrenocorticotropic hormone*), thyroid-stimulating hormone (TSH), and gonadotropins, such as luteinizing hormone (LH) and follicle-stimulating hormone (FSH). Secretion of trophic hormones stimulates the adrenal cortex, thyroid gland, and gonads. Hypothalamic hormones also stimulate the pituitary gland to release or inhibit the release of effector hormones, such as growth hormone (GH) and prolactin (PRL).

Hormones

Hormones are natural chemical substances secreted into the bloodstream from the endocrine glands that regulate and control the activity of an organ or tissues in another part of the body. A list of major hormones and endocrine glands is provided in Table 4–1. Hormones from the various endocrine glands work together to regulate vital processes of the body and include the following:

TABLE 4–1 Endocrine Glands and Their Hormones

Gland	Hormones
Hypothalamus	Releasing and inhibiting hormones, such as GnRH, GHRH, and TRH
Pituitary Anterior	Growth hormone (GH)
	Adrenocorticotropic hormone (ACTH)
	Thyroid-stimulating hormone (TSH)
	Luteinizing hormone (LH)
	Follicle-stimulating hormone (FSH)
	Prolactin (PRL)
Pituitary Posterior (hormone storage site)	Oxytocin (OT)
	Vasopressin (antidiuretic hormone – ADH)
Thyroid	Thyroid hormone (T_4 and T_3)
	Calcitonin
Parathyroid	Parathyroid hormone
Thymus	Thymosin
Pancreas (islets of Langerhans)	Insulin Glucagon
Adrenal Cortex	Cortisol (a glucocorticoid)
	Aldosterone (a mineralocorticoid)
	Androgens
Medulla	Epinephrine
	Norepinephrine
Testes	Testosterone
Ovaries	Estrogen
	Progesterone

1. Secretions in the digestive tract
2. Energy production
3. Composition and volume of extracellular fluid
4. Adaptation and immunity
5. Growth and development
6. Reproduction and lactation

Inactivation of hormones occurs enzymatically in the blood, liver, kidneys, or target tissues. Hormones are secreted primarily via the urine and, to a lesser extent, via the bile. In medicine, hormones generally are used in three ways: (1) for replacement therapy, (2) for pharmacologic effects beyond replacement, and (3) for endocrine system diagnostic testing.

Pituitary Gland

The hypothalamus controls the pituitary gland, which consists of two lobes, an anterior lobe (adenohypophysis) and a posterior lobe (neurohypophysis).

Anterior Pituitary Gland

The anterior lobe of the pituitary gland is particularly important in sustaining life as it secretes at least six hormones: growth hormone (somatotropin, GH), adrenocorticotropic hormone (ACTH), thyroid-stimulating hormone (TSH), follicle-stimulating hormone (FSH), luteinizing hormone (LH), and prolactin (PRL). Figure 4–11 illustrates the major hormones of the pituitary gland and their principal target organs.

Adrenocorticotropic Hormone. ACTH is another hormone from the anterior pituitary gland that stimulates the growth of the adrenal gland cortex and the secretion of corticosteroids. Under normal conditions, a diurnal rhythm occurs in ACTH secretion, with an increase beginning after the first few hours of sleep and reaching a peak at the time a person awakens.

Thyroid-Stimulating Hormone. TSH, a substance secreted by the anterior lobe of the pituitary gland, controls the release of thyroid hormone and is necessary for the growth and function of the thyroid

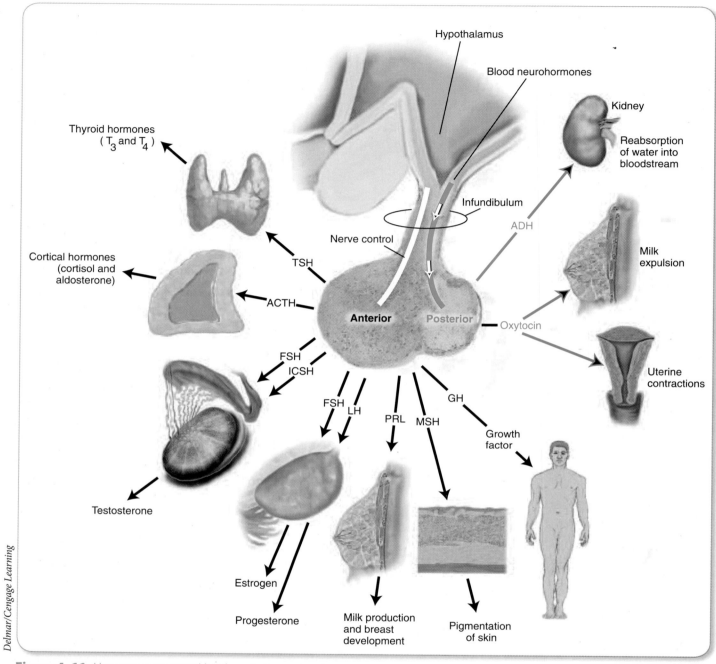

Figure 4–11 Hormones secreted by the pituitary gland.

gland. TSH stimulates the thyroid gland to increase the uptake of iodine and increase the synthesis and release of thyroid hormones. The hormone is prescribed for hypothyroidism and diagnostic tests.

Posterior Pituitary Gland

The posterior lobe of the pituitary gland, or the neurohypophysis, is the release point of antidiuretic hormone (ADH, or vasopressin) and oxytocin. When the hypothalamus stimulates it, the neurohypophysis releases ADH. The hormone acts on the distal and collecting tubules of the kidneys. Because of this action, kidneys will be more permeable to water and reduce the volume of the urine. Under appropriate stimulation from the hypothalamus, the neurohypophysis releases oxytocin, which produces powerful contractions of the uterus of pregnant women and causes milk to flow from their lactating breasts. Hypofunction of the posterior pituitary gland results in diabetes insipidus.

Thyroid Gland

Located in the anterior neck, the thyroid gland is the largest of the endocrine glands (see Figure 4–12) and secretes three hormones essential for proper regulation of metabolism. The thyroid gland, through its hormone, thyroxine, governs cellular oxygen consumption and, hence, energy and heart production. The thyroid gland secretes thyroxine (T_4), triiodothyronine (T_3), and calcitonin. Iodine is essential for thyroid hormone synthesis, and the hormone calcitonin has a very important role in calcium metabolism. Normally, calcitonin decreases the level of blood calcium.

Parathyroid Glands

Located on the posterior surface of the thyroid gland, four parathyroid glands secrete parathyroid hormone, which increases blood calcium concentration and decreases blood phosphate ion concentration. Parathyroid hormone affects the bones, intestines, and kidneys.

Adrenal Glands

The adrenal glands are located at the top of each kidney. They consist of two parts—the outer cortex and the inner medulla (see Figure 4–13). The adrenal cortex synthesizes three important classes of hormones: glucocorticoids (cortisol), mineralocorticoids (primarily aldosterone), and androgens. The cortex of the adrenal gland is one of the endocrine structures most vital for normal metabolic function. The medulla secretes two hormones, epinephrine and norepinephrine.

Pancreas

One of the accessory organs of the digestive system, the pancreas is located below the stomach. It produces digestive enzymes that are deposited in the small intestine. Islets of specialized cells (islets of Langerhans) exist throughout the pancreas. The α cells produce glucagon to raise blood glucose levels, whereas the β cells release insulin, which lowers blood glucose levels. When serum blood glucose levels decline, glucagon facilitates the breakdown of glycogen to glucose in the liver. The conversion of glycogen to glucose results in an increase in blood glucose. The release of glucagon stimulates insulin secretion, which then inhibits the release of glucagon.

Gonadal Hormones

Gonadal tissues produce three main classes of steroid hormones: estrogenic, progestational, and androgenic. The ovary is the primary site for synthesis and secretion of estrogen and progestin hormones in women. The menstrual cycle is regulated by the production of hypothalamic gonadotropin-releasing hormone (GnRH), which stimulates the release of FSH and LH from the anterior pituitary gland. In men and postmenopausal women, the principal source of estrogen is adipose tissue, in which the level of estrogens is regulated in part by the availability of androgenic precursors from the adrenal cortex. The most important androgenic hormone produced by the testes in men is testosterone, although the adrenal cortex also produces some androgenic hormones in both men and women. FSH and LH also regulate testosterone production by specific cells in the testes that control

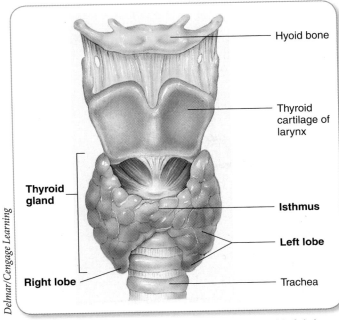

Delmar/Cengage Learning

Hyoid bone

Thyroid cartilage of larynx

Thyroid gland

Isthmus

Left lobe

Right lobe

Trachea

Figure 4–12 The thyroid consists of a right and left lobe joined by the isthmus.

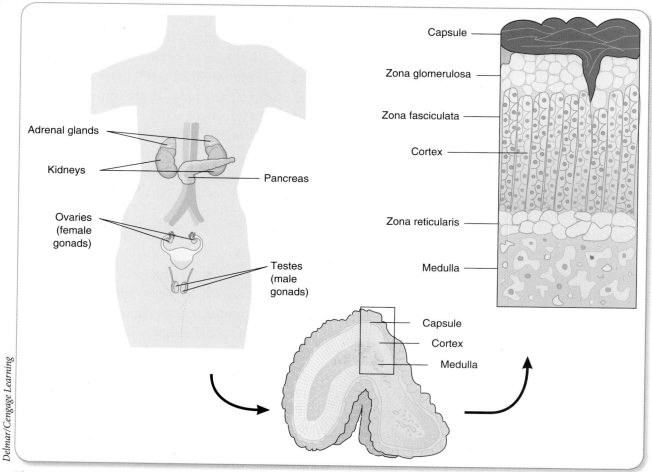

Delmar/Cengage Learning

Figure 4–13 The adrenal glands.

spermatogenesis and the development of primary and secondary sexual characteristics in men.

Ovarian Hormones

The reproductive system of the human female consists of the ovaries, fallopian tubes, uterus, and vagina. The ovaries, known as gonads, produce ova and form endocrine secretions that initiate and maintain the secondary sex characteristics in women (see Figure 4–14).

Estrogen. The ovaries are the primary source of various types of estrogen in nonpregnant females. When females reach puberty, the anterior pituitary gland influences the ovaries' secretion of increasing amounts of estrogen. This stimulates enlargement of accessory organs. The estrogen hormones also develop and maintain the *female secondary sex characteristics.*

Progesterone. During the female reproductive years, progesterone is secreted primarily by the ovarian cells in the corpus luteum. Only during the last two weeks of the menstrual cycle does the corpus luteum secrete progesterone. The greatest amount is secreted during the week after ovulation has taken place. Progesterone is responsible for the changes in the uterine endometrium during the second half of the menstrual cycle, development of the maternal placenta after implantation, and development of the mammary glands. Progesterone also causes an increase in the viscosity of cervical secretions, which impedes the movement of sperm.

Testicular Hormones

The hypothalamus, anterior pituitary gland, and testes secrete hormones that control male reproductive functions. These hormones initiate and maintain

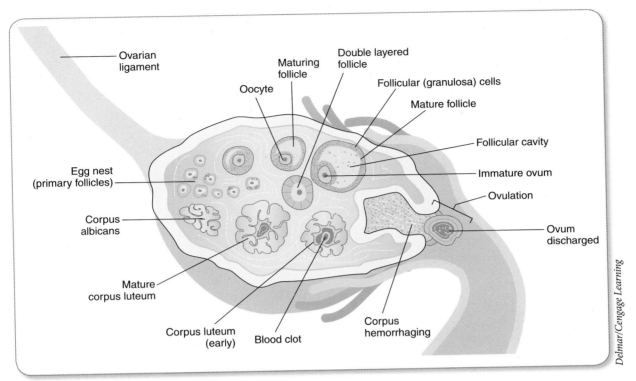

Figure 4–14 An ovary showing a developing ovum.

sperm cell production and oversee the development and maintenance of male secondary sex characteristics. Androgens are secreted mainly in the interstitial tissue of the testes in the male and secondarily in the adrenal glands of both sexes (see Figure 4–15). Androgens include testosterone and androsterone. Inadequate production of androgens in the male may be due to the result of pituitary malfunction. Testosterone stimulates the development of the male secondary sex characteristics, initiates the production of sperm, and enhances the functional capacity of the penis and accessory sex organs.

MUSCULOSKELETAL SYSTEM

Consisting of two different systems that work closely together for the frame and movement of the body, the musculoskeletal system includes a collection of connective tissue, muscles, bones, and joints (see Figures 4–16A, 4–16B, 4–16C, and 4–16D).

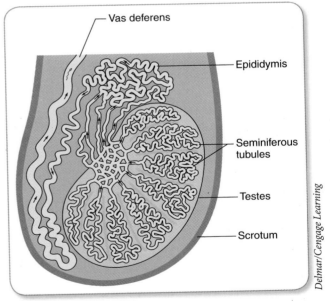

Figure 4–15 The testes.

The muscular system consists of three types of muscles: skeletal muscle, which attaches to bones and joints by connective tissue (tendons and ligaments), smooth muscle, and myocardium. Muscles require

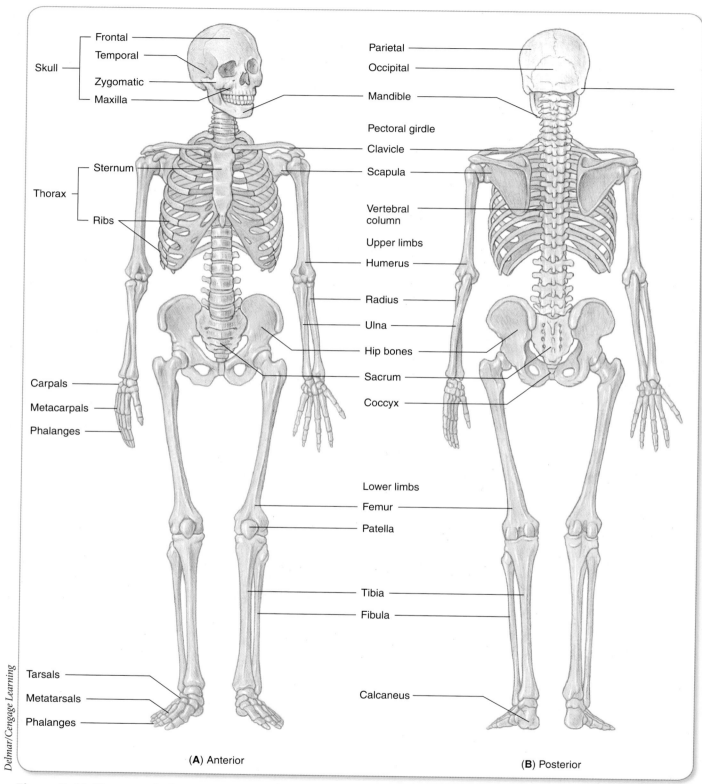

Delmar/Cengage Learning

Figure 4–16 The musculoskeletal system. A. Human skeleton, anterior view. B. Human skeleton, posterior view.

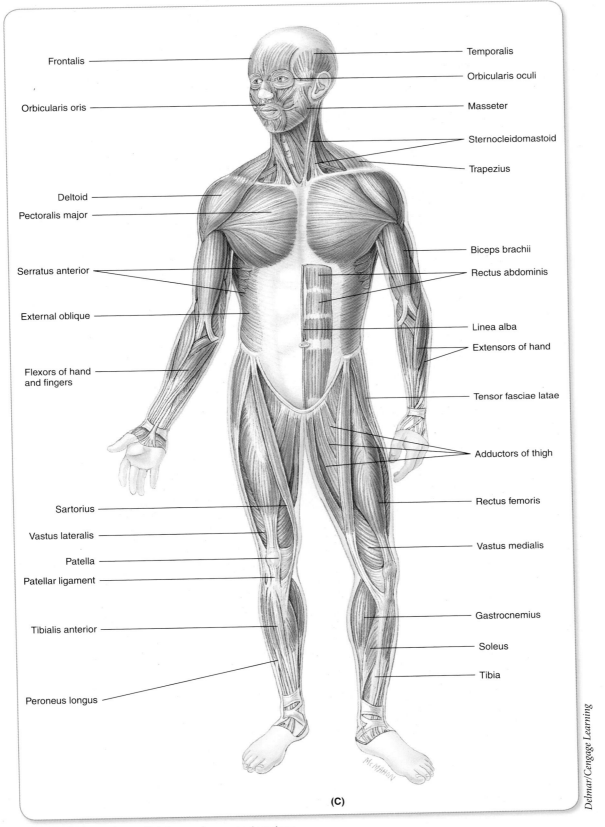

Frontalis

Orbicularis oris

Deltoid

Pectoralis major

Serratus anterior

External oblique

Flexors of hand
and fingers

Sartorius

Vastus lateralis

Patella

Patellar ligament

Tibialis anterior

Peroneus longus

Temporalis

Orbicularis oculi

Masseter

Sternocleidomastoid

Trapezius

Biceps brachii

Rectus abdominis

Linea alba

Extensors of hand

Tensor fasciae latae

Adductors of thigh

Rectus femoris

Vastus medialis

Gastrocnemius

Soleus

Tibia

(C)

Figure 4–16 C. Superficial muscles, anterior view.

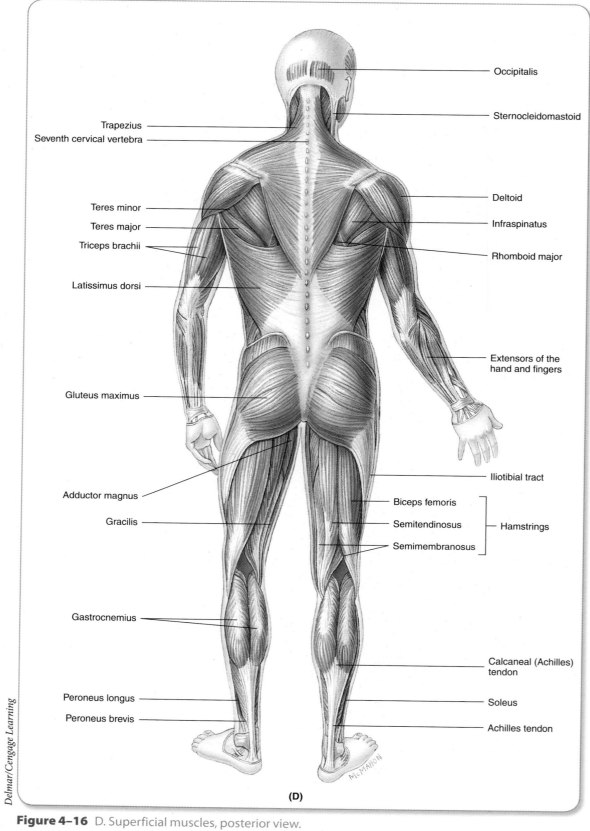

Occipitalis

Sternocleidomastoid

Trapezius
Seventh cervical vertebra

Teres minor
Teres major
Triceps brachii

Latissimus dorsi

Deltoid
Infraspinatus
Rhomboid major

Extensors of the
hand and fingers

Gluteus maximus

Iliotibial tract

Adductor magnus

Gracilis

Biceps femoris
Semitendinosus
Semimembranosus

Hamstrings

Gastrocnemius

Calcaneal (Achilles)
tendon

Peroneus longus
Peroneus brevis

Soleus

Achilles tendon

(D)

Figure 4–16 D. Superficial muscles, posterior view.

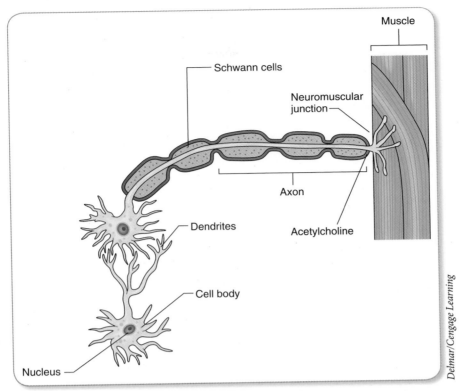

Figure 4–17 A neuron stimulating muscle.

Delmar/Cengage Learning

electrical impulses from motor nerves for stimulation (see Figure 4–17). When excited, muscles cause contraction and relaxation. Skeletal muscles also have other functions. They produce movement and heat, maintain body posture and temperature, and stabilize joints.

The skeletal system consists of bones and the joints where bones meet. Bone consists of a variety of very active, living tissues: bone tissue, cartilage, dense connective tissue, blood, and nervous tissue. The organs of the skeletal system, bones are also multifunctional and provide points of attachment for muscles. They protect and support softer tissues, house cells that produce blood, store inorganic salts, and form passageways for blood vessels and nerves.

The skeleton is divided into two major portions: an axial skeleton and an appendicular skeleton. Table 4–2 summarizes the divisions of the adult skeleton.

The joints allow the body to be mobile and flexible. The articulation sites are covered with cartilage.

URINARY SYSTEM

The *urinary system* removes certain salts and nitrogenous wastes, and helps maintain the normal concentrations of water and electrolytes in body fluids. It also regulates the pH and volume of body fluids, and helps control red blood cell production as well as blood pressure.

The urinary system consists of a pair of kidneys, which remove substances from the blood. The kidneys also form urine and help regulate certain metabolic processes. Other parts of the urinary system include the ureters, which are tubular structures that transport urine from the kidneys; a sac-like urinary bladder, (an expandable organ that stores urine); and a tubular urethra, which conveys urine to outside of the body (see Figure 4–18).

Nephrons

A kidney contains about one million nephrons, with each nephron consisting of a renal corpuscle and a

TABLE 4–2 Divisions of the Adult Skeleton

Type of Skeleton	Type of Bones	Total Number of Bones
Axial Skeleton	Skull –	22
	8 cranial bones: frontal (1), parietal (2), occipital (1), temporal (2), sphenoid (1), ethmoid (1)	
	14 facial bones: maxilla (2), zygomatic (2), palatine (2), inferior nasal concha (2), mandible (1), lacrimal (2), nasal (2), vomer (1)	
	Middle ear –	6
	Malleus (2), incus (2), stapes (2)	
	Hyoid –	1
	Hyoid bone (1)	
	Vertebral column –	26
	Cervical vertebrae (7), thoracic vertebrae (12), lumbar vertebrae (5), sacrum (1), coccyx (1)	
	Thoracic cage –	25
	Rib (24), sternum (1)	
Appendicular Skeleton	Pectoral girdle –	4
	Scapula (2), clavicle (2)	
	Upper limbs –	60
	Humerus (2), radius (2), ulna (2), carpal (16), metacarpal (10), phalanx (28)	
	Pelvic girdle –	2
	Hip bone (2)	
	Lower limbs –	60
	Femur (2), tibia (2), fibula (2), patella (2), tarsal (14), metatarsal (10), phalanx (28)	
	Total Bones in the Body: 206	

renal tubule (see Figure 4–19). Fluid flows through the renal tubules on its way out of the body. The nephron begins as a double-walled globule known as Bowman's glomerular capsule. A renal corpuscle is composed of a cluster of blood capillaries called a glomerulus. Glomerular capillaries filter fluid, which is the first step in urine formation.

The renal tubule leads away from the glomerular capsule and coils into a portion called the *proximal convoluted tubule*. The next section of this tubule is called the *descending limb of Henle*, which bends into a U-shaped structure known as the loop of Henle.

After this structure, the tubule becomes the distal convoluted tubule, which ends by merging with a large, straight collecting duct.

RESPIRATORY SYSTEM

The most important function of the respiratory system is the inspiration of oxygen and the expiration of carbon dioxide. Therefore, the respiratory tract must exchange gases and supply oxygen to the body. The effectiveness of the respiratory system affects the body's ability to function correctly and to be in

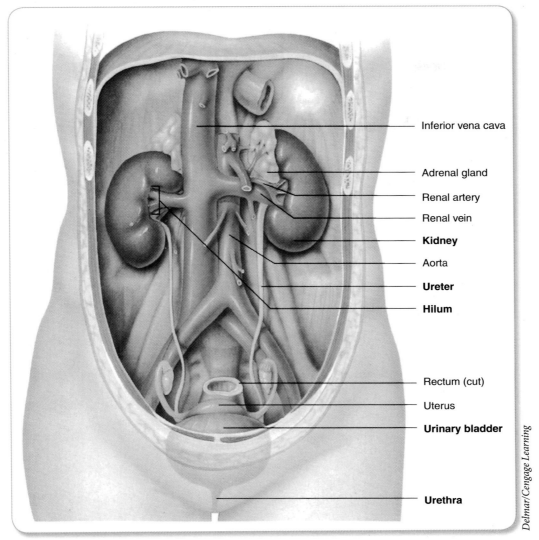

Inferior vena cava

Adrenal gland

Renal artery

Renal vein

Kidney

Aorta

Ureter

Hilum

Rectum (cut)

Uterus

Urinary bladder

Urethra

Delmar/Cengage Learning

Figure 4–18 The organs of the urinary system of a female.

homeostasis. The respiratory system consists of the nasal passages, mouth, pharynx, larynx, trachea, and lungs, as well as the accessory organs, such as the skeletal muscles of the chest wall and the diaphragm (see Figure 4–20).

The upper respiratory tract contains the nasal cavity, sinuses, mouth, and pharynx. The lower respiratory tract is essential for the exchange of oxygen and carbon dioxide. This system is made up of the larynx, trachea, and lungs. The lower end of the trachea separates into the right and left bronchi. As the bronchi enter the lungs, they subdivide into bronchial tubes and small bronchioles. At the end

of each bronchiole is an alveolar duct, which ends in a sac-like cluster called alveolar sacs (alveoli) (see Figure 4–21).

DIGESTIVE SYSTEM

A hollow tube extending from the mouth to the anus, the digestive system breaks down (digests) food into particles that are small and simple enough to be absorbed. The digestive system ingests food, digests it, absorbs the end products of digestion, and eliminates waste. Absorbed by movement across the lining of the digestive tract into the blood, digested

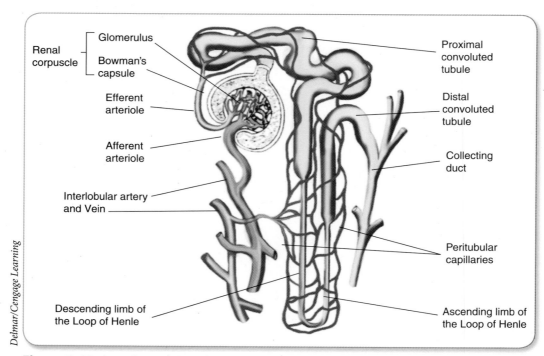

Figure 4–19 A nephron unit and its associated structures.

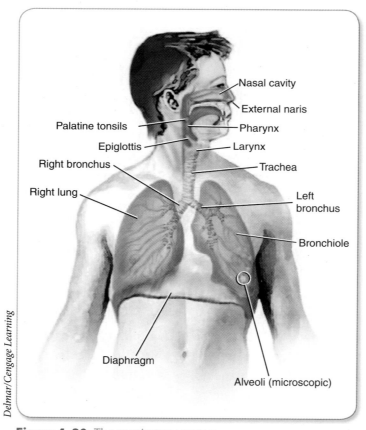

Figure 4–20 The respiratory system.

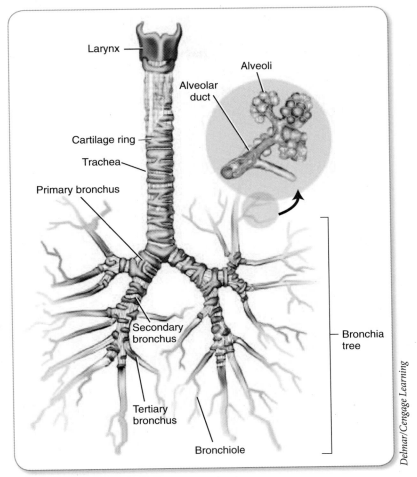

Figure 4–21 The bronchi and bronchioles.

Delmar/Cengage Learning

nutrients eventually reach every cell in the body. Elimination of waste products is the last stage of the digestive process. Some water is also eliminated in the feces. The gastrointestinal (GI) tract digests, stores and absorbs nutrients, and eliminates wastes. Figure 4–22 is an illustration of the digestive system.

Consisting of the digestive tract (several organs) and accessory glands of digestion, the digestive system contains the digestive tube of the body through which food passes from the mouth to the esophagus, stomach, and intestines. The intestines include the small intestine, the longest part of the digestive system, and large intestine (colon). The accessory glands include the salivary glands, liver,

gallbladder, and pancreas. The salivary glands and pancreas secrete digestive enzymes, which break down food substances in preparation for absorption into the bloodstream.

The **liver**, one of the largest organs of the digestive system (see Figure 4–23), has numerous and important functions. Humans cannot survive without this organ. Its major functions include the manufacture of plasma proteins; phagocytosis (eating) of certain bacteria and older, worn-out red blood cells; storage of glycogen (animal starch) and the vitamins A, D, E, and K; and the production of bile salts. The liver is also needed for the metabolism of medications.

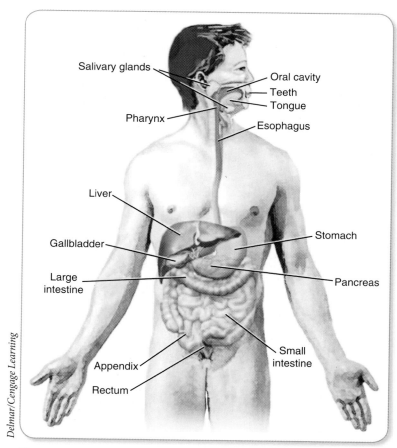

Delmar/Cengage Learning

Figure 4–22 The digestive system.

INTEGUMENTARY SYSTEM

The skin, and the various accessory structures that are associated with it, is the largest organ in the body by weight. The structures that make up the integumentary system include the hair, nails, sensory receptors, and glands.

The skin helps regulate body temperature, reduces water loss from deeper tissues, houses sensory receptors, synthesizes certain biochemicals, and excretes small amounts of waste. Skin cells also help to produce vitamin D, which is vital for normal bone and tooth development. Specialized cells in the epidermis called *melanocytes* produce melanin, a dark pigment that provides skin color that also absorbs the ultraviolet radiation in sunlight.

The skin includes two distinct layers (see Figure 4–24). The outer layer is called the *epidermis*. The inner layer, or *dermis*, is thicker than the epidermis and includes connective tissue consisting of blood, *collagenous* and *elastic* fibers, nervous tissue, smooth muscle, sebaceous glands, and sweat glands. Beneath the dermis is loose connective tissue (predominately consisting of adipose tissue) that binds the skin to the underlying organs forming the *subcutaneous layer*.

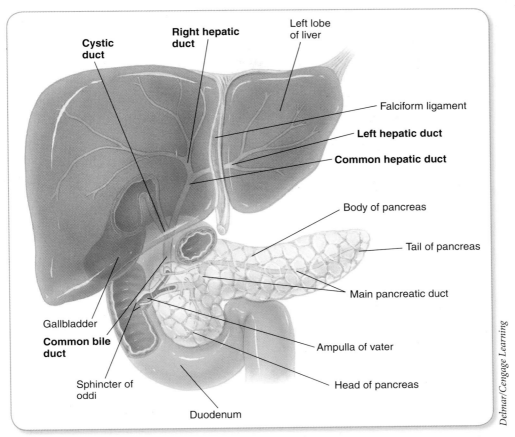

Figure 4–23 The anatomy of the liver.

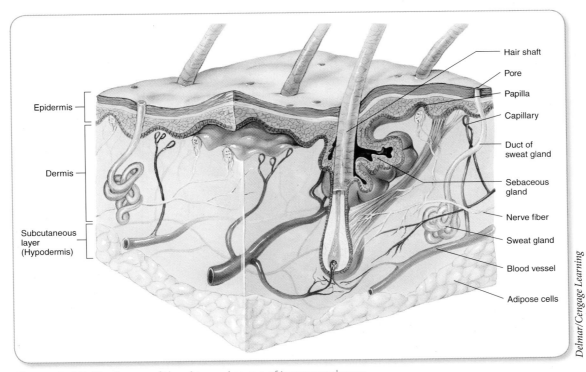

Figure 4–24 The layers of the skin and some of its appendages.

EXPLORING THE WEB

Visit http://www.innerbody.com; search for cardio-vascular system.

Visit http://www.human-body-facts.com; search for diseases.

Visit http://www.myeyeworld.com; follow the links to learn about eye structure and function.

Visit http://www.entmags.org; search for ears to learn more about how they function.

Visit http://www.human-biology.net; search for integumentary to learn more about this system.

Visit www.lymphomation.org to learn more about the lymphatic system, especially about lymphoma.

Visit http://www.webmd.com; search for Brain & Nervous System Health Center.

Visit http://www.umm.edu; search for urinary system anatomy to learn how the urinary system gets rid of waste.

REVIEW QUESTIONS

1. Which portion of the brain coordinates skeletal muscle activity?

   A. cerebellum
   B. pons
   C. medulla oblongata
   D. hypothalamus

2. Which endocrine gland releases glucagon?

   A. thyroid gland
   B. adrenal cortex
   C. pancreas
   D. anterior pituitary

3. The hypothalamus releases:

   A. prolactin
   B. testosterone
   C. vasopressin
   D. inhibiting hormones

4. The organs of the respiratory system include all of the following except:

   A. larynx
   B. pharynx
   C. trachea
   D. thoracic duct

5. An expandable organ that stores urine is the:

   A. urinary bladder
   B. kidney
   C. ureter
   D. urethra

6. The longest part of the digestive system is the:

   A. large intestine
   B. sphincter
   C. stomach
   D. small intestine

7. All of the following are neurotransmitters except:

   A. endorphins
   B. dopamine
   C. renin
   D. serotonin

8. Pulmonary arteries:

   A. send blood toward the heart
   B. transfer oxygenated blood away from the heart
   C. transfer low-oxygen blood away from the heart
   D. transfer blood to the brain

9. Which cell releases histamine?

   A. lymphocytes
   B. monocytes
   C. basophils
   D. erythrocytes

10. A synapse is:

   A. the junction between two bones
   B. the junction between two neurons
   C. a type of bone cell that supports, protects, and nourishes the bone
   D. a type of nerve cell that supports, protects, and nourishes the neuron

Common Disorders and Conditions

OUTLINE

GLOSSARY

Acromegaly – abnormal growth of the bones of the face, hands, feet, and soft tissue that occurs after puberty; it is caused by hypersecretion of growth hormone (hGH)

Allergens – nonparasitic antigens that can stimulate a hypersensitivity reaction in certain individuals; common allergens include dust, pollen, and pet dander

Antibiotics – drugs used to treat infections caused by bacteria and other microorganisms

Bacteria – single-celled microorganisms that can exist either as independent organisms or as parasites

Chancre – a painless, highly contagious lesion or ulceration that may form during the primary stage of syphilis

Conjunctivitis – an inflammation of the outermost layer of the eye and inner surface of the eyelid, usually due to an allergic reaction or an infection; commonly called "pink eye"

Diverticulum – a hollow or fluid-filled sac, many of which exist in the walls of the colon

Dwarfism – the abnormal underdevelopment of the body that occurs during childhood commonly because of hyposecretion of growth hormone; it may be caused by many other conditions, including kidney disease and metabolic disorders

Dysuria – painful or difficult urination, often with a burning or stinging sensation

Edema – tissue swelling due to interstitial fluid surrounding or accumulating in the cells

Emphysema – a chronic pulmonary disease characterized by loss of elasticity of the lung tissue often caused by exposure to toxic chemicals and smoke from tobacco products

Genitourinary – referring to the reproductive organs and the urinary system

Gigantism – abnormally large growth of body tissue as a result of an excess of growth hormone during childhood

Hyperpyrexia – extremely high temperature, which is considered a medical emergency

Hypertension – an abnormal increase in arterial blood pressure

Intrinsic factor – a glycoprotein produced by the parietal cells of the stomach; it is required for the body's absorption of vitamin B_{12}

Melanoma – malignant tumor of bottom-layer skin cells (melanocytes), which may also affect the eyes or bowels

Meningitis – inflammation of the meninges that cover the brain and spinal cord

Metastatic – relating to the spread of cancer from one body part to another

Metastasis – the process by which cancer spreads from one part of the body to a distant site or sites

Normal flora – the nonpathogenic microorganisms that exist externally and internally in humans

Osteoporosis – a bone disease characterized by reduced bone mineral density, leading to an increased risk of fracture

Parasites – organisms that live in or on another organism and take their nourishment from the host organism

Peritonitis – inflammation of the peritoneum (the membrane lining parts of the abdominal cavity and visceral organs)

Squamous cell carcinoma – malignant tumor of the flat, scale-like cells of the most superficial layer of the skin, mouth, esophagus, bladder, prostate, lungs, and vagina

Toxemia – the presence of toxins in the blood

Uremia – an illness accompanying renal failure involving urinary waste products contained in the blood

Urethritis – inflammation of the urethra caused by an infection such as chlamydia

Virus – the smallest of all microorganisms, it cannot grow or reproduce apart from a living cell

CANCER

The second leading cause of death in the United States, cancer can originate in almost any organ, with skin cancer being the most common type of cancer in U.S. patients. Excluding skin cancers, the prostate is the most common site of cancer in men; the breast, the most common site in women. The ability to cure cancer varies considerably, depending on the type of cancer and the extent of the disease at the time of diagnosis.

Cancer is a disorder of altered cell differentiation and growth. The resulting process is called *neoplasia,* meaning "new growth," and the new growth is called a *neoplasm.* Malignant neoplasms, which invade and destroy nearby tissue and spread to other parts of the body, tend to grow rapidly and spread widely. Malignant neoplasms can cause death.

There are two categories of malignant neoplasms: solid tumors and hematologic cancers. Solid tumors are initially confined to a specific tissue or organ. Metastasis is the ability of a solid tumor to progress and spread to distant sites. Hematologic cancers involve cells normally found in the blood and lymph, making them *disseminated* diseases from the beginning of their development.

Many cancers are related to specific environmental and lifestyle factors. These factors can predispose a person to develop cancer. Risk factors for cancer include air pollution, alcohol, tobacco, occupation, sexual and reproductive behavior, sunlight, hormones, diet, and X-rays. The most common cancers in the United States, skin cancers include *basal cell carcinoma,* squamous cell carcinoma, and melanoma.

Metastatic tumors develop from cancer cells that travel from an original (or *primary*) site to a second, more distant site. Metastasis commonly occurs via the blood vessels and lymphatic system. Table 5–1 lists some of the more common sites of metastasis for selected cancers.

INFECTIOUS DISEASES

The twentieth century saw astonishing advances in treating and preventing infection, including potent antibiotics, improved immunizations, and better

TABLE 5–1 Common Sites of Metastasis

Original Site	Metastasis Site
Breast	Axillary lymph nodes, lungs, liver, bones, brain
Colon, rectum	Liver, lungs, peritoneum
Lungs	Liver, brain, bones
Ovaries	Liver, lungs
Prostate	Bones
Testicles	Lungs, liver

sanitation. Even so, infection remains the most common cause of human disease. Even in countries with advanced medical care, infectious diseases cause many serious illnesses. In some developing countries, infection is one of the most critical current health problems.

Infection is the invasion and growth of microorganisms in or on body tissue that produces signs and symptoms of disease. Additionally, these microorganisms trigger an immune response. An *immune response* is the way the body recognizes and defends itself against bacteria, viruses, and substances that appear foreign and harmful to the body. Infectious diseases range from relatively mild illnesses to debilitating and lethal conditions, from the common cold through chronic hepatitis, to acquired immunodeficiency syndrome (AIDS). Very young and very old people are especially susceptible to infection.

A select group of microorganisms are called *pathogens*. Pathogens are also called *antigens*, which stimulate the immune system to produce antibodies to respond to them. Fortunately, there are few human pathogens in the microbial world. Most microorganisms are harmless *saprophytes*, free-living organisms that grow by utilizing dead or decaying organic material in the environment. All microorganisms can be opportunistic pathogens, including saprophytes and certain types of normal flora. The term "opportunistic" means that they are capable of causing an infectious disease when the host's health

and immunity have been greatly weakened by illness, malnutrition, or medical therapies. Various types of pathogenic microorganisms include viruses, bacteria, *fungi*, and parasites.

DISEASES AND CONDITIONS OF THE CARDIOVASCULAR SYSTEM

- **Arteriosclerosis** is the term used to describe degenerative changes in small arteries, commonly occurring in older individuals and individuals with diabetes. The arteries lose elasticity (the ability to change shape and return to normal), and their walls become thick and hard. The lumen gradually narrows and may become obscured. This leads to diffuse ischemia and death in various tissues such as those of the heart, kidneys, or brain.

- **Atherosclerosis** is differentiated by the presence of atheromas (plaques consisting of lipids, cells, and cell debris, often with attached thrombi, that form inside the walls of large arteries). Atheromas form primarily in large arteries such as the aorta and the coronary arteries. Figure 5–1 illustrates accumulation of lipids in blood vessels causing occlusion.

- **Angina pectoris** is an episodic, reversible oxygen insufficiency. This term is applied to varying forms of transient chest pain that are attributable to insufficient myocardial oxygen. Atherosclerotic lesions that produce a narrowing of the coronary arteries are the major cause of angina. However, tachycardia (increased heart rate), anemia, hyperthyroidism, and hypotension can cause an oxygen imbalance.

- **Myocardial infarction** is the sudden death of a segment of the heart muscle that is caused by an abrupt interruption of blood flow to part of the heart. Myocardial infarction is most often caused by a blood clot that occludes a

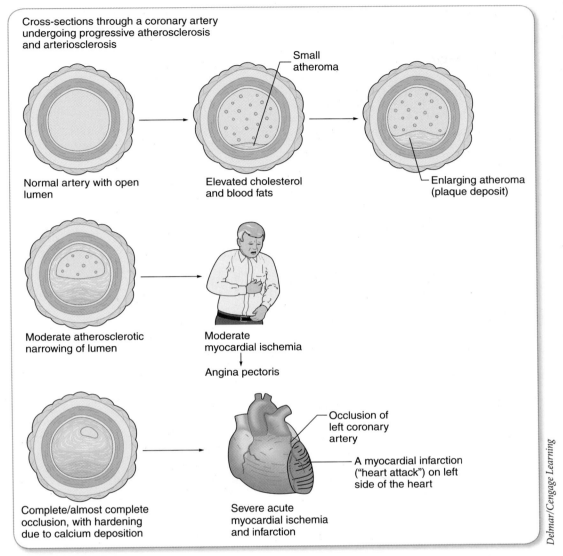

Cross-sections through a coronary artery undergoing progressive atherosclerosis and arteriosclerosis

Small atheroma

Normal artery with open lumen

Elevated cholesterol and blood fats

Enlarging atheroma (plaque deposit)

Moderate atherosclerotic narrowing of lumen

Moderate myocardial ischemia

Angina pectoris

Occlusion of left coronary artery

A myocardial infarction ("heart attack") on left side of the heart

Complete/almost complete occlusion, with hardening due to calcium deposition

Severe acute myocardial ischemia and infarction

Delmar/Cengage Learning

Figure 5–1 Atherosclerosis.

coronary artery. This occlusion cuts off blood flow and oxygen supply to an area of the heart. If thrombolytic medications are not started within a few hours, that section of the heart dies. Myocardial infarctions can range from relatively small types, causing few long-term effects, to massive infarctions that cause immediate death.

- Hypertension is defined as an abnormal increase in arterial blood pressure and can occur as two major types. Essential (primary) hypertension is the most common and results from unknown causes. Secondary hypertension results from renal disease or other identifiable causes such as complications from diabetes, kidney diseases, glandular tumors, thyroid conditions, defects of the aorta, sleep apnea, obesity, complications from pregnancy, and various medications or supplements. Hypertension is a major cause of cardiac disease, renal failure, and stroke. The risk of hypertension increases with age and is higher in African Americans than in Caucasians. It is also higher in people with less education and lower income. Men have a higher incidence of hypertension during young to early-middle adulthood. Thereafter, women have a higher incidence.

- **Arrhythmias** (dysrhythmias) are irregular heartbeats, or when the heart beats with an irregular rhythm. Some arrhythmias are harmless, whereas others are immediately fatal. Arrhythmias may result from damage to the heart's conduction system or from systemic causes such as electrolyte abnormalities, fever, hypoxia, stress, and drug toxicity. Table 5–2 summarizes various cardiac arrhythmias.

- **Congestive heart failure (CHF)** is one of the most common cardiovascular disorders. This condition occurs when the heart is not able to pump enough blood to meet the body's metabolic demands. CHF is characterized by a collection of fluid (congestion) in the lungs and extremities. Because there is no cure for heart failure, the treatment goals are to prevent, treat, or remove the underlying causes when possible. Drugs can relieve the symptoms of heart failure by a number of different mechanisms, including slowing the heart rate, increasing contractility, and reducing its workload.

- **Hyperlipidemia** is a general term indicating excessive levels of any specific fat or fats in the blood. Hyperlipidemia may be caused by excess cholesterol, triglycerides, or low-density lipoproteins (LDL). Dietary or drug

therapy of elevated plasma cholesterol levels can reduce the risk of atherosclerosis and subsequent cardiovascular disease. A patient with high serum cholesterol and increased LDL is at risk of atherosclerotic coronary disease and myocardial infarction. Atherosclerosis is a disorder in which lipid subgroups [total cholesterol, triglycerides, LDL, and high-density lipoproteins (HDL)] in various proportions indicate risk factors for the individual. HDL is commonly referred to as "good cholesterol," whereas LDL is commonly referred to as "bad cholesterol." Table 5–3 shows normal values of cholesterol and triglyceride levels.

TABLE 5–3   Normal Values of Cholesterol and Triglyceride Levels

Cholesterol Level	Cholesterol Category
Less than 200 mg/dL	Desirable
200–239 mg/dL	Borderline
≥ 240 mg/dL	High
HDL Cholesterol Level	**HDL Cholesterol Category**
Less than 40 mg/dL (for men) and less than 50 mg/dL (for women)	Low HDL cholesterol. A major risk factor for heart disease.
60 mg/dL and above	High HDL cholesterol. A High-density lipoproteins of 60 mg/dL and above are considered protective against heart disease.
LDL Cholesterol Level	**LDL Cholesterol Category**
Less than 100 mg/dL	Optimal
100–129 mg/dL	Above optimal
130–159 mg/dL	Borderline high
160–189 mg/dL	High
≥ 190 mg/dL	Very high
Triglyceride Level	**Triglyceride Category**
Less than 150 mg/dL	Normal
150–199 mg/dL	Borderline high
200–499 mg/dL	High
500 mg/dL and above	Very high

TABLE 5–2   Various Cardiac Arrhythmias

Type of Arrhythmia	Beats per Minute
Bradycardia	Less than 60
Tachycardia	150 to 250
Atrial flutter	200 to 350
Atrial fibrillation	More than 350
Ventricular fibrillation	Variable
Premature atrial contraction	Variable
Premature ventricular contraction	Variable

DISEASES AND CONDITIONS OF THE HEMATOLOGIC SYSTEM

- **Aplastic anemia** (hypoplastic anemia) is a condition wherein the bone marrow does not produce sufficient new cells to replenish blood cells. This condition results from injury to, or destruction of, stem cells in bone marrow, which causes *pancytopenia* (anemia, leukopenia, and thrombocytopenia). These disorders generally produce fatal bleeding or infection. Possible causes of aplastic anemia include radiation, drugs (antibiotics, anticonvulsants), toxicity (such as benzene or chloramphenicol), and hepatitis.

- **Folic acid deficiency**, occurring as a result of a lack of the essential nutrient known as folic acid, is a common, slowly progressive condition. It usually occurs in infants, adolescents, pregnant and lactating women, alcoholics, elderly people, and those with cancer. Folic acid deficiency anemia may result from alcohol abuse, poor diet, impaired absorption, overcooking of food, prolonged drug therapy, and increased folic acid requirements during pregnancy. It may also be caused by the rapid growth that occurs during infancy, childhood, and adolescence.

- **Iron deficiency anemia** is a disorder of oxygen transport in which hemoglobin synthesis is deficient. It is a common disease worldwide and occurs most in premenopausal women, infants (particularly premature babies), children, and adolescents (especially females). Possible causes of iron deficiency anemia include inadequate dietary intake of iron (less than 1 mg/day), iron malabsorption, blood loss caused by drug-induced GI bleeding (from aspirin, anticoagulants, and steroids), and heavy menses. It may also be caused by bleeding from trauma, peptic ulcers, and cancer. Pregnancy that diverts maternal iron to the fetus for production of red blood cells may cause iron deficiency anemia in the mother.

- **Pernicious anemia** is a disorder of red blood cells that causes them to develop into an enlarged, misshapen form. It is caused by the inability to absorb vitamin B_{12} from the diet. Pernicious anemia is characterized by decreased production of hydrochloric acid in the stomach and a deficiency of intrinsic factor, which is normally secreted by the inner layer of the stomach. This factor is essential for vitamin B_{12} absorption in the ileum (the final section of the small intestine). The resulting deficiency of this vitamin inhibits red blood cell growth, which leads to the production of fewer and deformed cells that have poor oxygen-carrying capacity. This also causes neurologic damage by impairing *myelin* formation.

- **Polycythemia vera** is a chronic disorder characterized by increased red blood cell mass and increased hemoglobin level. Also characterized by increased white blood cells and platelets, it usually occurs in people between ages 40 and 60, often among Jewish males of European descent. It seldom affects children. The cause of polycythemia vera is unknown.

- **Idiopathic thrombocytopenic purpura (ITP)** is a deficiency of platelets that occurs when the immune system attacks and destroys them. Acute (as in post viral thrombocytopenia) or chronic (as in essential thrombocytopenia), ITP may be caused by viral infection, immunization with a live virus vaccine, immunologic disorders, and drug reactions.

- **Thrombocytopenia** is a deficiency of platelets in circulating blood. Severe thrombocytopenia can involve spontaneous bleeding. The most common cause of thrombocytopenia is cancer chemotherapy, but it may be drug-induced by heparin or carbamazepine.

- **Thrombophlebitis** is defined as an inflammation inside a vein, along with the formation of a blood clot at the site. It is a dangerous situation because the thrombus may break away and lodge in a vital organ. Deep vein thrombophlebitis is characterized by aching or cramping pain, especially in the calf of the leg when the patient is walking.

DISEASES AND CONDITIONS OF THE NERVOUS SYSTEM

- **Schizophrenia** is a mental illness characterized by distortion of reality, disorganized thought patterns, social withdrawal, hallucinations, and poor judgment. Schizophrenia, one of the most devastating forms of mental illnesses, occurs in approximately 1% of the population. The cause of schizophrenia may be genetic, along with brain damage in the fetus caused by perinatal complications or viral infections in the mother during pregnancy. The onset of schizophrenia usually occurs between ages 15 and 25 in men and between 25 and 35 in women. Stressful events appear to initiate the onset and recurrence of the disorder.

- **Bipolar disorder** is a mental illness characterized by periods of extreme excitation or mania and deep depression. It is not commonly understood why it takes patients months to move from one of these extremes to the other. Some patients have predominantly manic episodes or predominantly depressive episodes. Few patients experience the classic swing from mania to depression and back. Bipolar disorder is also called *manic-depressive illness.*

- **Depression** is classified as a mood disorder, of which there are several subgroups. Major depression, or unipolar disorder, is a chemical deficit within the brain; and a precise diagnosis is based on biologic factors or personal characteristics. The causes of depression include genetic and psychosocial stressors. Depression may also occur as a reactive episode, a response to a life event,

or secondarily to many systemic disorders (including cancer, diabetes, heart failure, and AIDS). This condition is a common problem, and many patients with milder forms may be misdiagnosed and not receive treatment.

- **Anorexia nervosa** is a complex psychological state characterized by the fear of being overweight. Often, patients' perceptions are distorted to the extent that they believe they are overweight despite appearing emaciated to others.

- **Bulimia nervosa** is another eating disorder, which is characterized by recurrent (at least twice a week) episodes of binge eating, during which the patient consumes large amounts of food and feels unable to stop eating. Then to compensate for the binge eating and to avoid gaining weight, patients take inappropriate actions such as self-induced vomiting, laxative or diuretic abuse, vigorous exercise, or fasting.

- **Dementia** is a chronic deterioration of intellectual function and other cognitive skills severe enough to interfere with the ability to perform activities of daily living. Dementia may occur at any age and can affect young people as the result of injury or hypoxia. However, dementia is mostly a disease of the elderly.

- **Anxiety disorders** are the most common psychiatric illnesses in the United States, affecting 40 million people, with a higher incidence of anxiety seen in women than in men. Anxiety is an uncomfortable state that has both psychological and physical components. The psychological component can be characterized by emotions such as fear, apprehension, dread, and uneasiness. The physical component may exhibit as tachycardia, palpitations, trembling, dry mouth, sweating, weakness, fatigue, and shortness of breath. Fortunately, anxiety disorders respond well to treatment such as behavior therapy, psychotherapy, or drug therapy. Anxiety disorders may be classified as generalized anxiety disorder, panic disorder, obsessive-compulsive disorder, social anxiety disorder, or post-traumatic stress disorder.

- **Insomnia** is the inability to fall asleep or stay asleep. Difficulty in falling asleep or disturbed sleep patterns both result in insufficient sleep. Sleep disorders are common and may be short in duration or may be long-standing. They may have little or no apparent relationship to other immediate disorders. Sleep disorders can be secondary to emotional problems, pain, physical disorders, and the use or withdrawal of drugs. Excess alcohol consumed in the evening can shorten sleep and lead to withdrawal effects in the early morning.

- **Parkinson's disease** is a progressive degenerative disorder affecting motor function through the loss of extrapyramidal activity. This disease is characterized by muscle tremor, muscle rigidity, and bradykinesia; and disturbances of posture and equilibrium are often present (see Figure 5–2).

In this condition, a decreased number of neurons in the brain secrete dopamine, an inhibitory neurotransmitter, leading to an imbalance between excitation and inhibition in the basal nuclei. Although its cause is not fully understood, Parkinson's disease is believed to be associated with an imbalance of the neurotransmitters acetylcholine and dopamine in the brain (see Figure 5–3).

- **Alzheimer's disease** (senile disease complex) is one of the most common causes of severe cognitive dysfunction in older persons. Pathologically, the brain experiences atrophy (shrinkage) and exhibits senile plaques. Although the exact cause of Alzheimer's

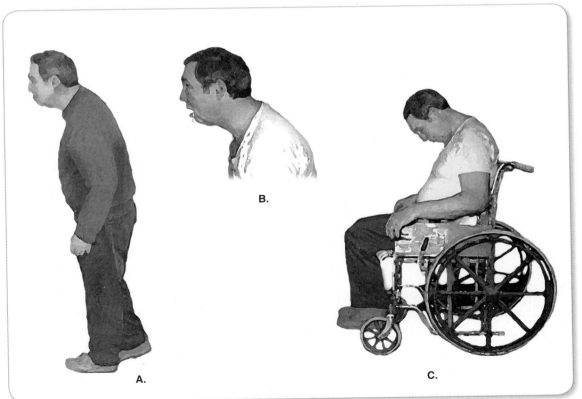

A.   B.   C.

Delmar/Cengage Learning

Figure 5–2 Parkinson's disease is characterized by shuffling gait and early postural changes.

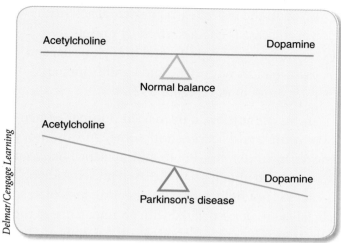

Delmar/Cengage Learning

Figure 5–3 Dopamine imbalance exhibited in Parkinson's disease.

TABLE 5–4 Classifications of Seizures

Partial Seizures (Focal)	Generalized Seizures
A. Simple	A. Tonic-clonic (grand mal)
1. Motor (includes Jacksonian)	B. Absence (petit mal)
2. Sensory (e.g., visual, auditory)	C. Myoclonic
3. Autonomic	D. Infantile spasms
4. Psychic	E. Atonic (akinetic)
B. Complex (impaired consciousness)	
1. Psychomotor	
C. Partial leading to generalized seizures	

disease is unknown, current theories include loss of neurotransmitter stimulation by choline acetyltransferase. Alzheimer's disease is a devastating illness characterized by progressive memory failure, impaired thinking, confusion, disorientation, personality changes, restlessness, speech disturbances, and the inability to perform routine tasks. Unfortunately, the disease is incurable.

- **Seizures** are a group of disorders that are characterized by hyperexcitability of neurons in the brain. The abnormal stimuli can produce many symptoms, from short periods of unconsciousness to violent convulsions. Usually brief, with a beginning and an end, seizures may be localized or generalized. Seizures may result acutely from any number of neurological disorders, as well as from metabolic disturbances, trauma, and exposure to certain toxins. Each seizure lasts for a few seconds or minutes, and the excessive activity of the neurons then ceases spontaneously. Seizure disorders are classified by their location in the brain and their clinical features. The international classification of seizures is summarized in Table 5–4. This is a commonly accepted classification that incorporates current terminology and divides seizures into two basic categories: generalized and partial.

Generalized seizures have multiple foci that may cause loss of consciousness, whereas partial seizures have a single or focal origin, often in the cerebral cortex (Figure 5–4). Partial seizures may or may not involve altered consciousness. However, partial seizures may progress to generalized seizures. The terms *epilepsy*, *convulsions*, and *seizures* are commonly used interchangeably, although they each have a slightly different medical meaning.

- **Meningitis**, an inflammation of one or more of the membranes (meninges) that cover the brain and spinal cord, may be caused by a viral or bacterial infection.

DISEASES AND CONDITIONS OF THE SENSORY SYSTEM

Changes in sensory function can cause dysfunctions of sight, hearing, smell, taste, balance, and coordination. The most common disorders of vision and hearing are discussed in this section.

Disorders of Vision

- A **cataract** is a clouding that develops in the lens of the eye or in the envelope that surrounds the lens. The development of a cataract is usually slow, causing vision loss and possible blindness if untreated. Certain

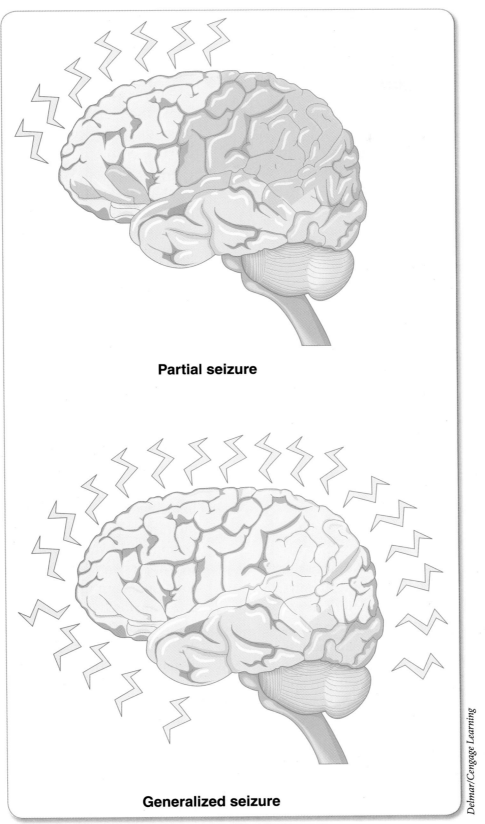

Partial seizure

Generalized seizure

Delmar/Cengage Learning

Figure 5–4 A partial seizure is characterized by chaotic firing occurring in one portion of the brain, whereas a generalized seizure is characterized by chaotic firing throughout the brain.

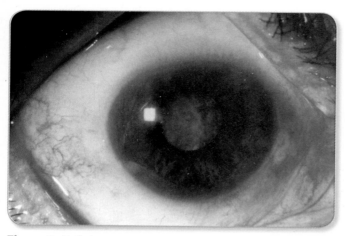

Figure 5–5 Cataract. (*Courtesy of the National Eye Institute, Bethesda, MD*)

cataracts can lead to glaucoma. Cataracts may be caused by long-term exposure to ultraviolet light, radiation exposure, diabetes, hypertension, advanced age, and loss of protein in the eye. Throughout the world, nearly half of all cases of blindness are caused by age-related cataracts. Cataracts are often corrected by surgery, and an artificial lens may be permanently implanted in the eye following removal of the original lens affected by the cataract (see Figure 5–5).

- The term **glaucoma** describes a group of diseases affecting the optic nerve. Raised intraocular pressure is a significant risk factor for the development of glaucoma. If untreated, glaucoma leads to permanent optic nerve damage, which can progress to blindness. It is the second leading cause of blindness throughout the world. Glaucoma affects 1 out of 10 people over the age of 80. Based upon its stage of development, the condition may be treated by eye drops and a variety of other types of medications.

Disorders of Hearing

- **External otitis**, also known as *otitis externa* or *swimmer's ear*, is an inflammation of the outer ear and ear canal. It is a common cause of earaches, and may be caused by

eczema (dermatitis), bacterial infection, or fungal infection. Symptoms include pain, ear discharge, itching, and conductive hearing loss. Contact with polluted water or water trapped within the ear may also cause the condition. Topical solutions or suspensions (in the form of ear drops) are commonly used to treat external otitis.

- **Otitis media** is inflammation of the inner ear. Like external otitis, it is a common cause of earaches; and both of these conditions are regularly referred to by the term *earache*. Otitis media is a common childhood condition. Viruses in the nose may infect the Eustachian tubes, which lead from the back of the nose to the inner ear. Although *acute otitis media* is of viral origin, *otitis media with effusion* is caused by a collection of fluid. *Chronic suppurative otitis media* is a condition wherein a hole in the eardrum exists, along with an active middle ear bacterial infection. Treatment usually involves antibiotics such as amoxicillin or other penicillin derivatives.

- **Tinnitus** is most commonly explained to as a "ringing in the ears." The sensation may differ in many ways, and has also been explained as intermittent or continuous "buzzing," "hissing," "humming," "whining," or "whistling" sounds. Actually a symptom of another underlying condition, tinnitus may be caused by ear infection, foreign objects, earwax, nasal conditions (such as allergies), and excessive noise exposure. It may also be caused by certain medications (such as aspirin) and by low levels of serotonin in the body. Tinnitus can result from conductive or sensorineural hearing loss, use of analgesics or antibiotics, chemotherapeutic and antiviral drug therapies, loop diuretics, psychedelic drugs, and other drugs.

- **Vertigo**, a type of dizziness wherein the patient experiences the sensation of spinning or swaying while the body is actually stationary, may induce nausea and vomiting. It is most often caused by an inner ear condition involving the balance mechanisms of the vestibular system, although it may also stem from brain or nerve disorders. Drug toxicity, strokes, or tumors are also potential causes of vertigo. Trauma (such as skull fractures), blood pressure conditions, and Ménière's disease may also trigger this condition.

- **Ménière's disease** is a chronic inner ear condition that causes dizziness, nausea, ringing in the ears, vomiting, and progressive hearing loss. Although the disease is usually treatable by rest and antihistamines, surgery may be required in severe cases.

- **Deafness** is the inability to hear (total deafness) or to hear clearly (partial deafness). Hearing loss may be determined to be *conductive* or *sensory*, temporary or permanent, and congenital or acquired. *Conductive hearing loss* is caused by an interruption in the transmission of sound waves to the inner ear. *Sensorineural hearing loss* is caused by damage to the inner ear, to the nerve from the ear to the brain, or to the brain itself.

Diseases and Conditions of the Respiratory System

- **Respiratory distress syndrome** is an acute lung disease in newborns. It occurs most often in premature babies and is caused by a deficiency of pulmonary surfactant. This deficiency results in overdistended alveoli and, at times, hyaline membrane formation. Respiratory distress syndrome is also called *hyaline membrane disease.*

- **Asthma** is a respiratory condition characterized by difficulty exhaling and by wheezing. Bronchial asthma, normally called simply *asthma*, is caused by smooth muscle spasms in the bronchi that reduce airflow. This condition causes inflammation and accumulation of mucus in the air passages.

Asthma is more common in children than in adults. In susceptible individuals, causes of asthma attacks include allergic reactions, exercise, changes in weather or altitude, and upper respiratory infection.

- **Chronic bronchitis** is inflammation of the bronchi caused by irritants or infection. A form of chronic obstructive pulmonary disease (COPD), bronchitis may be classified as acute or chronic. In chronic bronchitis, hypersecretion of mucus and chronic productive cough lasts for three months of the year and occurs for at least two consecutive years. Common causes of chronic bronchitis include exposure to irritants, smoking of tobacco products, genetic predisposition, exposure to noxious gases, and respiratory tract infection.

- **Chronic obstructive pulmonary disease** results from emphysema, chronic bronchitis, asthma, or a combination of these disorders. COPD is the most common lung disease, and its incidence is increasing. Smoking of tobacco products, recurrent or chronic respiratory tract infections, air pollution, allergies, and hereditary factors are common causes of COPD.

- **Pulmonary embolism** is caused by a blood clot or fat deposit formed in a peripheral blood vessel that breaks free from its site of formation and lodges in a blood vessel in the lung. This process is called *thromboembolism.* Pulmonary embolism is the most common pulmonary complication. Signs and symptoms include difficulty breathing, chest pain, unstable circulation, and collapse. Common causes of pulmonary embolism include extended confinement to bed rest, prolonged travel, recent surgery, trauma or injury, burns, and obesity.

- **Pulmonary tuberculosis** is an infection caused by *Mycobacterium tuberculosis.* Although it most commonly affects the lungs, it can also invade other parts of the body. Tuberculosis is usually transmitted by inhalation or ingestion of infected droplets.

DISEASES AND CONDITIONS OF THE IMMUNE SYSTEM

- **Human immunodeficiency virus (HIV)** infection may cause acquired immunodeficiency syndrome (AIDS). People with this disorder are at risk of fungal and protozoal infections and skin cancers that are not usually seen in people with intact immune systems. Although there is no known cure, the progression of AIDS can often be slowed or controlled by the use of antiviral drugs.

- **Allergic rhinitis** is a reaction to airborne (inhaled) allergens. Depending on the allergen, the resulting rhinitis and conjunctivitis may occur seasonally, such as in *hay fever*. The most common *atopic* (not in direct contact with an allergen) reaction, allergic rhinitis affects more than 20 million people in the United States.

- **Anaphylaxis** is an acute, potentially life-threatening type 1 (immediate) hypersensitivity reaction. It is marked by the sudden onset of rapidly progressive vascular swelling in the skin, accompanied by itching and respiratory distress. If promptly recognized and treated, the prognosis is good. A severe reaction may cause vascular collapse and lead to systemic symptoms and even death. The reaction typically occurs within minutes, but can occur up to one hour after reexposure to the antigen.

- **Latex allergy** is a hypersensitivity reaction to products that contain natural latex, which is derived from the sap of the rubber tree and is found in an increasing number of products at both home and work. Synthetic latex does not cause latex allergy. Hypersensitivity reactions can range from local dermatitis to life-threatening anaphylactic reaction.

DISEASES AND CONDITIONS OF THE ENDOCRINE SYSTEM

- **Hypopituitarism** is a condition caused by a deficiency or absence of any of the pituitary hormones, especially those produced by the anterior pituitary lobe. Hypopituitarism produces growth retardation in children. Dwarfism is the abnormal underdevelopment of the body that occurs in children. Hyposecretion of growth hormone results in growth retardation.

- **Hyperpituitarism**, a chronic and progressive disease, is caused by excessive production and secretion of pituitary hormones (particularly human growth hormone [hGH]). Excessive hGH produces one of two distinct conditions: gigantism or acromegaly, either of which depends upon the time of life at which the dysfunction begins. Gigantism describes an abnormal pattern of growth and stature. It occurs before puberty, resulting in a proportional overgrowth of all body tissue. Acromegaly is a chronic metabolic condition in adults caused by hypersecretion of hGH. It occurs after puberty, and results in an overgrowth of the bones of the face, hands, and feet (as well as an excessive overgrowth of soft tissue).

- **Diabetes insipidus** is a disturbance of water metabolism that results in extreme thirst and excessive secretion of dilute urine. A deficiency in the release of vasopressin (antidiuretic hormone) by the posterior pituitary gland, diabetes insipidus causes the excretion of larger than normal amounts of colorless, dilute urine.

- **Simple goiter** is an enlargement of the thyroid gland. Simple (nontoxic) goiter results from a shortage of iodine in the diet. Iodine is necessary for the synthesis of thyroxine (T_4), which is the major form of thyroid hormone in the blood.

- **Hashimoto disease** is a chronic disease of the immune system that attacks the thyroid gland. It is also referred to as *chronic Hashimoto's thyroiditis*. This condition occurs in women more than in men, is most common between ages 45 and 65, and is the leading cause of non-simple goiter and hypothyroidism.

- **Hyperthyroidism** is the overproduction of thyroid hormone, causing increased metabolism and changes of multiple body systems. *Graves' disease*, a condition of primary hyperthyroidism, occurs when the entire thyroid gland is enlarged, resulting in a diffuse goiter (see Figure 5–6).

- **Hypothyroidism** can strike either sex, at any age. Many people across the world are at high risk for hypothyroidism as a result of iodine-deficient diets. This can result in congenital hypothyroidism, which can lead to mental deficiency. *Cretinism*, a hypothyroidism developing in infancy or early childhood, is congenital and is typified by absence of the thyroid gland or the lack of thyroid hormone synthesis by the thyroid gland. This causes mental and physical retardation in infants and young children.

- **Myxedema** is caused by severe, prolonged hypothyroidism. It develops in older children or adults as a result of impairment of the thyroid gland's ability to form thyroxine. Symptoms of myxedema include skin thickening and other changes, mental problems, changes in the appearance of the face, weight gain, and thin, brittle hair.

- **Cushing's syndrome** is a condition of chronic hypersecretion of cortisol from the adrenal cortex, which results in excessive circulating cortisol levels. The patient experiences fatigue, muscular weakness, and changes in body appearance. Excessive cortisol levels can be caused by abnormal multiplication of the number of cells of the adrenal gland (see Figure 5–7).

- **Addison's disease** is caused by partial or complete failure of adrenocortical function. Symptoms include fatigue, weakness, lack of appetite, weight loss, and gastrointestinal disturbances. The onset of Addison's disease is usually gradual, with progressive destruction of the adrenal gland and the resulting reduction of many important hormones that it secretes.

- **Diabetes mellitus** is a chronic disorder of carbohydrate, fat, and protein metabolism caused by inadequate production of insulin by the pancreas or by faulty utilization of insulin by the cells. There are two primary forms of diabetes mellitus.

  1. Type 1 (formerly known as *juvenile onset* diabetes or *insulin-dependent diabetes mellitus* [IDDM]) has an early, abrupt onset, usually occurring before a person is 30 years of age. In this type of diabetes mellitus, the pancreas secretes little or no insulin. This condition can be difficult to control.

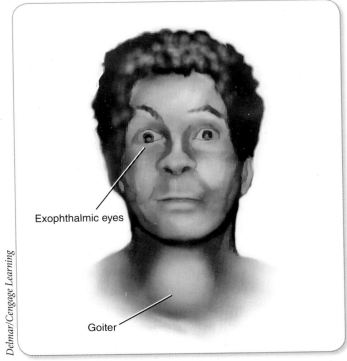

Delmar/Cengage Learning

Exophthalmic eyes

Goiter

Figure 5–6 Hyperthyroidism.

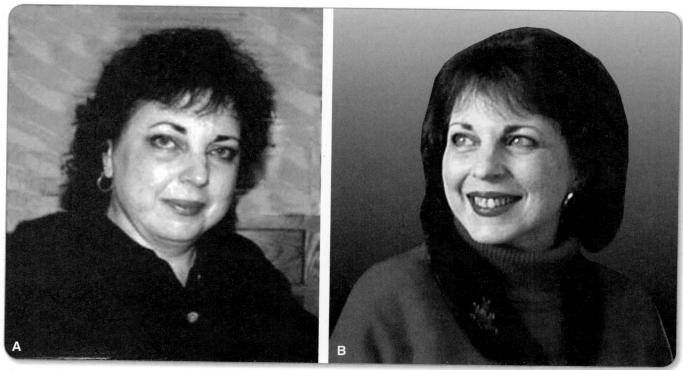

Figure 5–7 Cushing's syndrome A. Before treatment B. After treatment. (*Courtesy of R. Jones*)

2. Type 2 (formerly known as *adult onset diabetes* or *non-insulin-dependent diabetes mellitus* [NIDDM]) is the more common form. It has a gradual onset in adults older than age 30 and occurs more often in people over the age of 55. In this form, some pancreatic function remains, permitting control of symptoms by dietary management. In some cases, an oral hypoglycemic medication is required. According to the CDC, by the summer of 2008, as many as 24 million people in the United States were suffering from type 2 diabetes.

*   **Gestational diabetes mellitus (GDM),** or type 3 diabetes, is a condition of damaged ability to process carbohydrate that has its onset during pregnancy. Signs indicate that destruction of insulin by the placenta plays a role in causing GDM. Increased maternal insulin production results in increased placental production of human placental *lactogen* (which facilitates the energy supply

of the fetus). This is followed by the reduced effectiveness of maternal insulin.

The fetus receives its glucose from the mother, stressing the balance of glucose production and glucose utilization. Elevated levels of estrogen and progesterone block the action of insulin. Risk factors include a family history of diabetes, obesity, and age over 25 years.

DISEASES AND CONDITIONS OF THE MUSCULOSKELETAL SYSTEM

*   **Rheumatoid arthritis (RA),** a systemic inflammatory disease, attacks joints by producing inflammation of the synovial membranes that leads to the destruction of the articular cartilage and underlying bone. Women are affected by this condition two to three times more frequently than men. Although the disease occurs in all age groups, its prevalence increases with age. The

peak incidence among women is between the ages of 40 and 60 years, with the onset at 30 to 50 years of age.

- **Gout** is actually a group of diseases known as the gout syndrome. It includes acute gouty arthritis with recurrent attacks of severe joint inflammation and the accumulation of crystalline deposits in joint surfaces, bones, soft tissue, and cartilage. Gout also may cause gouty nephropathy or renal impairment and uric acid kidney stones. *Uric acid* is a waste product of purine metabolism, normally excreted through the kidneys. A sudden increase in serum uric acid levels usually precipitates an attack of gout. Gout often affects a single joint, such as in the big toe. When acute inflammation develops from uric acid deposits, the joint cartilage is damaged.

- **Osteoarthritis** is by far the most common form of arthritis among the elderly and is the greatest cause of disability and limitation of activity in older adults. It has been suggested that osteoarthritis begins at a very young age, expressing itself in the elderly only after a long period of latency.

- **Osteoporosis** is a metabolic bone disorder in which the rate of bone resorption accelerates as the rate of bone formation slows, causing a loss of bone mass. Bones affected by this disease lose calcium and phosphate salts and become porous, brittle, and abnormally vulnerable to fracture.

- **Osteomalacia** (in adults) and **rickets** (in children) are caused by vitamin D deficiency. Bones cannot calcify normally, and this abnormal calcification may cause bone deformity. Softening of bone tissue is because of loss of calcium. Osteomalacia is caused by either a dietary deficiency of calcium, phosphorus, and vitamin D or by an inability to absorb sufficient amounts of these nutrients from the digestive tract.

DISEASES AND CONDITIONS OF THE GASTROINTESTINAL SYSTEM

- **Gastroesophageal reflux disease (GERD)** refers to backflow of stomach contents into the esophagus and past the lower esophageal sphincter, without associated vomiting. GERD causes a burning sensation (known as heartburn), and the pain may radiate to the chest or arms and commonly occurs in pregnant or obese persons. Reclining after a meal also contributes to reflux.

- **Peptic ulcers**, lesions in the mucosal membrane, can develop in the lower esophagus, stomach, or duodenum. Ulcers may be acute or chronic. About 80% of all peptic ulcers are duodenal ulcers, which affect the proximal part of the small intestine. They occur most commonly in men ages 20 to 50. Gastric ulcers (which are peptic ulcers of the stomach) are most common in middle-aged and elderly men, especially in chronic users of nonsteroidal anti-inflammatory drugs (NSAIDs), alcohol, or tobacco. Peptic ulcers may be caused by *Helicobacter pylori* infection. Complications of peptic ulcers include hemorrhage, shock, gastric perforation, and gastric outlet obstruction.

- **Crohn's disease** is a condition of the intestinal tract characterized by patches of inflammation and even ulcers. Crohn's disease is also known as *regional enteritis* or *granulomatous colitis*. This disease is most prevalent in adults age 20 to 40. The exact cause is unknown. Signs and symptoms include fever, diarrhea, abdominal cramps, and weight loss.

- **Ulcerative colitis**, an inflammatory disease that affects the mucosa of the colon, is usually chronic. It produces edema and ulcerations. Severity ranges from a mild, localized disorder to a severe disease that may cause a perforated colon, progressing to potentially fatal **peritonitis** and **toxemia**. The disease cycles between exacerbation and remission. Ulcerative colitis occurs primarily in young adults, especially women. Onset of symptoms seems to peak between ages 15 and 20 and between ages 55 and 60. Although specific causes of ulcerative colitis are unknown, they may be caused by abnormal immune response in the gastrointestinal (GI) tract, possibly associated with food or **bacteria** such as *Escherichia coli*.

- **Diverticulitis** is an inflammation of a **diverticulum**, usually caused by entrapment of feces within the diverticulum. It occurs most commonly in the colon. Diverticulitis may cause potentially fatal obstruction, infection, or hemorrhage. Diverticulitis may also result from perforation, abscess, or fistulas.

Viral Hepatitis

- **Hepatitis A** is most common among male homosexuals and in people with human immunodeficiency virus (HIV) infection. It is commonly spread via the fecal-oral route by the ingestion of fecal contaminants.

- **Hepatitis B** (serum hepatitis) also is most common among HIV-positive persons. Routine screening of donor blood for hepatitis B has reduced the amount of post-transfusion cases. Transmission by drug users via the sharing of needles is still a serious problem.

- **Hepatitis C** accounts for most post-transfusion cases of hepatitis and accounts for about 20% of all cases of viral hepatitis.

- **Hepatitis D** (delta hepatitis) has a high mortality rate and is responsible for about half of all cases of fulminant hepatitis. In the United States, this type occurs only in those frequently exposed to blood and blood products (including IV drug users and hemophiliacs). This type develops only after patients have contracted acute or chronic hepatitis B.

- **Hepatitis E** is more common in young adults and those who have visited endemic areas such as Central America, Africa, Asia, or India. It is more severe when pregnant women contract it.

DISEASES AND CONDITIONS OF THE REPRODUCTIVE SYSTEM

- **Chlamydia**, one of the most commonly reported infectious diseases in the United States, causes **urethritis** in men, and urethritis and cervicitis (a common infection of the lower genital tract) in women. Sometimes referred to as the silent sexually transmitted infection (STI), chlamydia often has no symptoms. It causes *pelvic inflammatory disease (PID)* and is a major cause of female sterility. *Chlamydia trachomatis*, an intracellular bacterium, is the cause of chlamydia and is usually transmitted by sexual contact.

- **Gonorrhea**, a common STI, is an infection of the **genitourinary** tract. Caused by *Neisseria gonorrhoeae*, it is usually transmitted sexually.

- **Trichomoniasis** is a protozoal infection of the lower genitourinary tract. Initial symptoms for both male and female patients include urethritis with **dysuria** and itching. In addition, females may notice a profuse, greenish-yellow discharge from the vagina. Trichomoniasis is caused by a protozoa called *Trichomonas vaginalis* and is usually transmitted through sexual contact.

- **Genital herpes** is an infection of the skin of the genital area, with *ulcerations* spread by direct skin-to-skin contact, causing painful genital sores that are similar to cold sores. Genital herpes is caused by herpes simplex virus type 2 (HSV-2) and is a recurrent, incurable viral disease. One out of every six adults carries the highly contagious HSV-2. It is usually transmitted through sexual contact.

Cross-infection with herpes simplex virus type 1 (HSV-1) may result from oral-genital sex.

- **Syphilis** is a chronic, systemic, sexually transmitted infection that develops in four stages. Syphilis begins with the presence of a painless but highly contagious local lesion called a chancre on the male or female genitalia. Without early treatment during the primary stage, syphilis becomes a systemic, chronic disease that can involve any organ or tissue. It is caused by infection with the *Treponema pallidum* spirochete through sexual contact (or other direct contact) with infected lesions or infected body fluids. Congenital transmission of syphilis can occur during pregnancy.

- **Ovarian cysts**, fluid-filled or semi-fluid-filled sacs, form on or near the ovaries and can become large before any symptoms occur. The patient may report prolonged, excessive, or irregular *menses.*

- **Endometriosis** is a condition wherein tissue similar to that of the uterus lining forms in other parts of the body. This can cause painful cysts in the pelvic cavity or abdominal wall. The most common symptom of endometriosis is pelvic pain.

- **Pelvic inflammatory disease (PID)** is an infection of the uterine lining that may spread into the fallopian tubes. Signs and symptoms include foul-smelling vaginal discharge and abdominal pain. The most common causes of PID are gonorrhea and chlamydia.

- **Toxic shock syndrome** is a potentially fatal illness caused by certain strains of *Staphylococcus aureus* that secrete a unique toxin. The condition most commonly affects women who wear highly absorbent tampons for long intervals during their menstrual periods. It has also occurred in men and infants less commonly. The condition may progress to kidney failure, liver impairment, unstable blood pressure, mental confusion, and death.

- **Orchitis** is infection of the testes and is caused by viral or bacterial infection or injury. Orchitis may affect one or both testes, causing swelling, tenderness, and acute pain. It is often treated with oral antibiotics.

- **Prostatitis**, an acute or chronic inflammation of the prostate gland is more common in men over 50 years of age. In this condition, the prostate may become enlarged and tender. Although the cause of inflammation is usually infection, it is not always known. Infection may be either bacterial or nonbacterial.

- **Benign prostatic hyperplasia (BPH)** is nonmalignant, noninflammatory hypertrophy of the prostate gland. Enlargement of the prostate gland is a common condition in men over age 50, and frequency of this condition increases with age. BPH usually progresses to the point of causing compression of the urethra with urinary obstruction.

- **Hydronephrosis** is a distention of the pelvis and calyces (tubes) of the kidney by urine that cannot flow past an obstruction in a ureter. These obstructions may be caused by a tumor, a calculus (kidney stone), inflammation of the prostate gland, or edema caused by a urinary tract infection. The patient may experience pain in the flank and, in some cases, hematuria (blood in the urine), pyuria (pus in the urine), and hyperpyrexia. Prolonged hydronephrosis causes atrophy and eventual loss of kidney function (see Figure 5–8).

- **Pyelonephritis** is an inflammation usually as a result of bacterial infection of the kidney. In most cases, pyelonephritis results from a bladder infection that travels up one or both ureters to the kidneys. One of the most common renal diseases, pyelonephritis increases with age and is higher in sexually active women, pregnant women, and people with diabetes.

- **Acute renal failure** is a sudden interruption of renal function. It can be caused by obstruction,

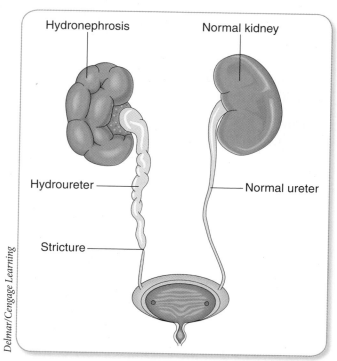

Delmar/Cengage Learning

Figure 5–8 Hydronephrosis.

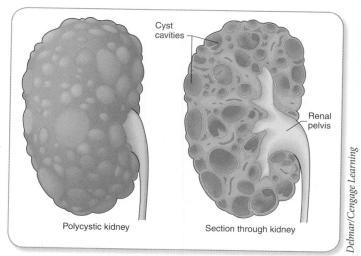

Delmar/Cengage Learning

Figure 5–9 Polycystic kidney.

poor circulation, or underlying kidney disease. The condition is usually reversible with treatment; but if not treated, it may progress to end-stage renal disease such as uremia and even death.

- **Chronic renal failure** is usually the end result of gradual tissue destruction and loss of renal function. It can also result from a rapidly progressing disease of sudden onset that destroys the nephrons and causes irreversible kidney damage.

- **Glomerulonephritis**, a bilateral inflammation of the glomeruli (capillary tufts in the kidney nephrons), typically occurs after a streptococcal infection. Acute glomerulonephritis is also called *acute poststreptococcal glomerulonephritis*. Acute glomerulonephritis is most common in boys between ages 3 and 7, but it can occur at any age. Most cases resolve within two weeks, and the patient experiences a spontaneous recovery. Chronic glomerulonephritis is a slowly progressive,

noninfectious disease that may result in irreversible renal damage and renal failure.

- **Polycystic kidney disease**, an inherited disorder, is characterized by multiple, bilateral, *grape-like clusters* of fluid-filled cysts (see Figure 5–9). These cysts enlarge the kidneys, compressing and eventually replacing functioning renal tissue. The disease affects males and females equally. No cure for polycystic disease is currently known.

- **Neurogenic bladder**, a dysfunction of urinary bladder control, consists of difficulty in emptying the bladder or urinary incontinence. The many factors that can cause neurogenic bladder include stroke, brain tumor, Parkinson's disease, and spinal cord diseases or injuries.

DISEASES AND CONDITIONS OF THE INTEGUMENTARY SYSTEM

- **Atopic dermatitis** (*eczema*) is a chronic or recurring skin lesion characteristic of an allergic reaction. The lesions usually itch intensely and are treated with a topical corticosteroid. The tendency of this condition to develop is inherited, and it may occur in

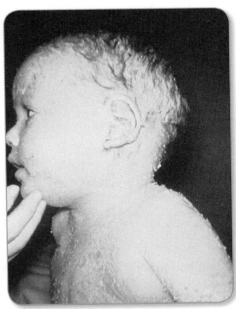

Figure 5–10 Seborrheic dermatitis. (*Courtesy of Robert A. Silverman, M.D. Pediatric Dermatology, Georgetown University*)

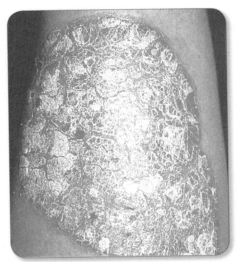

Figure 5–11 Psoriasis. (*Courtesy of Robert A. Silverman, M.D. Pediatric Dermatology, Georgetown University*)

some infants who are sensitive to milk, orange juice, or certain other foods.

- **Seborrheic dermatitis** is a common skin condition characterized by itchy, reddened, and oily patches of skin. The patches often shed large dandruff-like scales (see Figure 5–10). This condition is *idiopathic*. However, heredity may predispose an individual to the condition, and emotional stress may be a precipitating factor. Low-strength cortisone or hydrocortisone creams are the most effective methods of treatment.

- **Contact dermatitis**, an acute inflammation of the skin, is caused either by the action of irritants on the skin surfaces or by contact with a substance that causes an allergic reaction.

- **Psoriasis** is a chronic condition characterized by raised red patches covered with white scales (see Figure 5–11). The patches most often appear on the elbows, knees, scalp, genitalia, and trunk and may also appear at sites of trauma. Although its cause is unknown, psoriasis seems to be genetically determined and more common in Caucasians. Precipitating

factors for the development of psoriasis include hormonal changes (such as those occurring with pregnancy), climate changes, emotional stress, and a period of generally poor health.

- **Acne** is a skin condition characterized by inflammation of the oil-producing glands and ducts. It can occur on any skin surface and present itself at any age. Acne vulgaris, the most common type of acne and one that primarily affects adolescents during puberty, appears on the face, upper back, and chest. Resulting from blockage of follicles, acne can cause severe scarring of the skin. Available treatments include medications that prevent the blockage of follicles, those that kill the causative bacteria, those with anti-inflammatory effects, and those that change the hormonal balance of the skin.

- **Herpes zoster** (*shingles*) is an infection caused by the varicella-zoster virus, which is the same virus that causes chickenpox. Persons who have previously had chickenpox continue to harbor the varicella-zoster virus in their nervous systems, and the virus may emerge during times of physical stress or when the immune system is impaired. When the virus reactivates, it inflames nerves in the trunk and abdomen, causing blisters and severe pain (see Figure 5–12).

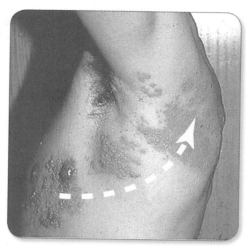

Figure 5–12 Shingles. (*Courtesy of Robert A. Silverman, M.D. Pediatric Dermatology, Georgetown University*)

- **Cellulitis**, an infection of the subcutaneous tissue, is usually caused by an injury that pierces the outermost layer of skin and allows bacteria to reach the lower layers. Cellulitis is usually painful, and is capable of spreading rapidly over a large area. This infection is often treated with intravenous antibiotics.

- **Impetigo** is a bacterial skin infection most commonly seen in children, although it is not limited only to their age group. It is highly contagious and spreads rapidly in schools where children have physical contact with each other, often during athletic events or during close play. Impetigo initially appears as a fluid-filled blister that may burst, leaving a crusty margin around the lesion. The condition often causes intense itching that may help spread the infection. Impetigo is usually treated with both oral and topical antibiotics.

- **Athlete's foot** is a fungal infection of the foot. It usually starts between two toes and can spread to other toes, the bottom of the foot, the toenails, or any other surface on the foot. Athlete's foot is clinically referred to as *tinea pedis*.

EXPLORING THE WEB

Visit http://cancer.stanford.edu/blood; search blood diseases to find information and resources on blood diseases.

Visit http://www.cardiovasculardiseases.org; search for cardiovascular diseases for more information about them.

Visit http://www.righthealth.com; search for ear and eye infections for more information about them.

Visit http://www.endocrineweb.com for more information about the endocrine system.

Visit http://www.gistalliance.com; search gastrointestinal diseases to learn more about them.

Visit http://www.hon.ch; search musculoskeletal diseases for more information.

Visit http://medlineplus.gov; search immune system and disorders to learn more about them.

Visit http://www.urologychannel.com; search kidney and urinary health for more information.

Visit http://www.nervous-system-diseases.com; search nervous system diseases to learn more about them.

Visit http://nursingcrib.com; the target are student nurses, but many topics on this site apply to all health-care professionals.

Visit http://www.web-books.com; search reproductive diseases to find sources of information about them.

Visit http://www.umm.edu/respiratory; search respiratory system and lung diseases to learn more about them.

REVIEW QUESTIONS

1. What is the condition caused by hypersecretion of growth hormone before puberty?

   A. myxedema
   B. dwarfism
   C. gigantism
   D. acromegaly

2. Which sexually transmitted infection is sometimes called "the silent STI"?

   A. syphilis
   B. moles
   C. genital warts
   D. chlamydial infection

3. Which respiratory condition is more common in children than in adults?

   A. chronic bronchitis
   B. atelectasis
   C. pneumoconiosis
   D. asthma

4. Deep thrombophlebitis occurs most commonly in the:

   A. lower legs
   B. lower arms
   C. lower abdomen
   D. lungs

5. Which skin condition is highly contagious and spreads rapidly, especially in schools?

   A. psoriasis
   B. eczema
   C. impetigo
   D. seborrheic dermatitis

6. Tumors that develop from cancer cells traveling from an original site to a more distant site are called:

   A. hemopoietic
   B. hepatoma
   C. hemostasis
   D. metastatic

7. Herpes zoster is also called:

   A. warts
   B. shingles
   C. gangrene
   D. impetigo

8. Diabetes insipidus results from the lack or deficiency of:

   A. thyroxine
   B. aldosterone
   C. thymosin
   D. antidiuretic hormone

9. The sudden onset of a disease marked by intensity is described as:

   A. critical
   B. aplastic
   C. acute
   D. chronic

10. When his or her bone marrow fails to produce sufficient new cells to replenish blood cells, a person has:

    A. leukemia
    B. aplastic anemia
    C. hemolytic anemia
    D. sickle cell anemia

OUTLINE

GLOSSARY

Aerosol – a liquid or fine powder that is sprayed in a fine mist

Ampule – a sealed glass container that usually contains a single dose of medicine; the top of the ampule must be broken off to open the container

Buccal – pertaining to the inside of the cheek

Caplet – a tablet shaped like a capsule

Capsule – a solid dosage form in which the drug is enclosed in either a hard or soft shell of soluble material

Cream – a semisolid emulsion of either the oil-in-water or the water-in-oil type, ordinarily intended for topical use

Elixir – a clear, sweetened, hydroalcoholic liquid intended for oral use

Emulsion – a preparation containing two liquids that cannot be mixed; one liquid is dispersed, in the form of very small globules, throughout the other

Enteral – passing through the gastrointestinal tract to be absorbed by the body

Gel – a jelly or the solid or semisolid phase of a colloidal solution

Gelcap – an oil-based medication that is enclosed in a soft gelatin capsule

Granule – a very small pill, usually gelatin- or sugar-coated, containing a drug to be given in a small dose

Implants (pellets) – implants or pellets are dosage forms that are placed intradermally, or under the skin, by means of minor surgery or special injections; the term *implant* may also mean a device inserted surgically under the skin for delivery of medications

Intradermal injection – an injection that is given between the layers of the skin; a dose of an agent administered between the layers of the skin

Intramuscular injection – an injection that is given inside a muscle; normally used in the context of an injection given into a muscle

Intravenous injection – an injection that is given into a vein; most commonly used in the context of an injection given directly into a vein

Lozenge (troche) – a small, disk-shaped tablet composed of solidifying paste containing an astringent, an antiseptic, or an oil-based drug used for local treatment of the mouth or throat; held in the mouth until dissolved

Medication – a substance used in the treatment or maintenance of an illness

Mixture – an incorporation of two or more substances, without chemical union, in which the physical characteristics of each component are retained

Ointment – a semisolid preparation that usually contains medicinal substances and is intended for external application

Oral – pertaining to the mouth; medication given by mouth

Parenteral – a dosage form usually intended to be administered intravenously, subcutaneously, or intramuscularly

Pill – a small, globular mass of soluble material containing a medicinal substance to be swallowed

Plaster – a solid preparation that can be spread when heated and that becomes adhesive at body temperature

Powder – a dry mass of minute separate particles of any substance

Solution – the incorporation of a solid, a liquid, or a gas into a liquid

Spirits – an alcoholic or hydroalcoholic solution of volatile substances

Subcutaneous injection – the administration of a medication by means of a needle and syringe into the layer of fat and blood vessels beneath the skin

Sublingual – pertaining to the area under the tongue

Suppository – a small, semisolid bullet-shaped dosage for ready insertion into a body orifice, other than the oral cavity (e.g., rectum, urethra, or vagina); made of a substance, usually medicated, that is semisolid at ordinary temperature but melts at body temperature

Suspension – a class of pharmacopeial preparations of finely divided, undissolved drugs dispersed in liquid vehicles for oral or parenteral use

Syrup – a liquid preparation in a concentrated aqueous solution of a sugar used for medicinal purposes or to add flavor to a substance

Tablet – a solid dosage form containing medicinal substances with or without suitable diluents

Tincture – an alcoholic solution prepared from vegetable materials or from chemical substances

Topical – pertaining to a drug that is applied to the surface of the body

Transdermal drug delivery (TDD) – pertaining to a passage through the skin; dosage forms that release minute amounts of a drug at a consistent rate

Vial – a small glass or plastic bottle intended to hold medicine

Water – a mixture of distilled water with an aromatic volatile oil

Wheal – a bump on the skin

MEDICAL USES OF DRUGS

A medication is a drug or other substance that is legally used to treat or maintain an illness or disease state. Drugs have six medical uses: therapeutic, diagnostic, replacement, anesthetic, prophylactic or preventive, and destructive.

Therapeutic Agents

Therapeutic use of a drug is intended to relieve signs and symptoms of a disease or, for curative purposes, to combat and remove the agent causing the disease. Therapeutic agents include prescription or over-the-counter (OTC) medications. For example, antibiotics are able to kill or destroy microorganisms. Cough medicines may relieve coughing, and painkillers may be prescribed to relieve pain.

Diagnostic Agents

Diagnostic agents are used to determine the location of a disease by specific radiologic procedures and other diagnostic imaging techniques. Examples of diagnostic agents include the radiopharmaceutical thallium chloride for computed tomographic scans and barium meals or enemas to facilitate x-ray observation of the gastrointestinal tract.

Replacement Agents

Replacement agents restore substances normally found in the body. Examples are vitamins, minerals, and hormones.

Anesthetic Agents

Used in procedures to induce an altered state of consciousness, anesthetics permit comfortable performance of moderately painful diagnostic procedures of short duration. These agents may also be used for local or general surgical procedures. Examples are lidocaine for local procedures and nitrous oxide (laughing gas), ether, and chloroform for general surgery.

Prophylactic or Preventive Agents

Drugs used as prophylactic or preventive agents are intended to prevent a disease or disorder from occurring. Examples are vaccines and gamma globulin.

Destructive Agents

Destructive agents are able to destroy bacteria or cancer cells. Specific types are antiseptics and antineoplastics. Chemotherapy with these drugs is used to destroy malignant tumors. An example is radioiodine, which is used to destroy thyroid cancer.

DRUG CLASSIFICATION

Drugs are classified according to clinical indication (the intended condition it is designed for) or action on a particular body system. The clinical indication is different from a drug's therapeutic classification, which is its drug category (based on its effects). Drugs may have a principal action on the body or can act in other ways upon specific body systems or organs. Table 6–1 lists common drug classifications by clinical indication.

TABLE 6–1 Common Classifications of Drugs and Their Actions

Classification	Action	Example
Analgesic	A drug that relieves pain without loss of consciousness	aspirin
Anesthetic	A drug that causes a lack of feeling	nitrous oxide
Antacid	A drug that neutralizes stomach acid	aluminum compounds (Rolaids®)
Antianemic	A drug that replaces iron	cyanocobalamin (Vitamin B$_{12}$)
Antiarrhythmic	A drug that corrects and controls cardiac arrhythmias	quinidine
Anticoagulant	A drug that prevents or reduces blood clotting	heparin
Anticonvulsant (see Antiepileptic below)	A drug that relieves or prevents convulsions	phenytoin
Antidepressant	A drug that reduces feelings of depression	bupropion
Antidiarrheal	A drug that relieves or prevents diarrhea	loperamide
Antidote	A drug that counteracts poisons and their effects	activated charcoal
Antiemetic	A drug used to treat vomiting	dimenhydrinate
Antiepileptic	A drug used to treat or prevent epileptic seizures	clonazepam
Antiflatulent	A drug intended to reduce intestinal gas	lactase
Antifungal	Kills or inhibits reproduction of fungi	nystatin
Antihistamine	Prevents histamine from interacting with its receptors	diphenhydramine
Antihypertensive	Reduces high blood pressure	atenolol
Anti-inflammatory	Reduces inflammation	ibuprofen
Antimalarial	Kills or inhibits the reproduction of malaria parasites	sulfadoxine
Antimanics	Used for the treatment of the manic episode of bipolar disorder	lithium
Antineoplastic	Kills or inhibits reproduction of cancer cells	doxorubicin
Antiparasitic	Kills or inhibits reproduction of parasites	rifampin
Antiparkinsonian	Helps to control symptoms of Parkinson's disease	levodopa
Antipruritic	Reduces itching	hydrocortisone
Antipsychotic	Relieves symptoms of schizophrenia and chronic brain syndrome	haloperidol
Antipyretic	Reduces fever	naproxen
Antitoxin	An antibody that forms in response to a toxin produced by an infecting microorganism	(Such as those used against diphtheria or tetanus)
Antitussive	Reduces coughing	dextromethorphan
Antiulcer	Relieves and heals ulcers	cimetidine
Antiviral	Kills or inhibits reproduction of a virus	valacylovir
Bronchodilator	Dilates the bronchi	albuterol
Contraceptive	Prevents pregnancy	ethinyl estradiol
Decongestant	Relieves nasal congestion due to infection or allergy and inflammation in the eyes	pseudoephedrine
Diuretic	Promotes urine formation and excretion of excess interstitial fluid	hydrochlorothiazide
Expectorant	Facilitates removal of mucus secretion in the lungs	guaifenesin
Hemostatic	Controls or stops bleeding	chitosan

(continued)

TABLE 6–1 (continued)

Classification	Action	Example
Hypnotic	Causes sleep; it is also called a sleeping pill or sedative	triazolam
Hypoglycemic	Lowers blood glucose level	insulin
Laxative	Promotes bowel movements	bisacodyl
Muscle relaxant	Reduces the contraction of muscles	carisoprodol
Sedative	Produces calm or sleep	zaleplon
Tranquilizer	Acts on the central nervous system to reduce anxiety or emotional stress	methotrexate
Vasodilator	Causes blood vessels to relax and lowers blood pressure	prazosin
Vasopressor	Causes vasoconstriction and raises blood pressure	benazepril
Virucide	Kills viruses either in a living organism or inanimate surfaces	tenofovir

Dosage Forms

Drugs may also be classified by the dosage form in which they are prepared (examples include liquids, solids, semisolids, etc). Drug preparations include four basic types: solid, semisolid, liquid, and gaseous. Certain drugs are soluble in water, some in alcohol, and others in a mixture of several solvents. The route for administering a medication depends on its form, its properties, and the effects desired. To achieve the desired effects, each medication form is designed for the most effective absorption by the body.

Solid Drugs

Solid drugs include tablets, pills, plasters, capsules, caplets, gelcaps, powders, granules, troches, or lozenges (see Figure 6–1). The oral route is the most common way to administer solid drugs. (This will be discussed later in this chapter.) Drugs that must pass through the gastrointestinal tract are called enteral medications.

Tablets

A tablet is a pharmaceutical preparation made by compressing the powdered form of a drug and bulk filling material under high pressure. Special forms of tablets include sublingual tablets (to be dissolved under the tongue) and enteric-coated tablets (to which a special outside layer has been applied to certain tablets or capsules to ensure that they are passed through the stomach into the small intestine, where their special coating will dissolve). Most tablets are intended to be swallowed whole for dissolution and absorption in the gastrointestinal tract. Some are intended to be dissolved in the mouth or dissolved in water. Many times mistakenly called "pills," tablets come in various sizes, shapes, colors, and compositions. Examples of various forms of tablets include enteric-coated (for absorption via the intestine), chewable, sublingual (dissolved under the tongue), buccal (dissolved between the cheek and gum), and buffered (to protect the stomach).

Pills

A pill is a medicine initially compounded or manufactured as a putty. Measured portions of the putty are rolled into spheres that may or may not be coated. Pills are intended for oral administration. Produced by an entirely different process, tablets are often mistakenly referred to as "pills." For example, birth control pills are actually tablets. The terms *tablet* and *capsule* have replaced the term *pill*, which is not commonly used in the medical field today. However, because most patients still regularly use the word "pill" to mean most oral medications, pharmacy technicians must understand the term.

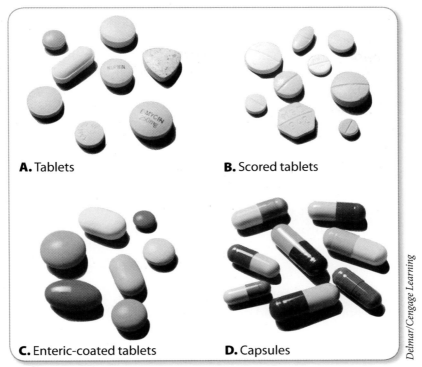

A. Tablets   B. Scored tablets

C. Enteric-coated tablets   D. Capsules

Delmar/Cengage Learning

Figure 6–1 Solid forms of drugs include tablets and capsules and are generally administered orally. A. Tablets. B. Scored tablets. C. Enteric-coated tablets. D. Capsules.

Plasters

Any composition of a liquid and a powder that hardens when it dries is a plaster. Plasters may be solid or semisolid. An example is the salicylic acid plaster used to remove corns.

Capsules

A medication dosage form in which the drug is contained in an external shell is a capsule. Capsule shells are usually made of hard gelatin and enclose or encapsulate powder, granules, liquids, or some combinations of these. Liquids may be placed in soft gelatin capsules. Examples include vitamin E capsules, Benadryl capsules, and cod liver oil capsules.

Caplets

A caplet is shaped like a capsule but has the consistency of a tablet. It is a coated, solid preparation for oral administration. An example is a Tylenol caplet.

Gelcaps

A gelcap is an oil-based medication that is enclosed in a soft gelatin capsule. An example is a vitamin A gelcap.

Powders

A drug dried and ground into fine particles is a powder. An example is potassium chloride powder (Kato powder).

Granules

A granule is a small pill, usually accompanied by many others, encased within a gelatin capsule. In most cases, granules within capsules are specially coated to gradually release medication over a period of up to 12 hours. An example of a granule is Metamucil, which is a popular bulk-forming laxative. Metamucil also comes in powder and wafer forms.

Troches or Lozenges

A hard or semisolid dosage form containing a medication intended for local application in the mouth or throat is called a troche or lozenge. Typically, a troche is placed on the tongue or between the cheek and gum and left in place until it dissolves. The medications most commonly administered by means of troches or lozenges include cough suppressants and medications used for relief of cough and sore throat. Many other drugs, such as nystatin or clotrimazole, are available in lozenge form. Examples of lozenges are cough drops or lozenges for the relief of a sore throat.

Semisolid Drugs

Semisolid drugs are often used as topical applications (applied to the surface of the body). Semisolid drugs include suppositories, ointments, creams, and gels (see Figure 6–2). These types of drugs can be used topically to treat burns, insect bites, and itching.

Suppositories

Intended to be inserted into a body orifice, a suppository is a semisolid bullet-shaped dosage that contains medication usually intended for a local effect at the site of insertion. Suppositories maintain their shape at room temperature but melt or dissolve when inserted. Although the most common sites of administration are the rectum and vagina, suppositories can also be inserted into the urethra. Rectal suppositories are often used for systemic administration of drugs because of the large number of blood vessels in the rectum. Suppositories are available in a variety of forms, including cocoa butter, glycerinated gelatin, and hydrogenated vegetable oils.

Ointments

An ointment is a semisolid, oil-based medication intended for external application, usually by rubbing. Medications that may be administered in ointment form include anti-inflammatory drugs, topical anesthetics, and antibiotics. Examples are zinc oxide and Ben-Gay ointments.

Creams

A pharmaceutical preparation that combines an oil with water, a cream is usually used topically and may or may not contain medication. Creams are usually dispensed in a tube or jar. Creams differ from lotions in that lotions contain more water and are more fluid.

Gels

A jelly-like substance that may be used for topical medication is a gel. Some gels have a high alcohol content and can cause stinging if applied to broken skin.

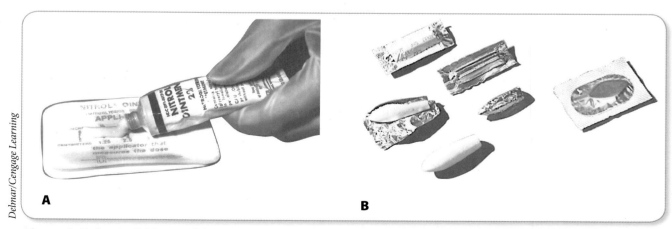

Delmar/Cengage Learning

A   B

Figure 6–2 Semisolid forms of drugs include creams and suppositories and are generally administered topically. A. Cream to be applied dermally. B. Suppositories to be applied rectally or vaginally.

Implants or Pellets

Implants or pellets are dosage forms that are placed intradermally, or under the skin, by means of minor surgery or special injections. This form of drug is used for the long-term, controlled release of medications, especially hormones. Radioactive isotopes, used in the treatment of cancer, may also be administered in the form of implants.

Liquid Drugs

Dissolved or suspended, liquid drugs include syrups, spirits, elixirs, tinctures, fluidextracts, liniments, emulsions, solutions, mixtures, suspensions, waters, sprays, and aerosols (see Figure 6–3). They are also classified by site or route of administration such as local (topical) on or through the skin, through the mouth, through the eye (ophthalmic), through the ear (otic), or through the rectum, urethra, or vagina. Liquid drugs may also be administered systemically by mouth or by injection (throughout the body).

Syrups

Consisting of a high concentration of a sugar in water, a syrup may contain additional flavorings, colors, or aromatic agents. Syrups come in two varieties. One type is medicated syrup that contains active ingredients such as simple syrup, lithium citrate syrup, or ipecac syrup. Another type is non-medicated syrup, such as cherry syrup or cocoa syrup, used as a vehicle because it does not contain alcohol.

Solutions

A solution is a drug or drugs dissolved in an appropriate solvent. An example of a solution is normal saline.

Spirits

An alcohol-containing liquid that may be used pharmaceutically as a solvent vehicle for medication or as a flavoring agent, a spirit is also known as an essence (e.g., essence of peppermint, aromatic ammonia spirit, and camphor spirit).

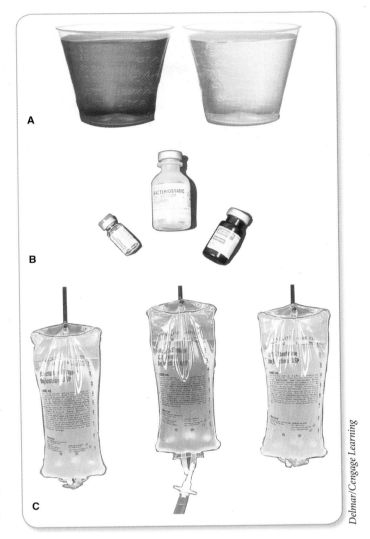

Delmar/Cengage Learning

Figure 6–3 Liquid drug forms include syrups and mixtures and can be administered via many different routes depending on the preparation.

Elixirs

A drug vehicle consisting of water, alcohol, and sugar, an elixir may or may not be aromatic and may or may not have active medicine. Its alcohol content makes an elixir a convenient liquid dosage form for many drugs that are only slightly soluble in water. In these cases, the drug is first dissolved in alcohol, and the other elixir components are then added. All elixirs contain alcohol (e.g., terpin hydrate elixir and phenobarbital elixir).

Tinctures

An alcoholic solution of a drug, a tincture may also contain water (e.g., iodine tincture and digitalis tincture).

Fluidextracts

A concentrated solution of a drug removed from a plant source by mixing ground parts of the plant with a suitable solvent, usually alcohol, and then separating the plant residue from the solvent is called a *fluidextract*. Typically, 1 mL (1 cc) contains 1 g of the drug. Fluidextracts are not intended to be administered directly to a patient. Instead, they are used to provide a source of drug in the manufacture of final dosage forms. Only vegetable drugs are used (e.g., glycyrrhiza fluidextract and ergot fluidextract). Although they are not commonly used today, fluidextracts are still important components of manufactured drugs.

Liniments

A mixture of drugs with oil, soap, water, or alcohol, a *liniment* is intended for external application with rubbing. Most liniments are counterirritants intended to treat muscle or joint pain by producing a feeling of heat in the area (e.g., camphor liniment and chloroform liniment). Although not as commonly used today as they were in the past, some medications are still available in liniment form.

Emulsions

An emulsion is a pharmaceutical preparation in which two agents that cannot ordinarily be combined are mixed. In the typical emulsion, oil is dispersed inside water. Most creams and lotions are emulsions (e.g., Haley's MO and Petrogalar).

Mixtures and Suspensions

In a mixture or a suspension, an agent is mixed with a liquid, but not dissolved. These preparations must be shaken before being taken by the patient. An example is milk of magnesia.

Waters

In pharmacy, a mixture of distilled water with an aromatic, volatile oil is called a water. Waters may be used for medicinal purposes (e.g., peppermint water and camphor water).

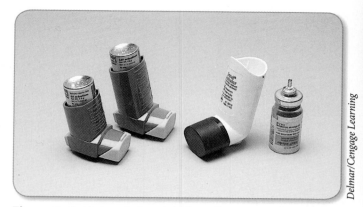

Figure 6–4 Metered-dose inhalers allow aerosolization of a liquid medication for inhalation.

Aerosolized Drugs

A liquid or fine powder that is sprayed in a fine mist, an aerosol is most commonly used in respiratory treatments for asthma and in skin sprays. Although most aerosolized medicines are liquids, some are powders whose particles are small enough to pass through the spray apparatus. An example is the inhaler in a metered-dose aerosol unit used in the treatment of asthma (see Figure 6–4).

Gaseous Drugs

Also known as "pharmaceutical gases," gaseous drugs are inhaled gases that contain medications. They include anesthetic gases, such as nitrous oxide and halothane. Compressed gases include oxygen and carbon dioxide.

Parenteral Medication Forms

Parenteral injections are those dosage forms usually intended to be administered intravenously, subcutaneously, or intramuscularly. Parenteral routes will be discussed later in this chapter.

PRINCIPLES OF DRUG ADMINISTRATION

When any medication is administered, the seven rights of drug administration—right patient, right drug, right dose, right time, right route, right technique, and right documentation—should always be followed.

MEDICATION ERRORS

Any incorrect or wrongful administration of a medication may result in serious effects for the patient. Mistakes may be made in prescribing, administering, or dispensing a medication. Causes of medication errors may include difficulty in reading handwritten orders, confusion about different drugs with similar names, differences between pharmaceutical and generic names, or lack of information about a patient's drug allergies or sensitivities.

When a medication error occurs, it is very important that the error be reported as soon as it is noticed and that the patient is monitored to see if any adverse reaction to the medication develops. Medication errors must be documented in the medical record with the signature of the person who made the error.

Pharmacists should consider reporting of errors as one of their professional duties. The U.S. Pharmacopeia (USP) and the Institute for Safe Medication Practices (ISMP) have developed a standardized form and method for reporting medication errors. Information about preventing medication errors can be obtained by calling 1-800-23-ERROR or by accessing the Web site for the USP (http://www.usp.org) or the ISMP (http://www.ismp.org). If pharmacists follow the seven rights of proper drug administration and dispensing guidelines, medication errors should not happen; but unfortunately, errors may be made periodically. When pharmacy technicians or nurses have doubts, they should delay administration of a drug until a physician makes confirmation.

METHODS OF ADMINISTERING MEDICATIONS

The route of a drug refers to how it is administered to the patient. Certain medications can be administered by more than one route, whereas others must be administered via a specific route. The route of administration is determined by a number of factors:

- The action of medication on the body
- The physical and emotional state of the patient, and
- The characteristics of the drug.

Other factors, such as age (pediatric and geriatric), the disease being treated, and the absorption, distribution, metabolism, and elimination of drugs, are important. There are generally three methods of administration: oral, topical, and parenteral.

Oral Route

The **oral** route is the safest and most convenient route chosen for most medications that are solid (tablet) or liquid (syrup). The presence or lack of food in the stomach affects absorption of many oral medications. Some drugs taken with food may have a slow absorption rate. Oral drugs may be swallowed or may be taken by the buccal or sublingual route.

Sublingual Route

Via the **sublingual** route, the drug is placed under the patient's tongue until it is completely dissolved. This method is used when rapid action is desired. For example, ergotamine tartrate (Ergostat) for migraines and nitroglycerin for angina pectoris can be administered by the sublingual route (see Figure 6–5).

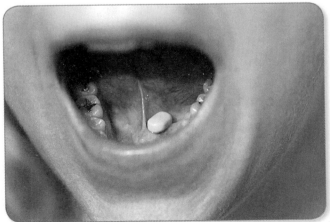

Figure 6–5 Nitroglycerin is a medication administered via the sublingual route.

Delmar/Cengage Learning

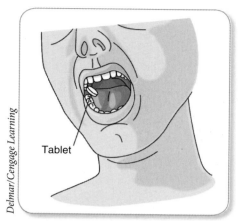

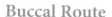

Figure 6–6 The medication is placed between the cheek and gum for administration via the buccal route.

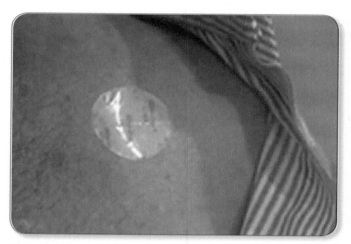

Figure 6–7 Transdermal patches deliver medication directly through the skin. (*Courtesy of 3M Pharmaceuticals*)

Buccal Route

Via the buccal route, the medication is placed between the gum and the mucous membranes of the cheek and left there until it is dissolved (see Figure 6–6). Drugs administered buccally are given for a local, rather than a systemic, effect and are absorbed slowly from the mucous membranes of the mouth. Drugs given buccally may be given as a tablet.

Topical Route

Via the topical route, medications are applied directly to the surface of the body. For instance, topical anesthesia is the application to the skin of a drug that temporarily deadens nerve sensations. Topical anesthetics are most commonly administered in aerosol, cream, or lotion form and may be used for conditions that include burns, insect bites, and itching. Other topical routes are transdermal absorption via mucous membranes, such as ophthalmic, otic, nasal, rectal, vaginal, and urethral membranes, for either local or systemic effects.

Transdermal Drug Delivery

In **transdermal drug delivery (TDD)**, medication passes through unbroken skin. For example, transdermal patches are dosage forms that release minute amounts of medication at a consistent rate (see Figure 6–7). The drug is released from the patch and absorbed into the skin and bloodstream. Examples of

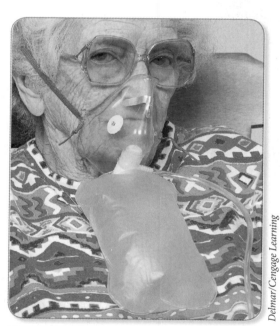

Figure 6–8 Gaseous administration of medications.

drugs administered transdermally include nicotine, nitroglycerin, estrogen, testosterone, and scopolamine.

Inhalation Administration

Drawing breath, vapor, or gas into the lungs is called inhalation. Inhalation therapy may involve the administration of medicines, water vapor, and gases such as oxygen, carbon dioxide, and helium. The medication is inhaled to achieve local effects within the respiratory tract through an aerosol, nebulizer, Spinhaler, or metered-dose inhaler (see Figure 6–8). Medications

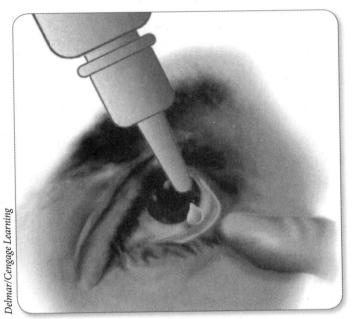

Delmar/Cengage Learning

Figure 6–9 Eyedrops are administered between the eyeball and lower lid.

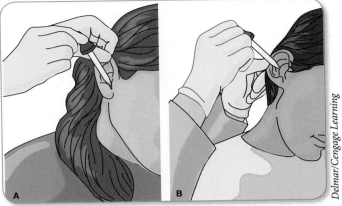

Delmar/Cengage Learning

Figure 6–10 A. Eardrops are administered in the adult by pulling the earlobe up and outward. B. In the child, eardrops are administered by pulling the earlobe down and back.

that are administered via an inhaler include bronchodilators, mucolytic agents, and steroids.

Ophthalmic Administration

Affecting only the area in contact, drops and ointments instilled into the eye, placed between the eyeball and the lower lid, are generally absorbed slowly (see Figure 6–9). Ophthalmic preparations and administration must be sterile to prevent eye infections and should be isotonic to minimize burning. Medications in ophthalmic preparations include antibiotics, antivirals, decongestants, artificial tears, and topical anesthetics.

Otic Route

Localized infection or inflammation of the ear is treated by dropping a small amount of a sterile or non-sterile medicated solution, depending on the condition, into the ear. Very low dosages of medication are required, and the manufacturer must indicate that the medication is meant for otic usage. In children younger than 3 years of age, gently pull the earlobe down and back; in adults, gently pull the earlobe up and out (see Figure 6–10). The patient must remain on that side for 5 minutes to allow the medication to coat the surface of the inner ear canal. The use of eardrops is usually contraindicated if the patient has a perforated eardrum.

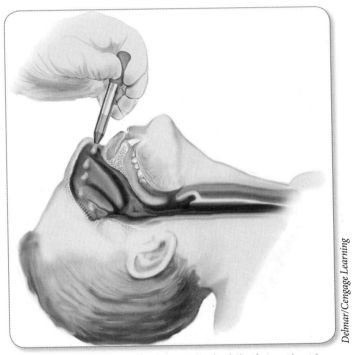

Delmar/Cengage Learning

Figure 6–11 Nose drops are instilled while the patient is lying down.

Nasal Route

Nasal solutions act locally to treat minor congestion or infection. The medication should be drawn up in the dropper and held just over one nostril; then the required number of nose drops should be administered (see Figure 6–11). If a nasal spray is used, the patient sits upright; blocks one nostril, and inserts the tip of the nasal spray into the other nostril. Taking a deep breath, the patient then squeezes a puff of spray into the nostril.

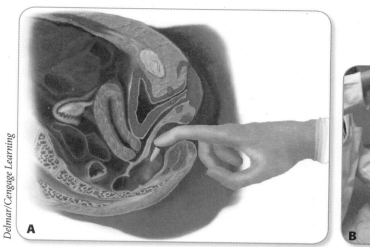
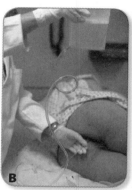

Delmar/Cengage Learning

Figure 6–12 Rectal suppositories can be administered to the patient who is nauseous, vomiting, or unconscious. A. Insertion of suppository. B. Administration of an enema.

Rectal Route

If the patient is nauseated, vomiting, or unconscious, rectal medications are useful. Manufacturers supply rectal medications in the form of gelatin- or cocoa butter-based suppositories, which melt in the warmth of the rectum and release the medication (see Figure 6–12A). Rectal medications also come in the form of enemas as a solution (see Figure 6–12B). Rectal medications may be used to soften the stool or stimulate evacuation of the bowel.

The best time to administer a rectal drug for a systemic effect is after a bowel movement or an enema. The means of delivering a solution or medication into the rectum and colon, an enema is also used to cleanse the lower bowel in preparation for radiography, proctoscopy, sigmoidoscopy, and surgery. Promoting bowel evacuation by softening the feces and stimulating peristalsis, Fleet Ready-To-Use Enema does not cause burning, irritation, or dehydration and does not interfere with the absorption of vitamins or the actions of drugs.

Vaginal Route

Vaginal suppositories, tablets, creams, and fluid solutions are used to treat local infections. Medications are deposited into the vagina. Douches may be used as anti-infectives, and creams (instilled with applicators) and foams are available as local contraceptives. Vaginal instillation is most effective if the patient is lying down.

Parenteral Route

Injection of medications into body tissues with a syringe and a needle for rapid effect and absorption, parenteral administration also refers to injection of medications from an intravenous (IV) bag that is connected via special tubing to the patient. IV bags are commonly used when medications, such as IV fluids or antibiotics, need to be infused over a longer time and when total parenteral nutrition (TPN) is required. According to the site of the infection, there are four main categories for parenteral administration. Drugs may be injected into muscles, veins, skin (intradermal or subcutaneous), and the spinal column.

Intradermal Injection

Intradermal injections are given within the skin. If drugs are injected correctly, a small wheal (bump) occurs on the skin. The angle of insertion is 15 degrees, almost parallel to the skin surface (see Figure 6–13). The common site of injection is the center of the forearm, but other sites, the upper chest and back areas, may also be used. Skin tests for allergies and tuberculin tests are the most common uses for intradermal injections.

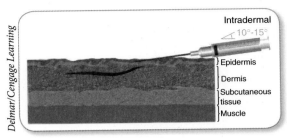

Figure 6–13 Proper angle of intradermal injection.

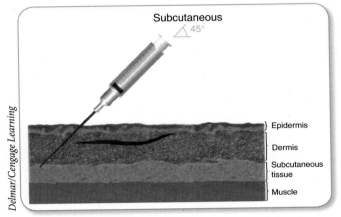

Figure 6–14 Proper angle of subcutaneous injection.

Subcutaneous Injection

Subcutaneous injections are given just below the skin and the layer of fatty tissue called *adipose tissue*. The most common sites for subcutaneous injections are the deltoid area, anterior thigh, abdomen, and upper back. The angle of insertion is 45 degrees for local anesthetics, allergy treatments, and epinephrine; however, insulin and heparin are usually injected at a 90-degree angle (see Figure 6–14). The amount of drug administered through the subcutaneous route should not be more than 2 mL.

Intramuscular Injection

An **intramuscular injection** is given into a large muscle, preferably in the gluteus, deltoid, and vastus lateralis muscles in adults (see Figure 6–15). Part of the quadriceps muscle in the thigh, the vastus lateralis is also considered the safest site of administration for infants. The deltoid site is acceptable for adults and older children. Muscles can absorb a greater amount of fluid than what is usually given by subcutaneous administration.

Dosage may vary from 0.5 to 5 mL. The needle should be 1 to 3 inches in length or may sometimes be longer. The gauge of the needle ranges from 18 to 23.

Drugs are injected into a muscle for the following reasons:

- The drug being given irritates skin tissues
- A more rapid absorption is desired
- The volume of the medication to be injected is large

Intravenous Injection

An **intravenous injection** is used during emergency situations, when immediate effects are required, or when drugs or fluids are being administered by infusion. Sometimes large doses of medication must be given, either every few hours or over a long period of time. The rate of absorption and the onset of action are faster by intravenous medication. Intravenous injections are generally inserted into the smallest veins and as close to the hands as possible. The metacarpal, dorsal, basilic, and cephalic veins are commonly used in adults. Veins commonly used in infants and children include the scalp vein in the temporal area and veins in the dorsum of the foot and the back of the hand. Peripheral veins used in adults include the back of the hand, arm and forearm, and dorsal plexus of the foot.

Implants

An *implant* is a device inserted surgically under the skin for the delivery of medications. For example, Ganciclovir, an ocular implant that treats cytomegalovirus eye infections in AIDS patients.

EQUIPMENT USED FOR ORAL ADMINISTRATION

Three measuring devices are used in the administration of oral medications: the medicine cup, the medicine dropper, and the calibrated spoon (see Figure 6-16). The medicine cup may be calibrated in fluid ounces (oz),

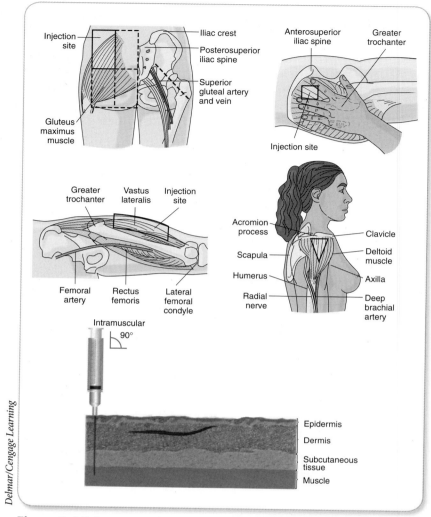

Delmar/Cengage Learning

Figure 6–15 Intramuscular injection sites and proper angle of injection.

fluidrams, cubic centimeters (cc), milliliters (mL), teaspoons (tsp), or tablespoons (Tbsp). The medicine dropper may be calibrated in milliliters (mL), minims (m), or drops (gtt).

EQUIPMENT USED FOR PARENTERAL ADMINISTRATION

Various types of equipment are used to administer medication via a parenteral route. Needles, syringes, intravenous devices, and unit- and multiple-dose forms of injections are some of the equipment with which pharmacy technicians should be familiar.

Pumps

Medication can be administered via a pump to provide continuous flow into the system. Electronic devices that force a precisely measured amount of intravenous fluid into a patient's vein over a predetermined amount of time (see Figure 6–17), pumps are a very popular way of administering a constant dose of insulin to a diabetic patient.

Needles

Two types of needles are available for parenteral medication administration: disposable (after one use) and reusable (for multiple injections). Disposable needles are used the most. Used when drawing medications out of ampules, filter needles have a filtration material

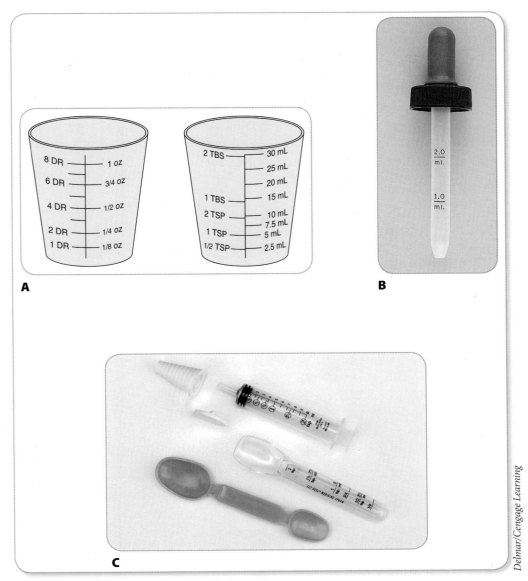

Delmar/Cengage Learning

Figure 6–16   A. Medicine cup. B. Calibrated dropper. C. Calibrated spoon.

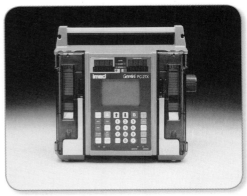

Figure 6–17   Medication Infusion Pump. *(Courtesy of Medtronic, Minneapolis, MN)*

inside them that does not allow particles to be drawn into the needle. Retractable needles are commonly used in the field of nursing and are also referred to as "easy cap" needles. They are very safe for use when patients are in close proximity. In the pharmacy, retractable needles are seldom used because only pharmacy staff members are allowed in the areas where they are handled.

The gauge of a needle is determined by the diameter of the lumen or opening at its beveled tip. Needle gauges range from 28 to 14 and needle lengths vary from 1/4-inch to 2 inches. The larger the needle gauge, the smaller the diameter of its lumen. Various sizes and types of needles are shown in Figure 6–18. Needles consist of five parts: the point, the lumen, the shaft, the hilt, and the hub.

Syringes

Both disposable and reusable syringes are available. Disposable syringes are sterilized, prepackaged, nontoxic, nonpyrogenic, and ready for use. Syringe sizes commonly vary from 1 mL to over 60 mL.

Syringes are named according to their sizes and uses. The component parts of a syringe consist of the plunger, barrel, flange, and tip (see Figure 6–19). In general, there are two types of syringes: hypodermic and prefilled. Hypodermic syringes are commonly available in sizes of 1, 3, 5, 10, 20, and 50 cc, with

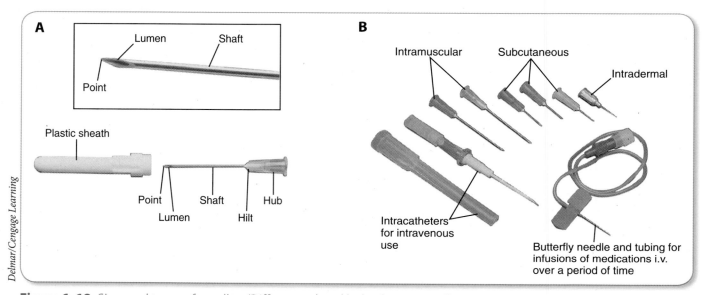

Figure 6–18 Sizes and types of needles. (Different colored hubs denote needle gauges.)

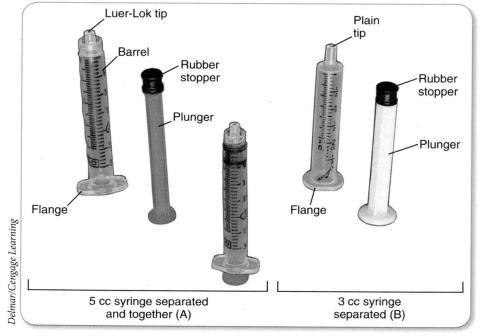

Figure 6–19 Parts of a syringe.

the sizes 1, 3, and 5 being used most often. These typically are used for intramuscular or subcutaneous injections. They are also used for venipuncture, medical or surgical treatment, aspiration, irrigations, and gavage (tube-to-stomach) feedings. There are several types of hypodermic syringes, including needleless, insulin, and tuberculin.

As required by OSHA standards, retractable needle syringes are used for prevention of needle sticks. These syringes come with retractable needle covers to prevent needle sticks from contaminated syringes (see Figure 6–20).

An *injector pen*, another type of syringe, is used most commonly for insulin administration. The insulin syringe is calibrated in units (U) specifically for use by diabetic patients. The common sizes of insulin syringes are U-30 (0.3 cc), U-50 (0.5 cc), and U-100 (1 cc) (Figure 6–21).

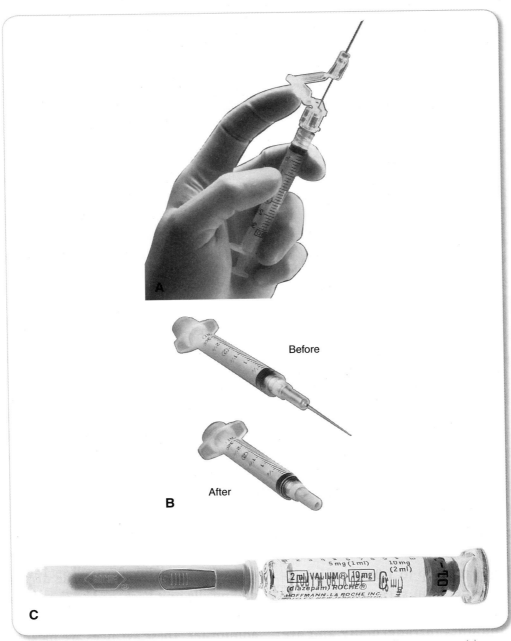

Figure 6–20 Syringes that have a safety device to slide over the needle or retractable needles are now preferred. *(Courtesy of Becton Dickinson, Courtesy of Retractable Technologies, Courtesy of Roche Laboratories, Inc.)*

GLOSSARY

Apothecary system – a very old English system of measurement that has been slowly replaced by the metric system; its basic units of measurement are the grain, dram, and minim

Arabic numbers – standard numerical numbers

Denominator – the total number of parts of the whole

Dividend – the number that is being divided; in 6 ÷ 3, the dividend is 6

Divisor – a number that is used to divide another; in 6 ÷ 3, the divisor is 3

Dram – a unit of weight in the apothecary system; 1 dram = 60 grains

Drip rate - the speed at which intravenous fluids are infused

Extremes – the two outside terms in a proportion

Fraction – an expression of division of a whole into parts

Grain – the basic unit of weight in the apothecary system

Gram – the basic unit of weight in the metric system

Liter – the basic unit of volume in the metric system

Means – the two inside terms in a proportion

Meniscus – the crescent-shaped curvature of the surface of a liquid standing in a narrow vessel such as a graduate

Meter – the basic unit of length in the metric system

Metric system – the preferred system of measurement throughout the world; it is based on the decimal system

Minim – the basic unit of volume in the apothecary system

Numerator – the number of the parts of the whole being considered

Ounce – a unit of weight in the apothecary system; 1 oz = 8 drams

Percent – a term referring to "hundredths"; a *percentage* is a fraction whose denominator is understood to be 100; for example, 25/100 is also expressed as 25 percent or 25%

Proportion – the equality of two ratios

Quotient – the answer to a division problem

Ratio – an expression that compares relative quantities

ARABIC NUMBERS AND ROMAN NUMERALS

Roman numerals use letters to designate numbers. If using the Roman numeral system, mathematical calculations would become extremely complicated. Most of the medications administered or ordered are measured by amounts expressed in Arabic numbers. The system of whole numbers (0 through 9), *fractions* (e.g., 1/5), and *decimals* (e.g., 0.7) is used widely in the United States and internationally. Table 7–1 shows some examples of Arabic numbers and Roman numerals.

FRACTIONS

Pharmacy technicians need to understand fractions to interpret and act on practitioners' orders, read prescriptions, and understand patient records and information used in pharmacy literature. Fractions are used in apothecary and household measures for dosage calculations. A fraction is a way of expressing

TABLE 7–1 Examples of Arabic Numbers and Roman Numerals

Arabic Number	Roman Numeral
1	I
2	II
3	III
4	IV
5	V
6	VI
7	VII
8	VIII
9	IX
10	X
20	XX
30	XXX
50	L
100	C
500	D
1000	M

division of a whole into parts. It can also be defined as "a part of a whole." For example, "three parts" out of a total of "four parts" can be expressed as "3/4."

Fractions can stand alone or can be part of a mixed number, which is a whole number and a fraction. A fraction has two parts. The bottom is referred to as the **denominator** and is the total number of parts. The **numerator** is the number of parts being considered.

Fractions can be converted into decimals by simple division. For example, 25/100 can be converted into a decimal by dividing the denominator 100 into the numerator 25.

$$25 \div 100 = 0.25$$

Also, a fraction may be converted into a percentage by performing the same calculation as shown above, and then multiplying the result by 100. So, the fraction 25/100 = 0.25, as we have shown. To find the equivalent percentage, multiply as follows:

$$0.25 \times 100 = 25\%$$

Example:

$$\frac{4}{6} = \frac{\text{Numerator}}{\text{Denominator}}$$

Comparing Fractions

When calculating some drug dosages, pharmacy technicians may need to know whether the value of one fraction is greater than or less than the value of another fraction. The size of a fraction can be determined by comparing the numerators when the denominators are the same or comparing the denominators if the numerators are the same. If the numerators are the same, the fraction with the smaller denominator has the greater value.

Example:

Compare $\frac{1}{2}$ tsp and $\frac{1}{3}$ tsp.

Numerators are both 1.
Denominator 2 is less than 3.

Therefore, ½ tsp has the greater value.

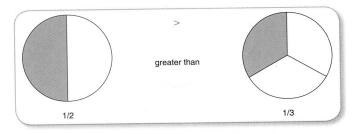

Conversely, if the denominators are both the same, the fraction with the smaller numerator has the lesser value.

Example:

Compare $\frac{2}{5}$ Tbsp and $\frac{4}{5}$ Tbsp.

Denominators are both 5.
Numerators: 2 is less than 4.

Therefore, 2/5 Tbsp has a lesser value.

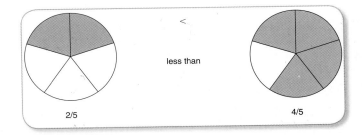

Adding Fractions

To add two fractions, it is necessary to find a common denominator first. Next, add the numerators, and keep the value of the common denominator the same. Finally, reduce the resulting value to its lowest terms.

Examples:

Add 1/6 and 4/12. To obtain a common denominator of 12, it is necessary to multiply the numerator and denominator of 1/6 by 2. An easier way to understand this is by multiplying 1/6 by 2/2, as follows:

$$\frac{1}{6} \times \frac{2}{2} = \frac{2}{12}$$

Now we have a common denominator and are able to simply add the numerators. Be sure to reduce the final answer:

$$\frac{2}{12} + \frac{4}{12} = \frac{6}{12} = \frac{1}{2}$$

The fraction 6/12 is reduced to its lowest terms, which is 1/2.

Subtracting Fractions

The first step in subtracting fractions is to find a common denominator. Then, subtract the numerator, and, finally, obtain the result by keeping the denominator the same and taking the difference of the numerators. Reduce the resulting value to its lowest terms to obtain the final answer.

Example:

Subtract 1/2 from 8/10. To obtain a common denominator, multiply the numerator and denominator by 5 to produce 10 as the common denominator:

$$\frac{1}{2} \times \frac{5}{5} = \frac{5}{10}$$

Subtract the numerators:

$$\frac{8}{10} - \frac{5}{10} = \frac{3}{10}$$

The answer cannot be reduced further. The final answer is 3/10.

Multiplying Fractions

To multiply fractions, first, multiply the numerators. Second, multiply the denominators; then place the product (the answer to a multiplication problem) of the numerators over the product of the denominators, and finally, reduce the resulting value to its lowest terms.

Example 1:

$$\frac{3}{4} \times \frac{2}{5} = \frac{6}{20} = \frac{3}{10}$$

Example 2:

$$\frac{2}{4} \times \frac{3}{4}$$

Reduce 2/4 to 1/2, then multiply:

$$\frac{1}{2} \times \frac{3}{4} = \frac{3}{8}$$

Dividing Fractions

To divide fractions, first, invert (or turn upside down) the divisor. Second, multiply the two fractions, and then reduce the resulting value to its lowest terms.

Example 1:

$$\frac{3}{4} \div \frac{2}{3} =$$
$$\frac{3}{4} \times \frac{3}{2} = 1\frac{1}{8}$$

Example 2:

$$\frac{3}{4} \div \frac{8}{9} =$$
$$\frac{3}{4} \times \frac{9}{8} = \frac{27}{32}$$

RATIOS

A **ratio** is a mathematical expression that compares two numbers by division. It is used to indicate the relationship of one part of a quantity to the whole. When written, the two quantities are separated by a colon (:). The use of the colon is a traditional way to write the division sign within a ratio and is expressed as "3 is to 7."

Example 1:

$\frac{3}{7}$ may be expressed as a ratio: 3:7

Example 2:

1:150 may be expressed as a fraction: $\frac{1}{150}$

PROPORTIONS

A **proportion** shows the relationship between two equal ratios. A proportion may be expressed as:

4:8 :: 1:2

or as:

4:8 = 1:2

In the first case, (::) is read as "so as." Hence, "4 is to 8 so as 1 is to 2." These are equal because multiplying

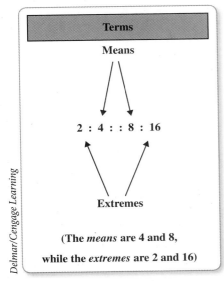

Terms

Means

$$2 : 4 :: 8 : 16$$

Extremes

(The *means* are 4 and 8,
while the *extremes* are 2 and 16)

Delmar/Cengage Learning

Figure 7-1 Means and extremes.

DECIMALS

Decimal fractions or decimals are used with the metric system, which is most often used in the calculation of drug dosages. Pharmacy technicians must manipulate decimals easily and accurately. Each decimal fraction consists of a numerator that is expressed in numerals, a decimal point placed so that it designates the value of the denominator, and the denominator that is understood to be 10 or some power of 10. In writing a decimal fraction, always place a zero to the left of the decimal point so that the decimal point can readily be seen. This also ensures that the decimal will not be mistaken for a whole number. Table 7-2 shows some examples.

For reading and writing decimals, observe Figure 7-2. Note that all whole numbers are to the left of the decimal point; all fractions, to the right.

To convert a decimal into a fraction, simply move the decimal point two spaces to the right, and place the resulting number as a numerator over a denominator of 100. For example, if you start with the decimal 0.33 and move the decimal point two spaces to the right, you are left with the number "33." Now, place 33 over the denominator 100, as follows:

$$\frac{33}{100}$$

Remember that converting a decimal into a percentage only requires you to multiply the decimal by 100, as follows:

$$0.33 \times 100 = 33\%$$

1 and 2 by 4 will result in 4 and 8, respectively. In a proportion, the terms have names. The **extremes** are the two outside terms, and the **means** are the two inside terms. This relationship is shown in Figure 7-1. In a proportion, the product of means is equal to the product of extremes.

Most of the time we know only three terms of a proportion. The term we do not know is the *unknown*; and in this text, the unknown is labeled X. To solve unknown proportion terms, first, multiply the extremes and the means. Their products are set as equal. Then, divide both sides of the equation by the number to the left of X.

Example 1:

$$2{:}4 = X{:}10$$
$$4X = 2 \times 10$$
$$4X = 20$$
$$X = \frac{20}{4} = 5$$

Example 2:

$$\frac{0.5}{X} = \frac{1}{8}$$
$$1X = 8 \times 0.5$$
$$X = 4$$

TABLE 7-2 Correct Usage of Decimals

Correct Usages	Incorrect Usages
One tenth = 0.1	One tenth = .1
One hundredth = 0.01	One hundredth = .01
Five = 5	Five = 5.0
Ten and one half = 10.5	Ten and one half = 10.50

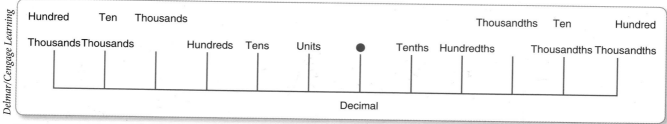

Figure 7–2 Decimal values.

Multiplying Decimals

To multiply decimals, first, find the product as usual. Second, count the number of decimal places in both the multiplicand (a number that is to be multiplied by another) and the multiplier (the number by which another number is multiplied). Finally, mark the total number of decimal places in the product and insert a decimal point.

Example:

Multiply 2.05 × 0.2

Step 1:

2.05 (multiplicand)
× 0.2 (multiplier)
0410 (product)

Step 2:

Count the number of decimal places in the multiplicand and the multiplier:

2.05 × 0.2 = Total of three decimal places

Step 3:

Mark off three decimal places in the product.
New decimal = 0.410

Dividing Decimals

To divide a decimal by a whole number, first, write the problem as usual. Second, place a decimal point in the quotient line directly above the decimal in the dividend, and then find the quotient. The **divisor** is the number performing the division. The action of division is expressed using several different symbols, such as:

A. ÷ (the standard "division symbol"), wherein the divisor appears on the right of this symbol, such as in the example "1 ÷ 2", with 2 being the divisor.

B. / (a "slash bar"), wherein the divisor also appears on the right of this symbol, such as in the example "1/2," which signifies "1 divided by 2," with 2 being the divisor—NOTE: This is also expressed as the fraction "one-half."

C. — (a "division bar"), wherein the divisor appears on the left of the symbol.

The answer to a division problem is called the **quotient**. The divisor must be a whole number (a number with no decimal point), and the decimal point must be correctly placed in the answer. When a decimal number is being divided by a whole number, the decimal point is placed directly above the decimal point in the **dividend** (number being divided). When a number is being divided by a decimal number, the decimal point in the divisor must be moved to the right as many places as needed to make the divisor a whole number. The decimal point in the dividend must be moved the same number of places to the right. The decimal point in the quotient is placed directly above the new position of the decimal point in the dividend.

Example:

3.25 ÷ 0.5

To divide decimal numbers, convert the divisor to a whole number. Move the decimal point in the dividend the same number of places to the right:

3.25 ÷ 0.5

Place the decimal point in the quotient directly above its new position in the dividend:

$$32.5 \div 0.5$$

Perform the calculation:

$$\frac{32.5}{5} = 6.5$$

Adding Decimals

To add decimals, write the decimals in a column, with the decimal points aligned. Then, add the numbers as you would when adding whole numbers, and place the decimal point in the sum (the answer to an addition problem) directly under the decimal points in the addends.

Example 1:

$$0.8 + 0.9 = \begin{array}{r} 0.8 \\ 0.9 \\ \hline 1.7 \end{array}$$

Example 2:

$$0.9 + 0.03 + 2 = \begin{array}{r} 0.90 \\ 0.03 \\ 2.00 \\ \hline 2.93 \end{array}$$

Subtracting Decimals

To subtract decimals, write the decimals in columns, keeping the decimal points aligned. Then, subtract as you do with whole numbers (zeros may be added after the decimal without changing the value), and place the decimal point in the difference (the answer to a subtraction problem), directly under the decimal point in the subtrahend (a number to be subtracted from another) and minuend (the number from which another number is to be subtracted).

Example 1:

$$0.80 - 0.423 = \begin{array}{r} 0.800 \\ -\ 0.423 \\ \hline 0.377 \end{array}$$

Example 2:

$$0.7 - 0.239 = \begin{array}{r} 0.700 \\ -\ 0.239 \\ \hline 0.461 \end{array}$$

PERCENTAGES

The term **percent** and its symbol % mean "hundredths." A percentage is a fraction whose numerator is expressed and whose denominator is understood to be 100. It can be changed to a decimal by moving the decimal point two places to the left to signify hundredths or to a fraction by expressing the denominator as 100.

Example 1:

$$7\% \text{ means } \frac{7}{100} \text{ or } 0.07$$

Example 2:

$$\frac{1}{5}\% \text{ means } \frac{1/5}{100} \text{ or } 0.002$$

When the percentage is unknown, you can use the formula of X.

Example 3:

What percent of 10 ounces are 3 ounces? You are looking for a percentage in this case.

$$3 = X \times 10$$
$$3 = 10X \text{ or } 10X = 3$$
$$X \text{ divided by } 10 = 3 \text{ divided by } 10$$
$$X = \frac{3}{10} \text{ or } X = 30\%$$

Therefore, converting a percentage into a fraction is as simple as dividing the percentage by 100. Using the above percentage, 30%, we find:

$$30 \div 100 = \frac{30}{100}$$

To convert a percentage into a decimal, simply add a decimal point two spaces to the left of the number in the percentage. Using the above percentage, 30%, we find that:

by adding a decimal two spaces to the left of the number 30,

we have the number ".30."

Proper mathematical expressions do not allow this number to be stated without a leading zero. Therefore, ".30" becomes "0.30." Because we do not need to use a trailing zero,

"0.30" becomes "0.3."
The decimal "0.3" is equivalent to "30%."

THE METRIC SYSTEM

Approximately 90% of the world's developed countries use the metric system. Today, the metric system is the system of choice when one deals with the weights and measures involved in the calculation of drug dosages. Its accuracy and simplicity is based on the decimal system, and the use of decimals can eliminate errors in measuring medications. The three basic units of the metric system are the following:

1. *Gram*: the basic unit for weight

2. *Liter*: the basic unit for volume

3. *Meter*: the basic unit for length

Parts of these basic units are named by adding a prefix. Each prefix has a numerical value, which is shown in Table 7–3. Pharmacy technicians must also be familiar with common metric abbreviations, which are shown in Table 7–4.

TABLE 7–3 Metric Prefixes

Prefix		Value
nano- (n)	=	1/1,000,000,000 (one-billionth of basic unit)
micro- (mc)	=	1/1,000,000 (one-millionth of basic unit)
milli- (m)	=	1/1000 (one-thousandth of basic unit)
centi- (c)	=	1/100 (one-hundredth of basic unit)
deci- (d)	=	1/10 (one-tenth of basic unit)
kilo- (k)	=	1000 (one thousand times basic unit)

TABLE 7–4 Common Metric Abbreviations

Metric Unit	Abbreviation
nanogram	ng
microgram	mcg
milligram	mg
kilogram	kg
milliliter	mL
deciliter	dL
liter	L
millimeter	mm
centimeter	cm
meter	m
kilometer	km

Gram

The gram (g) is the basic unit of weight in the metric system. Some medications are ordered as fractions of grams. The milligram is 1000 times smaller than a gram; medications may be ordered in milligrams. Table 7–5 shows the values of the gram.

Liter

The liter (L) is the basic unit of volume used to measure liquids in the metric system. It is equal to 1000 cubic centimeters (cc) of water. One cc is equivalent to 1 milliliter (mL); hence, 1 L = 1000 mL.

Meter

The meter is used for linear (length) measurements. Linear measurements (meter and centimeter) are commonly used to measure the height of an individual

TABLE 7–5 Gram Values

Gram		Value
1000 grams (g)	=	1 kilogram (kg)
1000 milligrams (mg)	=	1 gram (g)
1000 nanograms (ng)	=	1 microgram (mcg)
1000 microgram (mcg)	=	1 milligram (mg)

TABLE 7–6 Metric and Household Measurement Equivalents

Metric Measure		Household Measure
1 milliliter (mL)	=	15 drops (gtt)
5 milliliters (mL)	=	1 teaspoon (tsp)*
15 milliliters (mL)	=	1 tablespoon (Tbsp)*
180 milliliters (mL)	=	1 cup (c)*
240 milliliters (mL)	=	1 glass*
1 kilogram (kg) or 1000 grams (g)	=	2.2 pounds (lb)
2.54 centimeters (cm)	=	1 inch (in)

*Note: This unit is not standard—household measuring devices vary widely in size.

and to determine growth patterns and is not used in the calculation of doses. Therefore, only the units of weight and volume are discussed in this chapter.

HOUSEHOLD MEASUREMENTS

Household measurements are not accurate enough for health-care professionals to use in the calculation of drug dosages in the hospital or pharmacy. This system, however, is still used for doses given primarily at home, as indicated by the name. The household system is the least accurate of the three systems of measure. Capacities of utensils such as teaspoons, tablespoons, and cups vary from one house to another. Table 7–6 shows a list of approximate equivalents between the metric and household measurement systems.

THE APOTHECARY SYSTEM

Also called the "wine measure" or the "United States liquid measure," the apothecary system is a very old English system. The term "apothecary" used to refer to a pharmacist or pharmacy. Although it has slowly been replaced by the metric system, the apothecary system has a few units of measure that are used for medication administration. In the following paragraphs, some basic units for weight and volume in the apothecary system are discussed.

Weight

The basic unit for weight is the grain (gr). A dram (dr) is also a unit of weight; 1 dr = 60 gr. An **ounce (oz)** is larger than a dram; 1 oz = 8 dr.

Volume

The basic unit for volume is the minim (℥), which is extremely small, perhaps the size of 1 drop (gtt). Volume can also be measured by drams and ounces. In summary, the units of the apothecary system are as follows:

Weight:	grain (gr)
	dram (dr)
	ounce (oz)
Volume:	minim (℥)

CONVERTING WITHIN AND BETWEEN SYSTEMS

In pharmacy and medicine, the metric system currently dominates the other commonly used systems. Most prescriptions and medication orders are written in the metric system, and labeling on most prepackaged pharmaceutical products shows drug strengths and dosages described in metric units, replacing to a great extent the use of the other systems of measurement. Medications are usually ordered in a unit of weight measurement such as grams or grains.

Pharmacy technicians must convert and calculate the correct dosage of drugs, converting between units of measurement within the same system or converting units of measurement from one system to another. Also, pharmacy technicians must interpret the order and administer the correct number of tablets, capsules, tablespoons, milligrams, or milliliters.

Example:

To convert 25 grams to grains, you must first understand that 1 gram is approximately equivalent to 15 grains. Therefore, the conversion factor is 15. So:

$$25 \text{ g} = 25 \times 15 = 375 \text{ gr}$$

Example:

To convert 3 drams (ℨ) to milliliters, you must first understand that 1 dram is approximately equivalent to 3.69 mL. Therefore, the conversion factor is 3.69 So:

$$3 \times 3.69 = 11.07 \text{ mL}$$

Conversion of Weights

To convert units of weight, one must remember that 1000 mg = 1 g and that 1000 micrograms (mcg) = 1 mg. To convert grams to milligrams, always multiply by 1000 or move the decimal point three places to the right.

Example:

$$2 \text{ g} = 2000. \text{ mg}$$
$$0.2 \text{ g} = 200. \text{ mg}$$
$$0.02 \text{ g} = 020. \text{ mg}$$

Alternatively, to convert milligrams to grams, divide by 1000 or move the decimal point three places to the left.

Example:

$$250 \text{ mg} = 0.250 \text{ g}$$
$$50 \text{ mg} = 0.050 \text{ g}$$
$$5 \text{ mg} = 0.005 \text{ g}$$

To convert milligrams to micrograms, multiply by 1000 or move the decimal point three places to the right.

Example:

$$3 \text{ mg} = 3000. \text{ mcg}$$
$$0.5 \text{ mg} = 500. \text{ mcg}$$
$$0.08 \text{ mg} = 080. \text{ mcg}$$

To convert micrograms to milligrams, divide by 1000 or move the decimal point three places to the left.

Example:

$$1500 \text{ mcg} = 1.500 \text{ mg}$$
$$600 \text{ mcg} = 0.600 \text{ mg}$$
$$20 \text{ mcg} = 0.020 \text{ mg}$$

The microgram, milligram, and gram are the most commonly used measurements in medication administration. Tablets and capsules are most often supplied in milligrams. Antibiotics can be provided in grams, milligrams, or units. For small dosages or for very powerful drugs in pediatric and critical care patients, micrograms are used.

Conversion of Liquids

To convert and calculate the correct dosage of liquid medications, remember the units of the metric system for volume.

Example:

Convert 0.02 L to mL:
Equivalent: 1 L = 1000 mL
Conversion factor is 1000
Multiply by 1000:
$$0.02 \text{ L} = 0.02 \times 1000 = 20 \text{ mL}$$
Or move the decimal point three places to the right:
$$0.02 \text{ L} = 0.020. = 20 \text{ mL}$$

To convert milliliters to liters, one must divide. Remember that the equivalent of 1 L = 1000 mL. Then divide the number of milliliters by 1000.

Example

Convert 3000 mL to L:
Equivalent: 1 L = 1000 mL
Conversion factor is 1000.
Divide by 1000:
$$3000 \text{ mL} = 3000 \div 1000 = 3 \text{ L}$$
Or move decimal point three places to the left:
$$3000 \text{ mL} = 3.000 = 3 \text{ L}$$

Units and Milliequivalents

Certain products made from biologics (such as insulin, heparin, and vitamin E) are expressed in "units" or "International units." A *unit* represents an amount of activity within a particular system, and each pharmaceutical product is unique in regards to its amount of activity. Units represent specific concentrations and may be expressed as *units per tablet, units per milliliter (mL),* or in other ways.

A *milliequivalent* is one-thousandth of an equivalent weight of a chemical substance. Concentrations of serum electrolytes such as calcium, potassium, and sodium are expressed in milliequivalents (mEq). Because both units and milliequivalents are prepared and administered in the same system, there is no need to learn any conversions.

Concentration and Dilution

A substance's *concentration* is its strength, which can be expressed as a fraction (such as mg / mL), ratio (such as 1:100), or percentage (such as 30% or 60%). The dilution of a substance relates directly to its desired concentration. When pharmacy technicians receive an order to prepare a solution of a certain strength and volume, these terms are referred to as its *final strength (FS)* and *final volume (FV)*. The process involves choosing a product of an *initial strength (IS)*, and then determining the *initial volume (IV)* needed to prepare the compound. If a solid is to be compounded, instead of volume, the terms *final weight (FW)* and *initial weight (IW)* are used. The formula for either type of compounding is as follows:

Initial volume (or weight) × Initial strength = Final volume (or weight) × Final strength

In order to avoid errors, the initial strength must be larger than the final strength. Also, the initial volume (or weight) must be less than the final volume (or weight). The final volume (or weight), minus the initial volume (or weight), equals the amount of diluent that needs to be added.

Calculation of Dosages

The common practice in hospitals today is for pharmacy technicians to calculate and prepare the drug dosage form for administration to the patient. Most of the time, the drug is provided in a unit-dose package. However, pharmacy technicians must understand the concept of calculating medication dosages that patients receive. Learning to correctly calculate drug dosages is an extremely important skill, because it can often be the difference between life and death for the patient. Calculating incorrect dosages could result in undertreatment, with the patient's condition not improving or even worsening, or an overdose that causes the patient harm. The ability to calculate drug dosages is a skill that should not be taken lightly. In fact, all health-care professionals who deal with the preparation and/or administration of medications should aim for 100% success in performing this task. Recall the seven rights of drug administration discussed in Chapter 6: right patient, right drug, right dose, right time, right route, right technique, and right documentation.

The use of calculators is recommended for complex calculations of dosages to ensure accuracy and save time. These types of calculations require basic math skills to use calculators properly.

CALCULATION OF ORAL DRUGS

A variety of forms of drugs are commonly administered orally. Medications administered by mouth may be solid or liquid. Solid drugs are *generally* intended to be given in their entirety to achieve a specific effect in the body.

Dosing of Tablets and Capsules

Tablets and capsules are solid medications that are supplied in different strengths or dosages. Their dosages can be expressed in apothecary or metric measures, for example, grains or milligrams.

Depending on the conversion factor used, converting drug measures from one system to another and from one unit to another to determine the dosage to be administered can result in discrepancies. For example, one must remember the following:

- The label for Tylenol® may indicate 325 mg (5 gr). This is based on the equivalent 65 mg = 1 gr. On the other hand, the label for aspirin may indicate 300 mg (5 gr). Here the equivalent 60 mg = 1 gr was used. Both of the equivalents are correct. *Remember that equivalents are not exact.* Use the common equivalents when making conversions, for example, 60 mg = 1 gr.

- If the precise number of tablets or capsules is determined and administering the amount calculated is unrealistic or impossible, always use the following rule to avoid an error in administration: *No more than 10% variation should exist between the dose ordered and the dose administered.* For example, one may determine that a patient should receive 0.9 tablet or 0.9 capsule. Administration of such an amount accurately would be impossible. In this case, 1 tablet or 1 capsule could be safely administered.

- Capsules are not scored and cannot be divided. They are administered in whole amounts only. *Most* timed-release capsules should never be crushed, opened, or emptied into a liquid or food. (However, certain medications, such as Theo-Dur®, may be used in this fashion.) The reason for not crushing, opening, or emptying most timed-release capsules is because they should be taken as packaged. This is so the medication is absorbed slowly over time (often in the intestine, rather than in the stomach). Taking them in any other fashion may cause the absorbed dose to be higher, with absorption that may be too quick. Fluvoxamine is an example of a timed-release medication.

- In the calculation of oral doses, measures other than apothecary or metric may be encountered. For example, with electrolytes such as potassium the number of milliequivalents (mEq) per tablet will be indicated. Another measure that may be seen for oral antibiotics or vitamins is units. For example, the label for vitamin E capsules will indicate 400 units per capsule. Units and milliequivalent measurements are specific to the drugs for which they are being used. There is no conversion between these and apothecary or metric measures.

Dosing of Oral Liquids

Liquid medications include elixirs, syrups, tinctures, and suspensions. Certain liquid drugs are irritating to the stomach mucosa and must be well diluted before administration. An example is potassium chloride (KCl). Tincture medications are always diluted. Any liquid medication that may cause discoloration of the teeth should be diluted and taken through a drinking straw. In general, liquid cough medicines are not diluted. Liquid medications contain a specific amount of drug in a given amount of solution. Figure 7–3 shows examples of oral liquid labels.

When measuring a liquid medication, hold the transparent measuring device at eye level. The liquid curve in the center is called the meniscus. All liquid medication is measured at the meniscus level (see Figure 7–4).

For medications in liquid form, calculate the volume of the liquid that contains the ordered dosage of the medication. The label of drugs bottled

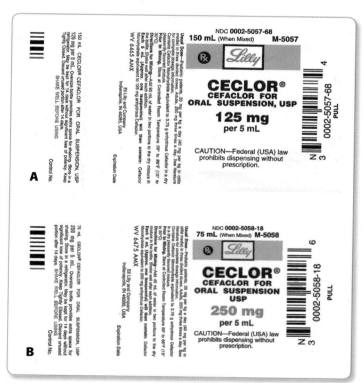

Figure 7–3 Labels typically found on an oral liquid. *(Courtesy of Eli Lilly and Company)*

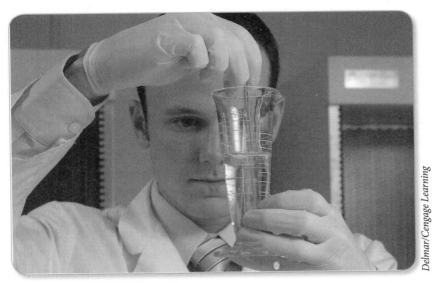

Figure 7–4 Reading the meniscus.

Delmar/Cengage Learning

may indicate the amount of drug per 1 mL or per multiple milliliters of solution, for example, 20 mg/5 mL, 250 mg/5 mL, or 1.4 g/30 mL. Liquid drugs must be calculated with the formula:

$$\frac{D}{H} \times V = X$$

In this formula, D represents the desired dosage or the dosage ordered; H, the dosage you have on hand per a quantity; and V, the volume of the drug. It is important to remember that, although a drug may be of a particular strength, the amount of fluid that it is contained in may differ, which alters its concentration.

For example, compare a solution of 5 mg/5 mL with a solution of 5 mg/10 mL. In this example, the medication is of 5 mg strength. However, the first solution is "stronger" because the fluid is only 5 mL. The second solution is "weaker" because the fluid is 10 mL. Although the drug is of the same strength in both solutions, the fluid amount is different, altering the concentration.

Example 1:

A prescription is written to give 100 mg of ampicillin with a dosage strength of 125 mg/5 mL. The following formula is used:

$$\frac{D}{H} \times V = \frac{100 \text{ mg}}{125 \text{ mg}} \times 5 \text{ mL} = X$$

$$\frac{4}{5} \times 5 \text{ mL} = \frac{20}{5 \text{ mL}} = 4 \text{ mL}$$

Example 2:

A prescription is written to give 100 mg of ampicillin. The medication is available with a dosage strength of 250 mg/5 mL. The following formula is used:

$$\frac{D}{H} \times V = \frac{100 \text{ mg}}{250 \text{ mg}} \times 5 \text{ mL} = X$$

$$\frac{2}{5} \times 5 \text{ mL} = \frac{10}{5} = 2 \text{ mL}$$

Alligation

Alligation is a method used to compound solutions and solids when the strength being mixed is different from the strength of the substance or substances in stock. In the example given below, one of the substances is more concentrated than the desired concentration and the other substance is less concentrated than the desired concentration. If pharmacists receive an order to prepare 5 ounces of a 15% solution using a 30% solution and a 10% solution, how much of each solution should they use?

Highest concentration: 30%		
	Desired concentration (5 ounces of 15%)	
Lowest concentration: 10%		

Using a table, it is easy to figure out the correct amounts for this mixture:

The next step is to subtract the desired concentration (15%) from the highest concentration (30%) and place the result in the lower right block to show the number of parts needed. Then, subtract the lowest concentration (10%) from the desired concentration (15%) and place the result in the upper right block to show the number of parts needed.

Highest concentration: 30%		5 parts
	Desired concentration (5 ounces of 15%)	
Lowest concentration: 10%		15 parts

Therefore, the total number of parts is: 5 parts + 15 parts, totaling 20 parts.

To determine the final amounts to use, set up a proportion as follows:

$$\text{Highest concentration (30\%)} = \frac{5}{20} \text{ parts} \times 5 \text{ oz}$$

$$= 1.25 \text{ oz of 30\% solution}$$

$$\text{Lowest concentration (10\%)} = \frac{15}{20} \text{ parts} \times 5 \text{ oz}$$

$$= 3.75 \text{ oz of 10\% solution}$$

To verify that the final amounts to use are correct, add the amounts of each concentration to see if they equal the amount to be compounded:

$$1.25 \text{ oz} + 3.75 \text{ oz} = 5 \text{ oz}$$

CALCULATION OF PARENTERAL DRUGS

Medications administered by injection can be given intradermally (within the skin), subcutaneously (SC, into fatty tissue or under the skin), intramuscularly (IM, into the muscle), and intravenously (IV, into the vein). Injectable drugs are ordered in grams, milligrams, micrograms, milliequivalents, grains, or units. The preparations of injectable drugs may be packaged in a solvent (diluent or solution) or in a powdered form.

Intramuscular injection is a common method of administering injectable drugs. The volume of solution for an intramuscular injection is 0.5 to 3.0 mL, with the average being 1 to 2 mL. A volume of drug solution greater than 3 mL causes increased muscle tissue displacement and possible tissue damage. Occasionally, 5 mL of certain drugs, such as magnesium sulfate or immunoglobulin (given after exposure to rabies), may be injected in a large muscle, such as the dorsogluteal. Dosages greater than 3 mL are usually divided and given at two different sites. Drug solutions for injection are commercially premixed and stored in vials and ampules for immediate use. The remaining drug solution in an ampule is *always* discarded after the ampule has been opened and used. For calculating intramuscular dosage, the following example can be used.

Example 1

An order is given for gentamicin 60 mg IM. The available dosage strength of gentamicin is 80 mg/2 mL in a vial. One of the following formulas may be used to determine the volume to withdraw:

$$\frac{D}{H} \times V = \frac{60}{80} \times 2 = \frac{120}{80} = 1.5 \text{ mL}$$

or

$$H:V::D:X$$

$$= 80 \text{ mg}:2 \text{ mL}::60 \text{ mg}:X \text{ mL}$$

$$= 80X = 120$$

$$X = \frac{120}{80} = 1.5 \text{ mL}$$

Example 2:

The physician's order is for atropine 0.2 mg SC stat. The drug is available at a dosage of 400 mcg/mL (0.4 mg/mL). The following formula is used:

$$\frac{D}{H} \times V$$

$$= \frac{0.2 \text{ mg}}{0.4 \text{ mg}} \times 1 \text{ mL}$$

$$= \frac{0.2}{0.4} \times 1$$

$$= 0.5 \text{ mL}$$

Drug Dosage in Standardized Units

Several drugs that are obtained from animal sources can be standardized in units according to their strengths, rather than on weight measures such as milligrams and grams. Some hormones such as insulin are too complex to be completely purified to obtain the exact weight of the drug per unit of volume. Therefore, insulin and many other drugs are measured in units for parenteral administration. The labels of such medications indicate how many units are needed per milliliter.

Insulin Dosage

To prevent errors, insulin orders must be written clearly and contain specific information. The order for insulin should include the type of insulin, supply dosage, number of units to be given, and the route and time or frequency of administration.

Example:

An order is given for Humulin R U-100®, 14 units SC stat or for Humulin U, U-100® 24 units SC 1/2 hour after breakfast.

Insulin is supplied in 10-mL vials labeled with the number of units per milliliter; hence, 100-unit insulin means there are 100 units/cc. In the past, insulin was administered in 40- and 80-unit dosage forms. Today, however, the 100-unit form has almost totally replaced the weaker strength forms. In addition to simplifying mathematical calculations, the smaller volume required per dose decreases local reactions at the injection site. Today, there are also concentrated insulins that contain 500 units, are long-acting, and are used for type I diabetes patients who need more than 200 units of insulin per day.

The simplest and most accurate method to measure insulin is within an insulin syringe. The syringe is calibrated in units, and the desired dose may be read directly on the syringe. Figure 7–5 shows several types of standard insulin syringes.

If an insulin syringe is not available, a tuberculin syringe may be used. The unit dosage may be converted to the equivalent number of cubic centimeters, using the proportion method.

Example:

Give 40 units of insulin, using 100-unit insulin and a tuberculin syringe. The amount administered is calculated as follows:

$$\frac{40}{100} \times 1 \text{ mL} = 0.4 \text{ mL}$$

Heparin Dosage

Heparin is also derived from animal sources and is standardized for its activity as an anticoagulant. It is obtained in unit-dose or multiple-dose vials and in strengths ranging from 1000 to 10,000 units/mL. There is often no set dose for the use of heparin; the patient's requirements are obtained from blood clotting studies done initially every four hours. Heparin is often given intravenously to produce a rapid effect and then is given in deep subcutaneous injections in larger and more infrequent doses. The normal adult heparin dosage is 20,000 to 40,000 units every 24 hours. When given IV, heparin is ordered in units per hour. Heparin is available in different strengths; therefore, it is important to read labels carefully when it must be administered.

Low molecular weight heparins (LMWHs) are now the drugs of choice for clotting disorders, which include acute myocardial infarction, coronary occlusion, and peripheral arterial embolism. LMWHs may produce fewer adverse effects than other types of heparin. They should be avoided, however, in patients with a hypersensitivity to the drug and in patients who have active bleeding or thrombocytopenia.

Example 1:

A physician's order is for heparin 7500 units SC. Heparin is available in a dosage of 10,000 units/mL. The amount administered is calculated as follows:

$$10{,}000 \text{ units}: 1 \text{ mL} = 7500 \text{ units}:X \text{ mL}$$
$$10{,}000X = 7500$$
$$X = \frac{7500}{10{,}000}$$
$$X = 0.75 \text{ mL}$$

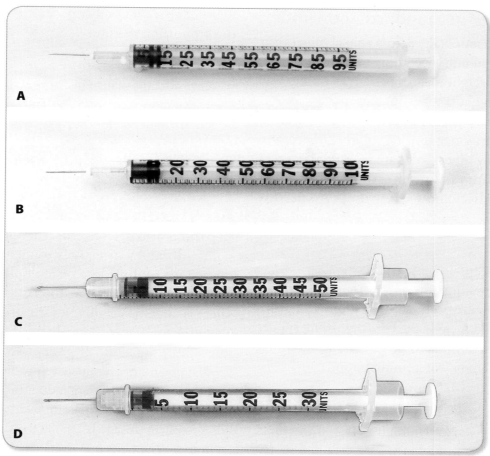

Figure 7–5 Insulin syringes. *(Courtesy of Becton Dickinson)*

Example 2:

A physician's order is for D5W (5% dextrose in water) 1000 mL containing 20,000 units of heparin, which is to be infused at 30 mL/hr. The dose of heparin the patient is to receive per hour is:

$$20,000 \text{ units}:1000 \text{ mL} = X \text{ units}:30 \text{ mL}$$

$$1000X = 20,000 \times 30$$

$$\frac{1000X}{1000} = \frac{600,000}{1000}$$

$$X = \frac{600 \text{ units}}{\text{hr}}$$

Antibiotic Dosage

The dosages of many antibiotics are still standardized in units. These may be prepared for injection in the form of a liquid containing a specified number of units per cubic centimeter. Antibiotics are also available in the form of a dry powder in a vial that must first be diluted with water or another diluent. The powder should be diluted so that the desired dose is in 1- or 2-cc (mL) amounts if the dose is to be given IM. If it is to be given IV, a larger amount of diluent may be used.

Example:

A vial of powdered penicillin G contains 1,000,000 units. The amount of diluent to be added to obtain a solution containing 100,000 units/mL is:

$$100,000:1 \text{ mL} = 1,000,000:X \text{ mL}$$

$$100,000X = 1,000,000 \times 1$$

$$X = \frac{1,000,000}{100,000}$$

$$X = 10 \text{ mL}$$

Dosing of Intravenous Medications

The term *intravenous* literally means "within a vein." Intravenous infusion is the slow introduction of a substance such as a solution, whole blood, plasma, or antibiotics into a vein. Intravenous solutions fall into four functional categories: replacement fluids, maintenance fluids, therapeutic fluids, and agents to keep the vein open. If patients are dehydrated and unable to eat or drink or if they have lost blood, physicians usually order replacement fluids. Maintenance fluids help patients maintain normal electrolyte and fluid balances. Therapeutic fluids deliver medication to the patient. Some intravenous lines provide access to the vein for emergency situations, and fluids prescribed to keep the vein open include 5% dextrose in water. Hence, pharmacy technicians must learn how to effectively calculate infusion rates and the administration of these agents.

Intravenous Solution Concentrations

Solutions may have different concentrations of dextrose (glucose) or saline (sodium chloride). For example, D5NS contains 5 g of dextrose and 0.9 g of sodium chloride per 100 ml. Figure 7–6 shows a label for a 5% dextrose solution.

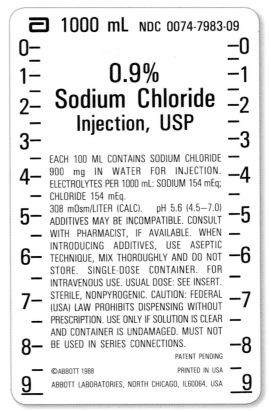

Figure 7–7 Label for 0.9% sodium chloride. *(Courtesy of Abbott Laboratories)*

In comparison, 0.9% sodium chloride (normal saline) contains 900 mg, or 0.9 g, of sodium chloride per 100 mL (see Figure 7–7).

Equipment for Intravenous Infusion

Equipment used to administer intravenous medications is available in several forms. They are either completely manual or electronic. The primary intravenous line may consist of a bag or bottle of solution and tubing. Bags for intravenous infusion come in different sizes. The solution of fluid to be infused is often 500 or 1000 cc (mL). The tubing, which is the primary line, usually includes a drip chamber, roller clamp, and injection ports (see Figure 7–8).

To measure the flow rate, the drip chamber must be squeezed until it is half full, making it easier to appropriately count the number of drops falling into the chamber. The roller clamp is used to adjust the speed of the infusion either up or down, as needed. The injection port is available to inject medications

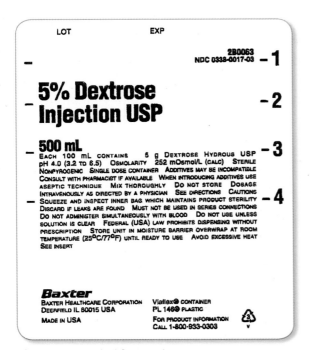

Figure 7–6 Label for 5% dextrose. *(Courtesy of Baxter)*

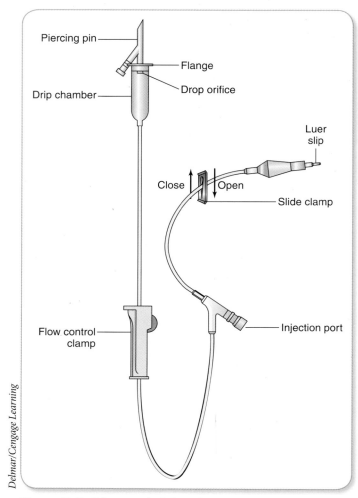

Figure 7–8   Primary administration set.

Delmar/Cengage Learning

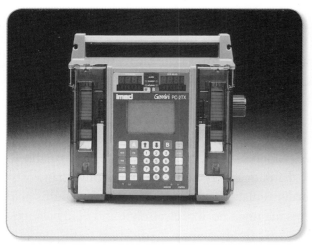

Figure 7–9   Electronic infusion pump. *(Courtesy of Alaris Medical System)*

into the primary line or to attach a second intravenous line. Two sizes of tubing are available: macrodrop and microdrop. Macrodrop tubing is used for fluids infused at a higher rate, for example, infusions that are set at 80 mL/hr or higher. For slower infusions for which accuracy of dosage delivery is essential, such as in the critical care or pediatric settings, microdrop tubing is used.

Monitoring the Intravenous Infusion

The infusion of intravenous fluids is monitored in many different ways. Most times, for manual monitoring, the bag containing the intravenous solution is hung 36 inches above the patient's heart so that gravity will draw the fluid through the tubing. When the infusion is monitored, the roller clamp is used to adjust the rate of delivery. Another method of monitoring is the use of an electronic infusion pump, which applies a set amount of pressure so that a set volume is infused over a set time period (see Figure 7–9). The flow rate is generally programmed into the device in milliliters per hour. The pumps do not rely on gravity but, rather, on pressure that the pump creates to force the solution through the tubing and into the patient's vascular system. Most electronic pumps are armed with sensors that sound when the bag of solution is empty or if the rate cannot be properly maintained. Despite advances in technology, there is no substitute for a vigilant health-care provider to ensure that the right patient is receiving the right medication, at the right time, and at the right infusion rate.

Calculation of Intravenous Flow Rates

A *flow rate* is the speed at which intravenous fluids are infused into a patient. If patients receive a prescribed fluid too fast or too slow, they can have adverse reactions. The pharmacy technician's ability to correctly and efficiently calculate flow rates of intravenous fluids is critical to the patient's well-being. Flow rates are generally prescribed or written as 125 mL/hr or 500 mL/2 hr, meaning that the fluids should be infused into the patient at a rate of 125 mL over a period of 1 hour or at a rate of 500 mL over a period of 2 hours, respectively. Flow rates can be regulated either by the use of an electronic pump or by manually adjusting the intravenous equipment to achieve the prescribed flow rate. When an electronic pump is used, the flow rate is calculated in milliliters per hour and can be arrived at by using the following formula:

$$\frac{\text{Total amount ordered (mL)}}{\text{Total number of hours (hr)}} = \text{mL/hr}$$

After it is successfully calculated, the flow rate is then programmed into an electronic infusion device.

Example:

Jane Doe is a patient for whom a *500-mL* bag of intravenous fluids to be infused over *2 hours* has been prescribed. To calculate the flow rate, use the preceding formula:

Total amount ordered (mL)/Total number of hours (hr)

$$= 500 \text{ mL/2 hr}$$

$$= 250 \text{ mL/hr}$$

Therefore, the infusion device is programmed for 250 mL/hr.

Another formula is especially helpful when flow rates that have a prescribed infusion time of $\frac{1}{2}$ hour or less are calculated.

Example:

J. P. Ellen is a patient for whom 500 mg of an IV antibiotic in a *100-mL bag* of fluid to be infused over *30 minutes* has been prescribed. To calculate the flow rate for this patient, use the following formula (remember that 60 min = 1 hr):

Total milliliters ordered/Total hours ordered

$$100 \text{ mL/ } 0.5 \text{ hr} = \text{X mL/hr}$$

$$100 \text{ mL/ } 0.5 \text{ hr} = 200 \text{ mL/hr}$$

Hence, the electronic infusion pump should be set at 200 mL/hr for the 100-mL bag of fluid to be infused over 30 minutes.

Manually Calculating Drip Rates

Depending on the setting, pharmacy technicians may have to calculate a drip rate of an intravenous fluid and then manually regulate the equipment to control the speed at which the fluid is being infused. To calculate the drip rate, technicians must determine how many drops (abbreviated as gtt) per minute should be infused over a prescribed time period. The number of drops per minute depends on the type of intravenous tubing used. Two types of tubing are available: standard, or macrodrop, and microdrop. Standard tubing has a drip factor of 10, 15, or 20 gtts/mL, whereas microdrop tubing has a drip factor of 60 gtt/mL. The drip factor is generally found on the outside packaging of the tubing.

The following formula is used to calculate flow rates in drops per minute:

$$\frac{V \text{ (total volume to be infused in mL)}}{T \text{ (total time in minutes)}} \times C$$
$$\left(\frac{\text{drip factor in gtt}}{\text{mL}}\right) = R \left(\frac{\text{rate of flow in gtt}}{\text{min}}\right)$$

Or the formula can also be written as:

$$\frac{V}{T} \times C = R$$

Example:

John Brown is to receive *200 cc* of intravenous fluids over *2 hours*. Macrodrop tubing has been selected, which has a drip factor of *20 gtt/mL*. (The technician's job is to calculate how many drops per minute are needed so that all 200 cc is infused over 30 minutes.)

Step 1:

Convert 2 hours into minutes (reminder: 1 hr = 60 min):

$$2 \times 60 = 120 \text{ min}$$

Step 2:

Set up the problem using the formula $\frac{V}{T} \times C = R$:

$$\frac{200}{120} \times 20 = 33.3 \text{ gtt/min}$$

Round the number of drops per minute to the nearest whole number. In this example, round down to 33 gtt/min.

Step 3:

Set the drip rate by adjusting the roller clamp and counting the amount of drops per minute that fall into the drip chamber.

You may believe that the ability to calculate and manually adjust drip rates is outdated. After all, electronic infusion pumps can be easily programmed to do these calculations. However, the opposite is true. Pharmacy technicians must know the math behind what electronic pumps do because an electronic pump may not always be available. In addition, emergency situations require immediate attention, and the ability to correctly determine intravenous infusion drip rates without the aid of an infusion pump is an invaluable skill.

Dosing of Total Parenteral Nutrition

Total parenteral nutrition (TPN), also called *hyperalimentation*, is an intravenous infusion that provides patients with all of their daily nutritional requirements in the form of a liquid infusion. TPN is generally prescribed for patients who, because of their disease process or surgical intervention, are unable to eat. It includes fluids such as dextrose, electrolytes, amino acids, trace elements, and vitamins. In some cases, other substances such as fat, insulin, or other drugs can be added to the infusion. The contents of TPN are determined by the patient's individual nutritional requirements. TPN is not infused through a peripheral vein (veins in the hands and arms) but, rather, through a central vein such as the subclavian vein or internal jugular vein.

Central lines are used to deliver TPN because its higher concentration of agents, such as concentrated dextrose solutions, could potentially damage peripheral veins. In addition, central lines, once established, can be left in place long-term, whereas peripheral lines are inserted for short-term use. The contents of TPN can be changed on a daily basis as the patient's physical and caloric needs change.

Usually administered through a peripheral intravenous catheter, partial parenteral nutrition (PPN) is normally prescribed for patients who can tolerate some oral feedings but cannot ingest adequate amounts of food to meet their nutritional needs. Two types of solutions commonly used in PPN are lipid emulsions and amino acid-dextrose solutions.

PEDIATRIC DOSAGE CALCULATIONS

Because infants and children cannot tolerate adult doses of drugs, their dosages must be measured accurately according to their age and weight. Several methods are used for calculating dosage for this group of patients. The dosage form per kilogram or pound of body weight is more accurate than the dosage calculated by age. The body surface area method is another way to measure the dosage for children. Charts are available to determine the body surface area in square meters, according to height and weight. These charts are called *nomograms,* and are shown in Figure 7–10.

Because they may have harmful side effects or because they have not been sufficiently tested in children to give a recommended dosage range, many drugs are not advised for administration to children. Three formulas are used to calculate dosage for infants and children: Clark's rule, Young's rule, and Fried's rule.

Clark's Rule

Clark's rule is calculated as follows:

$$\frac{\text{Weight of child}}{150} \times \text{Average adult dose} = \text{Child's dose}$$

Example:

Find the dose of cortisone for a 30-lb infant (adult dose = 100 mg). The calculation is:

$$\frac{30}{150} \times 100 \text{ mg} = 20 \text{ mg}$$

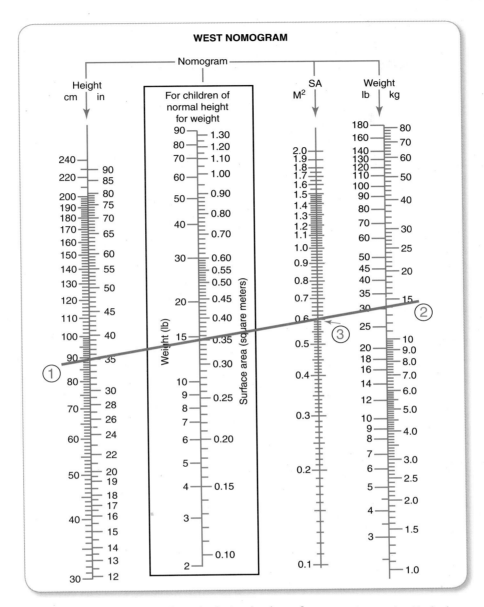

WEST NOMOGRAM

Figure 7–10 Nomogram for calculating body surface area. *(From Nelson Textbook of Pediatrics (16th ed.), by R. E. Behrman, R. M Kleigman, and H. B. Jenson, 2000, Philadelphia: Saunders. Reprinted with permission.)*

Young's Rule

Young's rule is calculated as follows:

$$\frac{\text{Age of child (expressed in years)}}{\text{Age of child (expressed in years)} + 12} \times \text{Average adult dose} = \text{Child's dose}$$

Example:

Find the dose of acetaminophen for a 4-year-old child (adult dose = 1000 mg). The calculation is as follows:

$$\frac{4}{4 + 12} \times 1000 \text{ mg} = \frac{4000}{16} = 250 \text{ mg}$$

Note that Young's rule is not valid after a child is 12 years of age. If the child is small enough to warrant a reduced dose after 12 years of age, the reduction should be calculated on the basis of Clark's rule.

Fried's Rule

Fried's rule is sometimes used for calculating dosages for infants younger than 2 years of age. The formula is as follows:

$$\frac{\text{Child's age (expressed in months)}}{150} \times$$

Average adult dose = Child's dose

Example:

Find the dose of phenobarbital for a 15-month-old infant (adult dose = 400 mg). The calculation is as follows:

$$\frac{15}{150} \times 400 \text{ mg} = 40 \text{ mg}$$

Pediatric drug dosages are calculated in three steps.

Example:

Amoxil® 25 mg/kg/day given every 12 hours is being ordered for a 24-lb infant.

Step 1:

The first step in calculating the correct dosage for this infant is to convert pounds to kilograms. The conversion rule is:

$$1 \text{ kg} = 2.2 \text{ lb}$$
$$\frac{1 \text{ kg}}{2.2 \text{ lb}} = \frac{X \text{ kg}}{24 \text{ lb}}$$

Cross-multiply this ratio:

$$2.2X = 24$$

$$X = 10.9 \text{ kg (round up to 11.0 kg)}$$

Step 2:

Calculate the drug dosage based on 25 mg/kg of body weight:

$$25 \text{ mg}/1 \text{ kg} = X \text{ mg}/11 \text{ kg}$$

Cross-multiply this ratio:

$$X = 275$$

$$X = 275 \text{ mg}/24 \text{ hr}$$

Step 3:

Calculate out how much Amoxil this patient receives per dose. Remember, the patient is to receive a dose once every 12 hours or 2 divided doses in one 24-hour period. The calculation is as follows:

$$\frac{275 \text{ mg}}{2} = 137.5 \text{ mg per dose}$$

Amoxil is available in 250 mg/5 mL dosages; so, the exact number of milliliters to give the patient per dose needs to be calculated:

$$\frac{250 \text{ mg}}{5 \text{ mL}} = \frac{137.5 \text{ mg}}{X \text{ mL}}$$

Cross-multiply this ratio:

$$250X = 687.5$$
$$X = \frac{687.5}{250}$$
$$X = 2.75 \text{ mL}$$

Therefore, the patient would receive 2.75 mL of Amoxil every 12 hours.

Calculating drug dosages for the pediatric patient is not as time-consuming as it initially appears. After pharmacy technicians have practiced doing several dosage calculations, they will soon become proficient.

TEMPERATURE CONVERSION

In the United States, temperatures are most often reported in Fahrenheit and occasionally in Celsius. Based on the differences between the freezing and boiling points of each scale (see Figure 7–11), a formula has been developed to convert temperatures between the two scales. To convert temperatures between Fahrenheit and Celsius, remember the following relationship between the two scales:

(9 × Celsius temperature) = (5 × Fahrenheit temperature) − 160 degrees

Therefore, the difference between the Celsius and Fahrenheit scales is based on the numbers shown above. The fraction 9/5 is equivalent to 1.8, and it

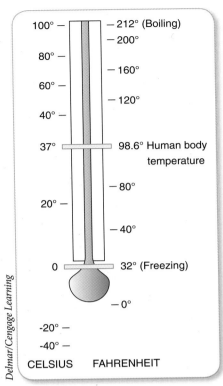

100° — — 212° (Boiling)
— 200°
80° —
— 160°
60° —
— 120°
40° —
37° — — 98.6° Human body
temperature
— 80°
20° —
— 40°
0 — 32° (Freezing)
— 0°
-20° —
-40° —
CELSIUS   FAHRENHEIT

Delmar/Cengage Learning

Figure 7–11 Comparison of Celsius and Fahrenheit scales.

Example:

You have a Fahrenheit temperature of 104 degrees. What is the equivalent Celsius temperature? Using the formula above, you find the following:

$$104 - 32/1.8 = 40 \text{ degrees Celsius}$$

EXPLORING THE WEB

Visit http://www.romannumerals.co.uk to learn more about Arabic numbers and Roman numerals and for a converter between the two numbering systems.

Visit http://www.dosagehelp.com; this site provides a dosage calculations tutorial, complete with explanations and examples.

Visit http://www.onlineconversion.com for more information on converting within and between systems of measurement.

Visit http://www.convert-me.com for more information on converting temperatures between Fahrenheit and Celsius.

Visit http://themetricsystem.info to learn more about the metric system.

is this decimal that is commonly used (below) to perform temperature conversions.

A Celsius temperature should be multiplied by 1.8 and then added to 32 to find a Fahrenheit temperature. This equation appears as follows:

$$(C \times 1.8) + 32 = F$$

Example:

You have a Celsius temperature of 35 degrees. What is the equivalent Fahrenheit temperature? Using the formula above, you find the following:

$$(35 \times 1.8) + 32 = 95 \text{ degrees Fahrenheit}$$

A Fahrenheit temperature should have 32 subtracted from it, with the result divided by 1.8, to find a Celsius temperature. This equation appears as follows:

$$F - 32/1.8 = C$$

REVIEW QUESTIONS

Calculations

Calculate the following numbers.

1. $0.021 + 0.88 =$ _____
2. $5.69 + 0.7 =$ _____
3. $17 + 0.009 + 4.8 =$ _____
4. $8.19 + 13.37 =$ _____
5. $5.47 - 0.39 =$ _____
6. $6.26 - 3.31 =$ _____
7. $0.684 - 0.89 =$ _____
8. $19.02 - 0.647 =$ _____
9. $5.3 \times 7.9 =$ _____
10. $0.67 \times 0.004 =$ _____
11. $9 \times 0.992 =$ _____
12. $12.09 \times 1.009 =$ _____
13. $48.62 \div 2.2 =$ _____
14. $6.876 \div 3.36 =$ _____
15. $4.4 \div 0.11 =$ _____
16. $1.6 \div 0.08 =$ _____

Conversions

Convert the following fractions into ratios.

1. $\frac{20}{100} =$ _____
2. $\frac{6}{8} =$ _____
3. $\frac{300}{900} =$ _____
4. $\frac{75}{1500} =$ _____
5. $\frac{20}{4000} =$ _____

Proportions

Solve for X in each proportion.

1. $2 : 9 = 3 : X$
2. $21 : 27 = 45 : X$
3. $32/128 = 4/X$
4. $8 : 72 : : 5 : X$
5. $X : 625 = 1 : 5$

Percentages

Solve the following problems and determine each whole number.

1. 60% of 20 _____
2. 50% of 1000 _____
3. 10% of 75 _____
4. 0.9% of 1200 _____
5. 15% of 400 _____

Equivalents

Convert the following amounts to their equivalent units.

1. 75 drops = _____ tsp
2. 24 oz = _____ cups
3. 3 Tbsp = _____ oz
4. 4 cups = _____ oz
5. 8 tsp = _____ Tbsp

Metric Conversions

Convert each metric unit into its equivalent unit.

1. 9 g = _____ mg
2. 20,000 mcg = _____ mg
3. 1500 mL = _____ L
4. 160 mm = _____ cm
5. 8.01 L = _____ mL

Apothecary Conversions

Convert each apothecary unit into its equivalent unit.

1. 24 oz = _____ glasses
2. 32 fl oz = _____ pt
3. 4.4 lb = _____ kg
4. 0.06 gr = _____ g
5. 120 mL = _____ tsp

Temperature Conversions

Convert between Celsius and Fahrenheit temperatures.

1. $37°C =$ _____ °F
2. $93°F =$ _____ °C
3. $62°F =$ _____ °C

4. 42.7°C = _____ °F

5. 104°F = _____ °C

6. 100°C = _____ °F

Multiple Choice

1. Which Arabic numeral is expressed by the letter "C" in the Roman system?

   A. 100   B. 1000
   C. 10   D. 5

2. What is the Roman numeral that stands for 29?

   A. XXIX   B. IIIX
   C. XXVIIII   D. IXXX

3. 5:12 = X:8. What does X stand for?

   A. 1.33   B. 3
   C. 2.65   D. 3.33

4. The prefix *milli-* (m) has a value of:

   A. $\dfrac{1}{1,000,000}$ B. $\dfrac{1}{1000}$

   C. $\dfrac{1}{100}$ D. 1000

5. What is the basic unit of weight in the metric system?

   A. nanogram   B. milligram
   C. kilogram   D. gram

6. One milliliter is equivalent to how many drops?

   A. 5   B. 15
   C. 25   D. 50

7. All are units of the apothecary system for weight and volume, except:

   A. minim   B. dram
   C. gram   D. grain

8. When you convert 0.3 g to mg, which of the following is the correct answer?

   A. 300   B. 0.003
   C. 0.03   D. 0.3

9. If the equivalent of 1 L is 1000 mL and the conversion factor is 1000, which conversion of 0.02 L to mL is the correct answer?

   A. 2 mL   B. 0.2 mL
   C. 20 mL   D. 200 mL

10. A patient should drink 48 oz of fluid every day. How many cups should the patient be advised to drink each day?

    A. 2   B. 4
    C. 6   D. 8

11. Approximately how many pounds are 79 kg equivalent to?

    A. 198.8 lb   B. 173.8 lb
    C. 163.8 lb   D. 143.8 lb

12. Approximately how many glasses are 360 mL of fluid equivalent to?

    A. $\frac{1}{2}$ glass   B. 1 glass

    C. $1\frac{1}{2}$ glasses   D. 2 glasses

13. How many milligrams are 400 grams equivalent to?

    A. 40   B. 4,000
    C. 40,000   D. 400,000

14. How many drops are 12 mL equivalent to?

    A. 192 gtt   B. 180 gtt

    C. 142 gtt   D. 135 gtt

15. How many teaspoons are equivalent to 45 mL?

    A. 9   B. 7
    C. 3   D. 2

16. How many grams are 529 mg equivalent to?

    A. 5.29 g   B. 0.529 g
    C. 0.029 g   D. 52.9 g

17. How many milligrams are 8.92 kg equivalent to?

    A. 8,920 mg   B. 80,920 mg
    C. 800,920 mg D. 8,920,000 mg

18. How many qt are in 4 gal?

    A. 4 qt   B. 8 qt
    C. 12 qt   D. 16 qt

19. How many milliliters are equivalent to five cups?

    A. 500 mL   B. 600 mL
    C. 700 mL   D. 900 mL

20. How many milliliters are approximately equivalent to one quart?

    A. 250 mL   B. 500 mL
    C. 800 mL   D. 1000 mL

21. How many milligrams are equivalent to one grain?

    A. 0.015 mg
    B. 0.15 mg
    C. 0.3 mg
    D. 60 mg

22. How many centimeters are equal to one inch?

    A. 1.54
    B. 2.54
    C. 2.84
    D. 3.84

23. Learning to correctly calculate _____ _____ is extremely important because it can often be the difference between life and death for a patient.

    A. unit doses
    B. common practices
    C. digital timings
    D. drug dosages

24. All these formulas are used to calculate drug dosage for infants and children, except:

    A. Clark's rule
    B. Fried's rule
    C. Franklin's rule
    D. Young's rule

25. In the formula $D/H \times V = X$, what does the D stand for?

    A. Diuretic
    B. Drug
    C. Desired dosage
    D. Drop

26. Insulin and many other drugs are measured in _____ for parenteral administration.

    A. units
    B. ampules
    C. milliliters
    D. cubic centimeters

27. Antibiotics are available in the form of a liquid and a/an _____ that must be reconstituted.

    A. elixir
    B. suspension
    C. grain
    D. powder

28. Normal saline is _____% saline. It contains 900 mg of sodium chloride.

    A. 0.9
    B. 90
    C. 9.09
    D. 10

29. To calculate flow rate, one formula requires dividing the total amount ordered (in milliliters) by:

    A. total number of drops.
    B. total number of minutes.
    C. total number of hours.
    D. total number of days.

30. A physician orders heparin 3500 U SC q12h. Heparin 5000 U/mL is available. The nurse must give which of the following amounts?

    A. 0.1 mL
    B. 0.3 mL
    C. 0.7 mL
    D. 1 mL

31. A nurse received an order from a physician for heparin 8000 U SC stat. The technician brought heparin 10,000 U/1 mL to the floor. Which of the following is the correct calculation of heparin for the patient?

    A. 0.2 mL
    B. 0.4 mL
    C. 0.6 mL
    D. 0.8 mL

32. A pediatrician ordered Ampicillin 50 mg/kg/day IV in equally divided doses every 6 hours for an infant who weighs 26 lbs. Ampicillin 125 mg/5 mL is available. How many mL of this medication should the infant receive?

    A. 1.9 mL
    B. 2.9 mL
    C. 3.9 mL
    D. 5.9 mL

33. A prescription is written for 1500 mL D5W over 12 hours. The drop factor is 15 gtt/mL. Which flow rate (in gtt/min) is correct?

    A. 11
    B. 21
    C. 31
    D. 41

34. Ceclor suspension 225 mg p.o., b.i.d. is prescribed. Ceclor suspension 375 mg per 5 mL is available. Which of the following is the right dose?

    A. 1.5 mL
    B. 3 mL
    C. 4.5 mL
    D. 6 mL

35. A patient needs Pepcid 20 mg p.o., q.i.d., but it is only available as 80 mg/10 mL. Which is the right dose?

    A. 1.5 mL
    B. 2.5 mL
    C. 3.5 mL
    D. 5 mL

36. A tablet contains 0.125 milligrams of medication. A patient receives three tablets a day for five days. How many milligrams of medication does the patient receive over the five days?

    A. 0.625
    B. 0.925
    C. 1.375
    D. 1.875

37. If you want to give a patient 1 1/2 teaspoons of cough syrup four times a day, how many teaspoons of cough syrup will you give each day?

A. 2.5   B. 4
C. 6   D. 7.5

38. Determine the amount to administer.

Ordered: Depakene syrup 125 mg p.o. q12h
On hand: Depakene syrup 250 mg/5 mL
Which of the following is the correct amount?

A. 1.25   B. 2
C. 2.5   D. 3

39. Determine the amount to administer.

Ordered: ranitidine HCL (Zantac) 35 mg, IM, q8h
On hand: ranitidine HCL (Zantac) 25 mg/mL
How many milliliters (mL) of Zantac should the patient receive every day?

A. 1.5   B. 4.2
C. 5.5   D. 6.2

40. Determine the amount to administer.

Ordered: Cedax susp 300 mg p.o. qd 2h after breakfast

On hand: Cedax oral suspension 90 mg/5 mL

Which of the following is the correct amount?

A. 1.7 mL   B. 5.7 mL
C. 13 mL   D. 17 mL

Biopharmaceutics and Factors Affecting Drug Activity

OUTLINE

GLOSSARY

Absorption – the movement of a drug from its site of administration into the bloodstream

Addition – the combined effect of two agents, which is equal to the sum of the effects of each drug taken alone

Agonist – a drug or other agent that mimics the effects of another substance or function; it may do this by interacting at a cellular receptor

Anaphylactic reaction – a life-threatening allergic reaction that is characterized by a drop in blood pressure and with difficulty in breathing

Antagonism – the combined effect of two drugs that is less than the effect of either drug taken alone

Antagonists – drugs or other agents that block the effects of other substances or functions

Arthus reaction – an acute local inflammatory reaction that occurs at the site of injection

Bioavailability – measurement of the rate of absorption and total amount of drug that reaches systemic circulation

Biotransformation (metabolism) – the conversion of a drug within the body

Cellular hypersensitivity reaction – the result of the activity of many leukocyte actions; the T1 lymphocytes become sensitized by their first contact with a specific antigen; subsequent exposure to an antigen stimulates multiple reactions aimed at destroying or inactivating the offending antigen

Cytotoxic reaction – severe damage to or destruction of cells by a substance

Dependence – the total psychophysical state of one addicted to drugs or alcohol who must receive an increasing amount of the substance to prevent the onset of withdrawal symptoms

Distribution – the process by which blood leaves the bloodstream and enters the tissues of the body

First-pass metabolism – the degree to which a drug is chemically altered as it circulates through the liver for the first time

Half-life – the time it takes for the plasma concentration to be reduced by 50%

Hypersensitivity – an unpredictable reaction to a drug due to the development of antibodies against it; also known as an allergy

Idiosyncratic reaction – experience of a unique, strange, or unpredicted reaction to a drug

Pharmacodynamics – the study of the biochemical and physiological effects of drugs

Pharmacokinetics – the study of the absorption, distribution, metabolism, and excretion of drugs

Placebo – an inactive substance or preparation used as a control in an experiment or test to determine the effectiveness of a medicinal drug

Placebo effect – a measurable improvement in a patient's health or condition after a placebo has been administered; it is thought to occur because of the patient's belief in the supposed drug administered

Potentiation – an effect that occurs when a drug increases or prolongs the action of another drug, the total effect being greater than the sum of the effects of each used alone

Receptor – the cell to which a drug has an affinity

Side effect – an outcome other than that intended; most commonly used in the context of drug therapy in which a side effect is an unwanted consequence of the drug in use

Specific affinity – the attraction a drug has for particular cells

Synergism – a combined action of two or more agents that produces an effect greater than would have been expected from the two agents acting separately

Tolerance – increasing resistance to the usual effects of an established dosage of a drug as a result of continued use; also, reduced responsiveness of a drug due to adaptation to it as the body becomes increasingly resistant

PROPERTIES AND ACTIONS OF DRUGS

The biochemical and physiological properties of drugs, as well as their mechanisms of action, differ widely. However, in clinical applications, drugs must penetrate, be absorbed by, and be distributed among the body tissues. The usual route of drug administration and mode of discontinuance should also be considered. Certain general principles help explain these differences. These principles have both pharmaceutic and therapeutic implications. For action, a drug must be absorbed, transported to the target tissue or organ, and then must penetrate into the cell membranes and their organelles and alter the ongoing processes. The drug may be distributed to a number of tissues, bound or stored, and metabolized to inactive or active products. Then the drug must be excreted.

PHARMACOKINETICS

Pharmacokinetics is the study of the absorption, distribution, metabolism, and excretion of drugs.

Drug Absorption

The movement of a drug from its site of administration into the bloodstream is called absorption. This process depends upon the drug's lipid solubility.

Agents that are relatively lipid-soluble diffuse more rapidly than do less lipid-soluble drugs.

Generally, absorption takes place through the digestive system unless an agent is administered directly into the bloodstream by injection into the veins, arteries, muscles, and other sites of injectable administration. The most convenient, economical, and common route of administration, the digestive system is generally safe for most drugs. Lipid-soluble drugs and weak acids may be absorbed directly from the stomach. The small intestine is the primary site of absorption because of the very large surface area across which drugs may diffuse. Many factors may influence gastrointestinal tract absorption of drugs. These factors include physical and chemical properties of the drugs, acidity of the stomach, presence of food, dosage of drugs, and the route of administration.

Drugs can also be absorbed via the following routes:

- Sublingual – under the tongue
- Buccal – through the inner lining of the cheeks
- Rectal – within the rectum

These routes are logical to protect the drugs from chemical decomposition, which might occur in the stomach or liver (through first-pass effect if the drugs were given orally). The choice of the route of administration is crucial in determining the suitability of a drug for each patient.

Absorption of drugs may occur via veins, arteries, muscles, or subcutaneously. The rate of absorption is most rapid via the blood vessels. In the muscles, absorption depends on the blood circulation and is not as fast as it is through the blood vessels.

Topical drugs may be absorbed through several layers of skin for local absorption. Sometimes, a drug may initially be administered in large doses that temporarily exceed the body's capacity to absorb them.

Drug Distribution

Distribution is the process by which a drug leaves the bloodstream and enters the tissues of the body. In this case, lipid solubility is important for effective distribution. A drug's initial rate of distribution is heavily dependent on the blood flow to various organs. Lipid-soluble drugs enter the central nervous system rapidly. Because of the nature of the blood-brain barrier, ionized drugs are distributed poorly to their desired site because they must pass through this barrier. The clinician must always consider the possibility that drugs administered to the mother may cross the placenta and reach the fetus.

Drugs are often bound to plasma proteins, particularly albumin. Drugs that are bound to albumin are known as *pharmacologically inactive drugs*, whereas those that are unbound are called *pharmacologically active drugs*. A drug that is bound to a protein will not pass through the membrane in the bound form. Only the unbound form can pass among the various compartments of the body. Drug administration and its effect on drug action are shown in Figure 8–1.

Biotransformation (Metabolism) of Drugs

The overwhelming majority of drugs undergo metabolism after they enter the body. In most cases, biotransformation can terminate the pharmacological action of the drug and increase removal of the

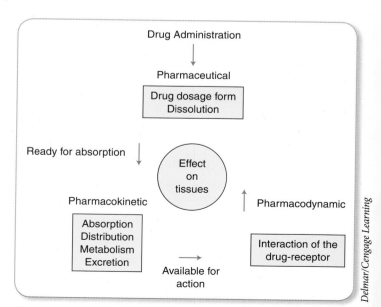

Figure 8–1 Drug administration and its effect on drug action.

drug from the body. Enzymes in the body act on most drugs and convert them to metabolic derivatives during metabolism. The process of conversion is called *biotransformation*.

Involving numerous enzymes in the metabolic process, the liver is the major site of biotransformation. These drug-metabolizing enzymes are often called *microsomal enzymes*. One of these enzymes is cytochrome P-450, which has a very important role in drug metabolism. The products produced by the metabolic action of these enzymes are known as *metabolites*, the majority of which are inactive and toxic.

Drug Excretion

Excretion is the process of elimination. The body excretes fluid wastes in the form of urine, solid wastes as feces, and gaseous wastes as *flatus* or breath. Drugs may be excreted from the body by many routes, including urine, feces (unabsorbed drugs and those secreted in the bile),

saliva, sweat, milk, lungs (alcohols and anesthetics), and tears. Although any route may be important for a given drug, the kidney is the major site of excretion for most drugs. Renal excretion of drugs and their metabolites may include three processes: (1) filtration, (2) secretion, and (3) reabsorption. The most common is the filtration of the agent through the glomerulus into the renal tubule (see Figure 8–2).

Available as sodium or potassium salts, penicillins or barbiturates are weak acids and can be better excreted if the urine pH is less acidic. On the other hand, any drug that is available as a sulfate, hydrochloride, or nitrate salt, such as atropine or morphine, can be excreted better if the urine is more acidic. By altering the pH of urine, elimination of certain drugs can be facilitated, hence preventing prolonged action or overdosage of a toxic compound. Another technique to alter the rate of a drug's excretion is to produce a competitively blocking effect. For example, probenecid may be used to block the renal excretion

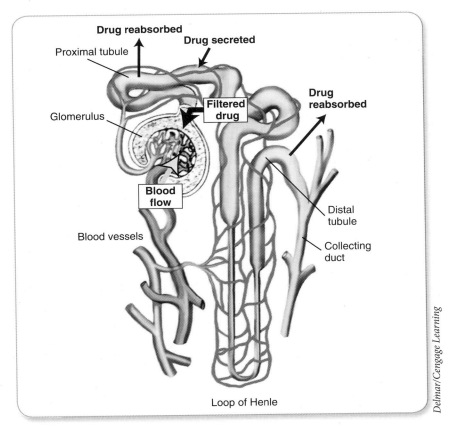

Figure 8–2 The excretion process of drugs.

of penicillin. This prolongs the effect of the antibiotic by maintaining a higher therapeutic plasma level.

As active transport systems, secretions of drugs require energy and may become saturated. Reabsorption may occur throughout the tubules of the nephrons. The mechanism is *passive diffusion*; therefore, only the un-ionized form of a drug is reabsorbed. Reabsorption depends on its lipid solubility.

PHARMACODYNAMICS

The study of the biochemical and physiological effects of drugs is called pharmacodynamics. It is also defined as the study of the mechanism of action of drugs. A basic understanding of the factors that control drug concentration at the site of action is important for the optimal use of drugs. This is the area of study referred to as *pharmacokinetics*, as discussed earlier. Drugs must dissolve before being absorbed, and they must pass across many lipoid barriers and some metabolizing systems before reaching the site of action.

Usually, the links between pharmacokinetics and pharmacodynamics demonstrate the relationship between drug dose and blood or other biological fluid concentrations. The pharmacological response by itself does not provide information about some very important determinants of that response, for example, dose or drug concentration in plasma or at the site of action. Pharmacokinetics and pharmacodynamics can determine the dose-effect relationship (see Figure 8–3).

Drug Action

Drugs produce their effects by altering the normal function of the body's cells and tissues. A drug chooses the correct cells because it has a specific affinity for a particular cell. The specific cell recipient is called a receptor, and the drug that has the affinity for it and produces a functional change in the cell is known as the agonist (see Figure 8–4). Not all drugs that bind to specific cells cause a functional change in the cell. Acting as antagonists to the natural process, these drugs work by blocking a sequence of biochemical

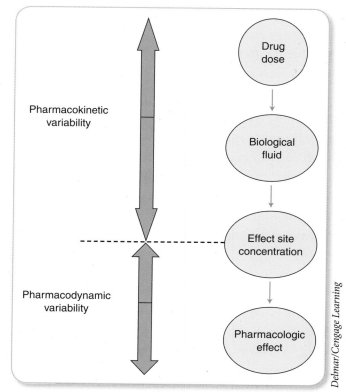

Figure 8–3 The dose-effect relationship.

Delmar/Cengage Learning

events. Some drugs may act by affecting the body's enzyme functions. When metabolized in the liver, drugs produce antimetabolites.

In determining the correct drugs for a patient, various factors are important. These factors include the drug's half-life; the patient's age, sex, and body weight; the time of day of administration (diurnal); the patient's illnesses and psychological factors; tolerance; drug toxicity; idiosyncratic reactions; and interactions with other drugs.

Drug Half-Life

The half-life of a drug is the time it takes for the plasma concentration to be reduced by 50%. This is one of the most common methods used to explain drug actions. The half-life of each drug may be different; for example, a drug with a short half-life, such as 2 or 3 hours, will need to be administered more often than one with a long half-life, such as 8 hours. Another method of describing drug action is a graphic representation of the plasma concentration of the drug versus time (see Figure 8–5).

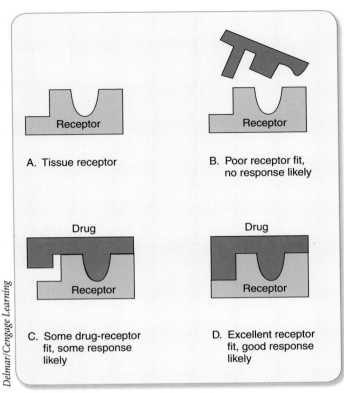

Figure 8–4 Drug-receptor interaction.

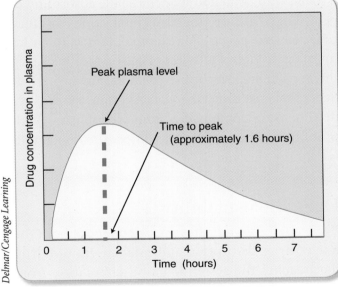

Figure 8–5 The half-life of a drug.

Age

Because of their ages, newborns and elderly patients are more sensitive to medications that affect the central nervous system and are at greater risk for development of toxic drug levels. Drug dosages for these two groups must be carefully measured, and treatment usually starts with very small doses.

Sex

Men and women respond differently to drugs. Some medications pose a risk in pregnant women because of damage to the developing fetus. In addition, certain drugs may have side effects that can stimulate uterine contractions, causing premature labor and delivery. Men absorb drugs administered intramuscularly more quickly than women do. Because of their higher body fat percentage, women retain drugs in their tissues longer than men do.

Body Weight

Basically, the same dosage has less effect in a patient who weighs more and a greater effect in one who weighs less. Pediatric medications are designed for children's body weight or body surface. If adult medications are used for children, the correct dosage must be calculated and adjusted for the child's body weight.

Time of Day

Diurnal (during the day) body rhythms play an important part in the effects of some drugs. For example, sedatives given in the morning will not be as effective as those administered before bedtime. On the other hand, the preferred time for corticosteroid administration is the morning, because this best mimics the body's natural pattern of corticosteroid production and elimination.

Presence of Illnesses

Because their bodies cannot detoxify and excrete chemicals properly, patients with liver or kidney disease may respond to drugs differently.

Psychological Factors

Psychological factors involve how patients feel about the drug(s) prescribed for them and the different ways they respond to them. If an individual believes in the therapy, even a placebo (sugar pill or sterile water that the patient believes is a drug) may help to bring relief. Some patients cooperate in following the directions for a specific drug, and a patient's mental attitude can reduce or increase an expected response to a drug.

Tolerance

Tolerance is the phenomenon of reduced responsiveness to a drug. Becoming so adapted to the presence of the drug, the body cannot function properly without it.

Drug Toxicity

Almost all drugs are capable of producing toxic effects. A range between the therapeutic dose of a drug and its toxic dose exists. This range is measurable by the therapeutic index, which is used to explain the drug's safety in the form of a ratio:

$$\text{Therapeutic Index (TI)} = LD_{50}/ED_{50}$$

where LD_{50} is the lethal dose of a drug that will kill 50% of animals tested and ED_{50} is the effective dose that produces a specific therapeutic effect in 50% of animals tested.

The greater the therapeutic index, the safer a drug is likely to be. There are four general mechanisms by which drugs can change the physiology of the body's cells or tissues. These mechanisms include the following:

1. Nonspecific chemical or physical interactions

2. Alterations in the level of the activity of enzymes

3. Action as antimetabolites

4. Interaction with receptors.

The final effect of a drug may be removed from its site of action.

Idiosyncratic Reactions

An idiosyncratic reaction occurs when a patient has a unique, strange, or unpredicted reaction to a drug. Idiosyncratic reactions may be caused by underlying enzyme deficiencies resulting from genetic or hormonal variation.

Drug Interactions

Plasma protein binding can be a source of drug interaction if several drugs compete for binding sites on protein molecules. Drug interactions may result in elevated concentrations of drugs by displacement of protein-bound drugs or by reduced rates of drug disposition that result in toxic drug concentrations.

A drug interaction may also cause more rapid drug disappearance, with plasma concentrations decreasing to below minimum effective values. Drug interactions often take place during the process of metabolism in the liver and result from the cytochrome P-450 enzyme pathways each person inherits. The cytochrome P-450 system may alter actions of many drugs when they are taken with other drugs. Examples include many antidepressants, cimetidine, ciprofloxacin, codeine, isoniazid, ketoconazole, morphine, phenobarbital, phenytoin, rifampin, tolbutamide, and warfarin.

Some medications are given together because the drug interactions are helpful. For example, probenecid is given with penicillin to increase the absorption of penicillin. There are other drug interactions that may cause adverse effects. For example, some antibiotics make birth control pills less effective. Multiple-drug therapy should never be used without convincing evidence that each drug is beneficial beyond the possible detriments of combined administration or without proof that a therapeutically equivocal combination is definitely harmless.

Drug Bioavailability

Bioavailability indicates measurement of both the rate of drug absorption and total amount of drug that reaches the systemic blood circulation from an administered dosage form. The route of drug administration is essential for this measurement. If administered by intravenous injection, all of a drug's dose enters the blood circulation. This is not true for drugs administered by other routes, especially for drugs given orally. Solid drugs such as tablets and capsules must dissolve. Hence, route of administration is a major source of difference in drug bioavailability.

Poor solubility or incomplete absorption of a drug in the gastrointestinal tract and rapid metabolism of a drug during its first pass through the liver are other factors that influence bioavailability.

FACTORS AFFECTING DRUG ACTIVITY

Certain factors may influence drug activity, such as age, gender, weight, time and route of drug administration (oral or parenteral routes), diet, pregnancy, psychological state, polypharmacy, and diseases. When writing the prescription, the prescribing physician must consider all of these factors. Pharmacy technicians must be familiar with these factors as well. The presence or absence of certain functional groups will determine the necessity, route, and extent of metabolism.

Age

The patient's age may influence a drug's effects. Infants and young children need to receive smaller doses of drugs than adults to avoid toxic side effects. Liver function is poorly developed in infants and young children. In this group, drugs are excreted slowly, which increases the risk of drug toxicity. In older children, some drugs may be less active than they are in adults, particularly if the dosage is based on weight. This effect occurs because the liver develops faster than general body weight increases, and, hence, it represents a greater fraction of total body weight. In the elderly, the effectiveness of metabolizing enzyme systems declines. The lowered level of enzyme activity slows the rate of drug elimination, causing higher plasma drug levels per dose than those found in young adults.

Gender

Several hormones such as androgen, estrogen, and adrenocorticotropin might affect the activity of certain enzymes in men or women. Metabolism of prednisolone, acetaminophen, diazepam, and caffeine is slightly faster in women. Oxidative metabolism of lidocaine, propranolol, and some steroids is faster in men than it is in women. Men may require a larger dose of some drugs than women because women are generally smaller than men.

Weight

In general, dosages are based on a weight of approximately 150 pounds, which is calculated to the "average" weight of men and women. A drug dose may sometimes be increased or decreased because the patient's weight is significantly higher or lower than this average. With narcotics, for example, higher or lower than average dosages, depending on the patient's weight, may be necessary to produce relief of pain.

Time and Route of Drug Administration

During the night (nocturnal), plasma levels of drugs, such as theophylline and diazepam, are lower than plasma levels during the day (diurnal). The time of drug administration is an important factor that affects drug activity. Some drugs should be taken before or after meals, and other medicines must be used in the early morning or before bedtime.

Oral Routes

Drugs administered orally are absorbed from the gastrointestinal tract and transported to the liver before they enter the systemic circulation. Hence, the drug is subject to hepatic metabolism before it reaches its site of action. This effect is known as first-pass metabolism, which is the degree to which a drug is chemically altered as it circulates through the liver for the first time.

Most orally administered drugs are absorbed into the blood vessels within the intestinal tract. The blood in these vessels flows directly to the liver, the body's primary site for drug metabolism, before it goes anywhere else in the body. Some drugs are totally destroyed the first and only time they pass through, whereas other drugs are hardly affected at all. The oral route of administration is not suitable for most drugs for which a high degree of first-pass

TABLE 8–1 Examples of Drugs that Undergo First-Pass Metabolism

acetaminophen	nortriptyline
alprenolol	oxprenolol
aspirin	pentazocine
cortisone	progesterone
cyclosporin	propoxyphene
estradiol	propranolol
imipramine	salbutamol
isoproterenol	terbutaline
lidocaine	testosterone
meperidine	verapamil

metabolism occurs because those drugs are quickly deactivated. Nitroglycerin tablets, for example, are dissolved under the tongue, rather than being swallowed, because nitroglycerin is completely inactivated during its first pass through the liver (see Table 8–1).

Parenteral Routes

Intravenous administration of drugs produces the most rapid drug action. Next in order of time of action is the intramuscular route, followed by the subcutaneous route. With parenteral administration, drugs bypass the liver. First-pass effect is named so because the drug does get metabolized in the liver. The liver is also bypassed with sublingual and rectal administration.

Diet

Food can increase, decrease, or not affect the absorption of drugs, and diet can influence the bioavailability of a drug from a modified release dosage form. Absorption of the drug in the gastrointestinal tract with another food element is a common drug interaction that reduces the extent of drug absorption. For example, tetracycline complexes with calcium (found in milk products), and alcohol can increase or decrease the activity of hepatic drug-metabolizing enzymes. Chronic alcoholism can increase the rate of metabolism of tolbutamide, warfarin, and phenytoin. Even in individuals who are not addicted to alcohol, acute alcohol intoxication can inhibit hepatic enzymes.

Pregnancy

Drugs present in their active forms in the maternal circulation probably pass unchanged into the fetal circulation. In general, lipid-soluble drugs administered to pregnant women will usually pass through the placenta. In pregnant women who smoke, the nicotine and carcinogenic substances in cigarettes will pass into the fetus through the bloodstream. Fetal metabolic activities vary and depend upon a number of factors, including fetal age. A major deficiency in the fetus is lack of glucuronic acid-conjugating activity when a drug, which may have local or systemic effects, is applied to the surface of the body such as the skin. In both the fetus and the neonate, these drugs produce slow drug action.

Psychological State

Patients' attitudes, whether positive or negative, about the drugs they receive have been proven to play a major role in the effect of drugs. The more positive patients feel about the drug they are taking, the more positive their physical response to the drug. A decreased drug effect is possible when patients feel negative about the medication. This is called the placebo effect.

A placebo is an inactive substance, such as saline solution, distilled water, sugar, or a less than effective dose of a harmless substance such as a water-soluble vitamin. Used in experimental drug studies to compare the effects of the inactive substance with those of the experimental drug, placebos are also prescribed for patients who cannot be given the medication they requested or who, in the judgment of the health-care provider, do not need the medication. Health-care professionals should realize that their attitudes and the impressions they create at the time of drug discussion or administration may influence the therapeutic result.

Polypharmacy

The combined effect of drugs taken concurrently may result in antagonism or synergism and, consequently, may be lethal in some patients. Health-care professionals need to be aware of the potential interactions of drugs that they prescribe, as well as those that the patient may be self-administering. Many patients, especially elderly patients, may take several medicines each day. The chance for these individuals to develop an undesired drug interaction increases rapidly with the number of drugs used. It is estimated that if a patient uses eight or more medications, there is a 100% chance of interaction. One drug may interact with another to increase, decrease, or stop the effects of the other drug. The following terms are used to describe drug interactions:

- **Synergism**: A combined action of two or more agents that produces an effect greater than would have been expected from the two agents acting separately. For example, the combination of the antibacterial drugs trimethoprim and sulfamethoxazole is more effective for treating infections than either drug acting alone.

- **Antagonism**: The combined effect of two drugs that is less than the effect of either drug taken alone. For example, ibuprofen reduces the effects of furosemide when the two drugs are taken simultaneously.

- **Potentiation**: An effect that occurs when a drug increases or prolongs the action of another drug with the total effect being greater than the sum of the effects of either drug used alone. For example, alcohol potentiates the sedating effects of the tranquilizer diazepam when a patient ingests the two drugs at the same time.

- **Addition**: The combined effect of two agents, which is equal to the sum of the effects of each drug taken alone. For example, psychological and physiological dependence on a chemical substance such as alcohol, heroin, or cocaine is additive.

- **Tolerance**: Increasing resistance to the usual effects of an established dosage of a drug as a result of continued use.

- **Dependence**: The total psychophysical state of one addicted to drugs or alcohol who must receive an increasing amount of the substance to prevent the onset of withdrawal symptoms.

Diseases

The presence of disease may influence the action of some drugs. Any disease or condition in the body and the severity of its symptoms may affect the type and dose of drug administered. The presence of cardiovascular, hepatic (liver), or renal (kidney) dysfunctions will interfere with the normal processes of drug action. In liver disease, for example, the ability to metabolize or detoxify a specific type of drug may be impaired. If the average or normal dose of the drug is given, the liver may be unable to metabolize the drug at a normal rate. Therefore, the drug may be excreted from the body at a much slower rate than normal.

SIDE EFFECTS

A secondary response to a medication other than the primary therapeutic effect for which the drug was intended is called a side effect. Side effects can range from mild, which disappear when a patient discontinues the drug, to debilitating diseases that become chronic.

Hypersensitivity

Resulting from previous sensitizing exposure and the development of an immunologic mechanism, a drug allergy is an altered state of reaction to a drug. Nearly 10% of patients have hypersensitivity reactions. All types of reactions from a simple rash to anaphylaxis can occur within two minutes or up to three days after administration.

Anaphylactic Reaction

There are four types of anaphylactic reactions, which are defined in the following paragraphs.

Type I—Anaphylactic

An anaphylactic reaction is an immediate reaction that may be severe and may result in death if not treated quickly. Signs and symptoms of the most severe reactions include severe bronchospasm, vasospasm, hypotension, and rapid death. Drugs that may be associated with type I hypersensitivity include penicillins and cephalosporin.

Type II—Cytotoxic

A cytotoxic reaction, an autoimmune response, may cause hemolytic anemia (methyldopa- or penicillin-induced), thrombocytopenia (quinidine-induced) or systemic lupus erythematosus (procainamide-induced).

Type III—Arthus

An Arthus reaction (also known as *serum sickness* or *Arthus phenomenon*) is associated with an acute local inflammatory reaction, usually in the skin and marked by edema, hemorrhage, and necrosis, which occurs at the site of injection. Penicillins, sulfonamides, and phenytoin can cause this delayed reaction.

Type IV—Cellular Hypersensitivity

A cell-mediated or delayed hypersensitivity reaction is responsible for defense against certain bacterial, fungal, and viral pathogens or malignant cells. Allergic (contact) dermatitis is an example of a cell-mediated immune response. A type IV reaction is also called a cellular hypersensitivity reaction.

EXPLORING THE WEB

Visit http://www.aafp.org to learn more about the American Academy of Family Physicians, one of the largest national medical organizations, with more than 94,600 members.

Visit http://www.fda.gov; the Food and Drug Administration's site has information on drugs and medical devices, among other topics.

Visit http://www.medscape.com; Medscape has many specialty sites, including one for pharmacists.

Visit http://www.nida.nih.gov; the National Institute on Drug Abuse (NIDA) gives strategic support to and conducts research across a broad range of disciplines and uses those results to improve prevention, treatment, and policy as it relates to drug abuse and addiction.

Visit http://www.nlm.nih.gov; the National Library of Medicine, the world's largest medical library, collects materials and provides information and research services in all areas of biomedicine and health care.

Visit http://www.pharmpedia.com; Pharmpedia is a free content, open source pharmaceutical encyclopedia that is written collaboratively by people from all around the world.

REVIEW QUESTIONS

1. Which statement correctly applies to the routes of administration?

   A. Sublingual: must take place in first-pass metabolism
   B. Intramuscular: generally offers poor absorption
   C. Rectal: poor compliance may limit
   D. Intravenous: complete bioavailability

2. Decreasing the pH of the intestinal contents is more likely to increase the absorption rate of a drug that is a:

   A. weak acid
   B. weak base
   C. neutral (not acidic or basic)
   D. strong acid

3. The greater the therapeutic index, the more likely a drug will be:

   A. more lethal
   B. more safe
   C. less safe
   D. less expensive

4. A term that indicates measurement of both the rate of drug absorption and the total amount of drug that reaches the bloodstream from an administered dosage form is called:

   A. idiosyncratic reaction
   B. drug toxicity
   C. drug bioavailability
   D. drug side effects

5. Which factor is the most important for effective distribution of a drug?

   A. lipid solubility
   B. water solubility
   C. glomerular filtration rate
   D. half-life of a drug

6. At what time of day is the plasma level of diazepam or theophylline lower?

   A. early morning
   B. at noon
   C. during the afternoon
   D. during the night

7. The first-pass metabolism effect occurs when the:

   A. drug passes through the membrane wall of the small intestine
   B. drug enters the systemic circulation
   C. drug is transported to the liver before entering the blood
   D. drug plasma level disappears

8. Type III hypersensitivity is known as:

   A. cytotoxic reaction
   B. anaphylactic reaction
   C. serum sickness or Arthus reaction
   D. cellular hypersensitivity reaction

9. An effect that occurs when a drug increases or prolongs the action of another drug is called:

   A. synergism
   B. tolerance
   C. dependence
   D. potentiation

10. Which hypersensitivity is called an autoimmune response?

    A. cellular hypersensitivity reaction
    B. cytotoxic reaction
    C. anaphylactic reaction
    D. Arthus phenomenon

Pharmacology

OUTLINE

GLOSSARY

Angina pectoris – also called *angina*, this condition describes chest pain as a result of lack of blood and oxygen supply to the heart muscle, usually because of vessel obstruction or spasm

Antibiotics – therapeutic agents that slow or stop the growth of microorganisms

Antihistamines – drugs that counteract the action of histamine

Anxiety – a physiological state consisting of fear, apprehension, or worry

Arrhythmias – various conditions of abnormal electrical heart activity; the heart may beat too fast, too slow, or irregularly

Antitussive – a drug that reduces coughing, also called a *cough suppressant*

Bacteriostatic – capable of stopping the growth and reproduction of bacteria; a term that is typically used to describe antibiotics that inhibit bacterial growth without killing the bacteria

Bactericidal – capable of killing bacteria; a term that is typically used in reference to antiseptics, disinfectants, or antibiotics

Bronchodilators – agents that relax the smooth muscle of the bronchial tubes

Cation – a positively charged atom

Centrally acting skeletal muscle relaxants – also known as *spasmolytics*, these agents alleviate musculoskeletal pain and spasms to reduce spasticity (continual muscular contraction)

Convulsion – an intense, involuntary muscle contraction or spasm, as is commonly seen during a seizure condition

Corticosteroids – the most potent and consistently effective anti-inflammatory agents that are currently available for relief of respiratory conditions

Dry powder inhaler (DPI) – a device used to deliver medication in the form of micronized powder into the lungs

Hormones – chemical messengers that move through the blood or through cells that carry signals; examples include estrogen, testosterone, melatonin, epinephrine, dopamine, and insulin

Hyperlipidemia – the presence of raised or abnormal levels of lipids (fatty molecules) or lipoproteins (biochemicals containing proteins and lipids) in the blood

Hypertension – high blood pressure; a chronic elevation of the blood pressure equivalent to or greater than 140/90

Hypnosis – a trance-like state, resembling sleep, or an increased tendency to sleep

Hypnotic – a drug that induces sleep; often used to treat insomnia and in surgical anesthesia

Metered dose inhaler (MDI) – a hand-held pressurized device used to deliver medications for inhalation

Nebulizer – a device used for inhalation that uses a small machine to convert a solution into a mist that a patient inhales through a facemask or a mouthpiece

Neuromuscular blocking agents – drugs that block neuromuscular transmission at the neuromuscular junction; they cause paralysis of specific skeletal muscles

Opiates – narcotic alkaloids found in opium

Opioids – chemical substances that have morphine-like action in the body; commonly used for pain relief

Parkinson's disease – a degenerative disorder of the central nervous system that usually impairs motor skills, speech, and other functions

Sedation – the use of a sedative agent to reduce excitement, nervousness, or irritation; commonly prior to a medical procedure

Sedatives – substances that suppress the central nervous system and induce calmness, relaxation, drowsiness, or sleep

Seizure – a temporary, abnormal electrical brain condition that results in abnormal neuronal activity; it can affect mental ability and cause convulsions; recurrent, unprovoked seizures are called *epilepsy*

PHARMACOLOGY AND THE CARDIOVASCULAR SYSTEM

Cardiovascular disorders such as angina pectoris, hypertension, myocardial infarction, and hyperlipidemia are among the most common causes of death in the United States.

Antianginal Drugs

Angina pectoris often causes a sharp pain that patients usually feel in their chests or arms and most commonly after exertion. The pain occurs when the heart does not receive a sufficient amount of oxygen to support its workload. Three groups of medications can help achieve the treatment goals for angina pectoris:

1. Nitrates
2. Beta blockers
3. Calcium channel blockers

Examples of commonly used antianginal drugs are listed in Table 9–1.

Antihypertensive Drugs

Hypertension is defined as an abnormal increase in arterial blood pressure. Approximately 90% of patients have essential hypertension that is of an unknown cause. Untreated hypertension may lead to heart attack, kidney damage, stroke, and blindness.

Many classes of drugs are used to treat hypertension, including:

- Diuretics
- Beta blockers (also commonly referred to as *betablockers*, beta-adrenergic blockers, and ß-blockers)
- Angiotensin-converting enzyme inhibitors (ACE inhibitors)
- Angiotensin II receptor blockers
- Calcium channel blockers
- Alpha-adrenergic blockers

Most often prescribed to treat hypertension and congestive heart failure, most diuretics work by causing the kidneys to eliminate more sodium than they normally would. Three types of diuretics

TABLE 9–1 Examples of Commonly Used Antianginal Drugs

Generic Name	Trade Name	Available Dosage Form	Major Adverse Effects
Nitrates			
isosorbide	Imdur	Capsule, tablet	Weakness, restlessness, postural hypotension, and flushing
nitroglycerin	Nitro-Bid, Nitrodisc, Nitro-Dur, Transderm	Spray, tablet Capsule, ointment, IV, transdermal patch	Blurred vision, vertigo, hypotension, circulatory collapse, and anaphylactoid reaction
Beta Blockers			
acebutolol	Sectral	Capsule	Insomnia, confusion, hypotension, agranulocytosis, hypoglycemia, bronchospasm, and pulmonary edema
atenolol	Tenormin	IV, tablet	Syncope, drowsiness, insomnia, bradycardia, and bronchospasm
nadolol	Corgard	Tablet	Laryngospasm, bradycardia, hypotension, and impotence
propranolol	Inderal	Capsule, IM, IV, tablet	Anaphylactoid reaction, dermatitis, depression, confusion, insomnia, bradycardia, and dry mouth
Calcium Channel Blockers			
diltiazem	Cardizem	Capsule, tablet	Nervousness, insomnia, flushing, syncope, hypotension, and impaired taste
nifedipine	Adalat	Tablet	Sore throat, mood changes, blurred vision, hypotension, hepatotoxicity, and sexual difficulties
verapamil	Calan	Capsule, IV	Dizziness, depression, hypotension, bradycardia, and pulmonary edema

TABLE 9–2 Examples of Diuretics

Generic Name	Trade Name	Dosage Form	Major Adverse Effects
Thiazide Diuretics			
chlorothiazide	Diuril	IM, IV, tablet	Anaphylactic reaction, hypotension, hypokalemia, hypercalcemia, and hyponatremia
hydrochlorothiazide	Esidrix	Capsule, oral solution, tablet	Mood changes, hypotension, pancreatitis, jaundice, agranulocytosis, aplastic anemia, hyperglycemia, hyperuricemia, and hypokalemia
Loop Diuretics			
ethacrynic acid	Edecrin	Injection	Hypotension, hyponatremia, hypokalemia, hypocalcemia, thrombocytopenia, and severe neutropenia
furosemide	Lasix	IM, IV, oral solution, Tablet	Hypotension, circulatory collapse, hyponatremia, hypokalemia, hypocalcemia (tetany), renal failure, and aplastic anemia (rare)
Potassium-Sparing Diuretics			
spironolactone	Aldactone	Tablet	Mental confusion, gynecomastia (both sexes), inability to achieve or maintain erection, hirsuitism, and electrolyte imbalance
triamterene	Dyrenium	Capsule	Dry mouth, anaphylaxis, photosensitivity of skin, hyperkalemia, and other electrolyte imbalances

are used to treat hypertension: thiazide, loop, and potassium-sparing diuretics. Table 9–2 lists some examples of diuretics.

Examples of other antihypertensive agents are listed in Table 9–3.

Antiarrhythmics

Arrhythmias are deviations from the normal pattern of the heartbeat. They may occur because of improper impulse generation, conduction, or both. Common arrhythmias originating in the upper and lower chambers of the heart include the following: atrial fibrillation, atrial flutter, premature ventricular contractions, ventricular tachycardia, and ventricular fibrillation. Antiarrhythmic drugs are classified according to their effects on the conduction of impulses through the heart and on their mechanism of action. Table 9–4 shows examples of antiarrhythmic drugs.

Drug Therapy for Heart Failure

Heart failure is the inability of the heart muscle to contract with enough force to properly circulate blood. The most common form of heart failure is often referred to as *congestive heart failure*. Heart failure may be treated with a variety of drugs and methods, including cardiac glycosides, diuretics, ACE inhibitors, beta blockers, fluid restriction, and a low-sodium diet. Two currently available cardiac glycosides are as follows:

- Digoxin (Lanoxin®)
- Digitoxin

Antihyperlipidemic Drugs

Diseases associated with plasma lipids can manifest as an elevation in triglyceride levels, hyperlipidemia, or as an elevation in the cholesterol level. Medications are not the first line of treatment for hyperlipidemia.

TABLE 9–3　Examples of Beta Blockers, ACE Inhibitors, and ARBs

Generic Name	Trade Name	Dosage Form	Major Adverse Effects
Beta Blockers			
atenolol	Tenormin	IV, tablet	Bronchospasm and syncope
bisoprolol	Zebeta	Tablet	Vertigo, bradycardia, hypotension, asthma, and acne
carvedilol	Coreg	Tablet	Increased sweating, chest pain, hypertension, bronchitis, hyperglycemia, gout, and weight increase
nadolol	Corgard	Tablet	Bradycardia and laryngospasm
ACE Inhibitors			
benazepril	Lotensin	Tablet	Hypotension, hyperkalemia, and bronchitis
captopril	Capoten	Tablet	Hypotension, weight loss, hyperkalemia, and impaired renal function
enalapril	Vasotec	IV, tablet	Insomnia, hypotension, and hyperkalemia
fosinopril	Monopril	Tablet	Hyperkalemia and fatigue
lisinopril	Prinivil, Zestril	Tablet	hypotension, chest pain, cough, dyspnea, and hyperkalemia
Angiotensin II Receptor Blockers (ARBs)			
candesartan	Atacand	Tablet	Arthralgia, back pain, and pharyngitis
irbesartan	Avapro	Tablet	Anxiety, chest pain, cough, and pharyngitis
losartan	Cozaar	Tablet	Insomnia, muscle cramps, and nasal congestion
olmesartan	Benicar	Tablet	Back pain, hypotension, hyperglycemia, hematuria, and pharyngitis
valsartan	Diovan	Capsule	Hyperkalemia, cough, and arthralgia
Calcium Channel Blockers			
amlodipine	Norvasc	Tablet	Peripheral or facial edema, chest pain, syncope, and sexual dysfunction
diltiazem	Cardizem	Capsule, IV, tablet	Insomnia, syncope, and hypotension
felodipine	Plendil	Tablet	Peripheral edema and tachycardia

Antihyperlipidemic drugs are used only if diet modification and exercise programs fail to lower low-density lipoprotein (LDL), or "bad cholesterol" levels, to normal. Table 9–5 shows examples of lipid-lowering drugs.

Anticoagulant Drugs

To prevent bleeding from cuts and other injuries, clot formation is vital. Without clotting, one can bleed to death. Sometimes, however, clot formation is not desired. Anticoagulants are agents that prevent formation of blood clots (thrombi). Warfarin and heparin are common examples of anticoagulants. Warfarin is an oral anticoagulant that affects the liver to prevent formation of vitamin K-dependent clotting factor, and heparin is a natural anticoagulant that is produced by basophils. Protamine sulfate is a heparin antagonist derived from fish sperm, which

TABLE 9–4   Examples of Antiarrhythmic Drugs

Generic Name	Trade Name	Dosage Form	Major Adverse Effects
Class I			
flecainide	Tambocor	Tablet	Chest pain, blurred vision, dyspnea, and edema
lidocaine	Xylocaine	IV	Dyspnea, psychosis with high dose, convulsions, respiratory depression and arrest, and cardiovascular collapse
mexiletine	Mexitil	Capsule	Exacerbated arrhythmias, syncope, and hypotension
procainamide	Pronestyl	Capsule, injection, tablet	Severe hypotension, pericarditis, and agranulocytosis
Class II (Beta Blockers)			
acebutolol	Sectral	Capsule	Insomnia, confusion, agranulocytosis, hypoglycemia, and bronchospasm
esmolol	Brevibloc	IV	Somnolence, agitation, cold hands and feet, and bronchospasm
propranolol	Inderal	Capsule, IV, tablet	Anaphylactic reactions, dermatitis, depression, insomnia, visual hallucinations, and bradycardia
Class III (drugs that interfere with potassium outflow)			
amiodarone	Cordarone	Injection, tablet	Cardiogenic shock, hepatotoxicity, and pulmonary toxicity
bretylium	Bretylium	IM, IV	Respiratory depression and syncope
Class IV (calcium channel blockers)			
diltiazem	Tiazac	Capsule, IM, IV, tablet	Hypotension, nervousness, and impaired taste
verapamil	Calan, Isoptin	Capsule, IV, tablet	Depression, hypotension, and pulmonary edema

is an antidote for heparin. Table 9–6 shows examples of anticoagulants.

PHARMACOLOGY AND THE CENTRAL NERVOUS SYSTEM

Drug classifications affecting the central nervous system (CNS) include sedatives, hypnotics, anti-anxiety drugs, anticonvulsants, anti-Parkinson drugs, antidepressants, antipsychotics, narcotic analgesics, and anesthetics.

Sedatives, Hypnotics, and Anti-anxiety Drugs

Sedatives and hypnotic drugs are used to treat anxiety and sleep disorders. Sedation is characterized by decreased anxiety, motor activity, and mental acuity. Anxiety is defined as a persistent and irrational fear of a specific object, activity, or situation. Sedation induces calmness or sleep and, as a result, reduces anxiety. Hypnosis is defined by an increased tendency to sleep. Hypnotic drugs are used to induce sleep or drowsiness. Some examples of anti-anxiety drugs are shown in Table 9–7.

TABLE 9–5 Examples of Lipid-Lowering Drugs

Generic Name	Trade Name	Dosage Form	Major Adverse Effects
Bile Acid Sequestrants			
cholestyramine	Questran	Powder, tablet	Constipation, fecal impaction, increased libido, and weight loss or gain
colesevelam	Welchol	Tablet	Abdominal pain, sinusitis, and pharyngitis
colestipol	Colestid	Powder, tablet	Joint and muscle pain, shortness of breath, constipation, dermatitis, and urticaria
Fibric Acid Derivatives			
clofibrate	Atromid-S	Capsule	Gastritis, stomatitis, cholelithiasis, and agranulocytosis
fenofibrate	Lofibra, Tricor	Capsule, tablet	Arthralgia, insomnia, arrhythmia, constipation, and rhinitis
gemfibrozil	Lopid	Tablet	Blurred vision, painful extremities, muscle cramps, and swollen joints
Niacin (Nicotinic Acid)			
niacin (extended release)	Niacor, Niaspan	Capsule, tablet	Transient headache, syncope, nervousness, panic, blurred vision, postural hypotension, dry skin, and pruritus
Statins			
atorvastatin	Lipitor	Tablet	Back pain, myalgia, rhabdomyolysis, sinusitis, and pharyngitis
fluvastatin	Lescol	Capsule, tablet	Headache, fatigue, and abdominal pain
lovastatin	Altoprev, Mevacor	Tablet	Generally well tolerated, insomnia, and blurred vision
pravastatin	Pravachol	Tablet	Nausea, diarrhea, and abdominal pain
rosuvastatin	Crestor	Tablet	Insomnia, depression, hypertension, angina, myalgia, and dyspnea
simvastatin	Zocor	Tablet	Dizziness, fatigue, insomnia, constipation, and rhinitis

TABLE 9–6 Examples of Anticoagulants

Generic Name	Trade Name	Dosage Form	Major Adverse Effects
heparin	Hep-Lock	IV, SC	Spontaneous bleeding, bronchospasm, and anaphylactoid reactions
lepirudin	Refludan	IV	Intracranial bleeding, heart failure, ventricular fibrillation, hematoma, and bronchospasm
warfarin	Coumadin	IV, Tablet	Minor or major bleeding from any organ, and anorexia
Low Molecular-Weight Heparin			
dalteparin	Fragmin	SC	Allergic reactions, arthralgia, insomnia, hemorrhage, and dyspnea
enoxaparin	Lovenox	SC	Allergic reactions, angioedema, arthralgia, and hemorrhage

TABLE 9–7   Examples of Anti-anxiety Drugs

Generic Name	Trade Name	Dosage Form	Major Adverse Effects
Benzodiazepines			
alprazolam	Xanax	Tablet	Drowsiness, sedation, syncope, depression, and tremor
chlordiazepoxide	Librium	Capsule	Respiratory depression, orthostatic hypotension, tachycardia, nightmares, and hallucinations
diazepam	Valium	Injection, tablet	Confusion, amnesia, slurred speech, hypotension, and cardiovascular collapse
estazolam	Prosom	Tablet	Impaired coordination and syncope
lorazepam	Ativan	IM, IV, tablet	Sedation, amnesia, depression, sleep disturbances, and hypertension or hypotension
oxazepam	Serax	Capsule, tablet	Confusion, vertigo, syncope, hypotension, and leukopenia
Nonbenzodiazepines			
buspirone	BuSpar	Tablet	Numbness, dizziness, dream disturbances, mood changes, urinary frequency, and hyperventilation
phenobarbital	Luminal	Capsule, injection, liquid, tablet	CNS depression, coma, respiratory depression, and death
secobarbital	Seconal	Tablet	Hangover, respiratory depression, and laryngospasm
zolpidem	Ambien	Tablet	Drugged feeling, depression, double vision, and amnesia

Anticonvulsants

Epilepsy is a group of disorders characterized by hyperexcitability within the CNS. A seizure is a term for all epileptic events, whereas a convulsion refers to abnormal motor movements. Antiepileptic drugs prevent or stop a convulsive seizure. Classifications of epileptic events are shown in Table 9–8.

The major drugs used to control seizures are phenytoin, carbamazepine, and valproic acid. Some additional examples of anticonvulsants are listed in Table 9–9.

Anti-Parkinson Drugs

Parkinson's disease is characterized by resting tremor, resistance to passive movement, akinesia (inability to initiate movements), loss of postural reflexes, and behavioral manifestations. Table 9–10 shows some examples of drugs used to treat Parkinson's disease.

TABLE 9–8   Classifications of Epileptic Events

I. Focal or partial seizures	II. Generalized seizures
A. Simple seizures	**A. Nonconvulsive** 1. Absence or petit mal seizures
B. Complex partial seizures	**B. Convulsive** 1. Tonic/clonic or grand mal seizures 2. Tonic/psychomotor seizures 3. Status epilepticus

Antidepressants

Depression, one of the most common psychiatric disorders in the United States, is characterized by feelings of intense sadness, helplessness, worthlessness, impaired functioning, inability to experience pleasure in activities, loss of energy, changes in sleep habits, and sudden weight gain or loss. Examples of drugs used to treat depression are shown in Table 9–11.

TABLE 9–9 Examples of Anticonvulsants

Generic Name	Trade Name	Dosage Form	Major Adverse Effects
carbamazepine	Tegretol, Tegretol XR	Chewable tablet, suspension, tablet	Arthralgia, leg cramps, edema, syncope, and arrhythmias
diazepam	Valium	IM, IV, rectal gel, tablet	Drowsiness, vertigo, amnesia, vivid dreams, slurred speech, tremor, and hypotension
ethosuximide	Zarontin	Capsule, syrup	Euphoria, restlessness, aggressiveness, night terrors, agranulocytosis, and aplastic anemia
lorazepam	Ativan	Injection, oral solution, tablet	Amnesia, sedation, hallucinations, blurred vision, and depressed hearing
phenytoin	Dilantin	Capsule, IV, suspension, tablet	Nystagmus, mental confusion, insomnia, cardiovascular collapse, agranulocytosis, and aplastic anemia
tiagabine	Gabitril	Tablet	Somnolence, depression, insomnia, hostility, hallucinations, dyspnea, and nosebleed
valproic acid	Depakene	Capsule, IV, syrup, tablet	Sedation, hallucinations, aggression, liver failure, pancreatitis, leucopenia, bone marrow depression, and pulmonary edema (with overdose)

TABLE 9–10 Examples of Anti-Parkinson Drugs

Generic Name	Trade Name	Dosage Form	Major Adverse Effects
amantadine	Symmetrel	Capsule, syrup	Anxiety, irritability, confusion, hallucinations, insomnia, and nightmares
benztropine	Cogentin	Injection, tablet	Tachycardia, blurred vision, photophobia, and dry mouth
bromocriptine	Parlodel	Capsule, tablet	Orthostatic hypotension, shock, arrhythmias, heart attack, vertigo, nightmares, and depression
carbidopa/levodopa	Sinemet	Tablet	Dyskinesias, nausea, chest pain, asthenia, cardiac irregularities, darkened saliva, agranulocytosis, angioedema, back pain, psychotic episodes, and others
levodopa	Dopar	Capsule, tablet	Increased hand tremor, grinding of teeth, confusion, hallucinations, hepatotoxicity, and dysphagia
trihexyphenidyl	Artane	Elixir, tablet	Blurred vision, photophobia, insomnia, agitation, tachycardia, and hypotension

Antipsychotics

Psychosis, a mental disorder in which a person's capacity to recognize reality is distorted, is characterized by the following symptoms:

- Hallucinations (hearing or observing things that are not real)

- Delusions (fixed beliefs that are false)

Antipsychotics can be classified as conventional and atypical agents. Conventional antipsychotics are thought to act by blocking the action of the neurotransmitter dopamine. Atypical agents appear to block not only dopamine, but also serotonin. Examples of drugs used to treat psychosis are shown in Table 9–12.

Narcotic Analgesics

Narcotic analgesics are also referred to as opioids, which is the general term for drugs with morphine-like activity that reduce pain and induce tolerance and physical dependence. Drugs made from opium

TABLE 9–11   Examples of Drugs Used to Treat Depression

Generic Name	Trade Name	Dosage Form	Major Adverse Effects
Tricyclic Antidepressants			
amitriptyline	Elavil	Injection, tablet	Sedation, dizziness, seizures, orthostatic hypotension, and blurred vision
imipramine	Tofranil	Capsule, tablet	Sedation, lack of coordination, exacerbation of psychoses, and urinary retention
nortriptyline	Pamelor	Capsule, oral solution	Blurred vision, urinary retention, dry mouth, and orthostatic hypotension
Second-Generation Cyclic Antidepressants			
bupropion	Wellbutrin	Tablet	Weight loss, weight gain, seizures, insomnia, dry mouth, and blurred vision
Monoamine Oxidase Inhibitors			
phenelzine	Nardil	Tablet	Dizziness, orthostatic hypotension, respiratory depression, coma, and hypertensive crisis
Selective Serotonin Reuptake Inhibitors			
citalopram	Celexa	Oral solution, tablet	Hypotension, dizziness, insomnia, and increased sweating
fluoxetine	Prozac	Capsule, tablet	Anxiety, insomnia, dry mouth, sweating, and sexual dysfunction
fluvoxamine	Luvox	Tablet	Insomnia, agitation, and seizures
paroxetine	Paxil	Oral suspension, tablet	Postural hypotension, tremor, anxiety, insomnia, urinary frequency, and blurred vision
sertraline	Zoloft	Oral liquid, tablet	Chest pain, hypertension or hypotension, edema, aggressive behavior, hallucinations, and gynecomastia
Medications for Bipolar Disorder			
lithium carbonate	Eskalith	Capsule, tablet	Slurred speech, seizures, confusion, recent memory loss, hypotension, and weight gain
valproic acid	Depakene, Depakote	Capsule, injection, syrup, tablet	Hallucinations, aggression, deep coma, liver failure, pancreatitis, bone marrow depression, and death (with overdose)

(such as morphine and heroin) are referred to as opiates. Table 9–13 shows some examples of common narcotic analgesics.

Anesthetics

Anesthesia, literally, is the unique condition of reversible unconsciousness or a loss of sensation and is characterized by four reversible actions: unconsciousness, analgesia, immobility, and amnesia. There are four stages of general anesthesia: Stage I (analgesia, euphoria, perceptual distortions, amnesia), Stage II (delirium, hypertension, tachycardia), Stage III (surgical anesthesia), and Stage IV (medullary depression). See Table 9–14.

Anesthetics are agents that generally act on the nervous tissue. By depressing the excitability of excitable tissues, local anesthetics act to produce a loss of sensation from a local area of the body. General anesthetics produce a state affecting overall body function. In anesthetic concentrations, they do not produce detectable generalized effects on all nerves. Examples of local anesthetics are shown in

TABLE 9–12 Examples of Antipsychotics

Generic Name	Trade Name	Dosage Form	Major Adverse Effects
Conventional Antipsychotics			
High-Potency			
haloperidol	Haldol	Injection, oral solution, tablet	Parkinsonian symptoms, mental depression, hyperthermia, laryngospasm, and respiratory depression
thiothixene	Navane	Capsule, oral solution	Cerebral edema, convulsions, sudden death, impotence, and blurred vision
trifluoperazine	Stelazine	Injection, tablet	Insomnia, dry mouth, blurred vision, agranulocytosis, and gynecomastia
Intermediate-Potency			
loxapine succinate	Loxitane	Capsule, injection, oral solution	Orthostatic hypotension, hypertension, ptosis, and urinary retention
perphenazine	Trilafon	Tablet	Sedation, convulsions, orthostatic hypotension, blurred vision, and urinary retention
Low-Potency			
thioridazine	Mellaril	Oral solution, tablet	Sedation, blurred vision, amenorrhea, breast engorgement, and galactorrhea
Atypical Antipsychotics			
clozapine	Clozaril	Tablet	Orthostatic hypotension, cardiomyopathy, agranulocytosis, and seizures
olanzapine	Zyprexa	Injection, tablet	Weight gain, chest pain, insomnia, Parkinsonism, increased salivation, and diabetes mellitus
quetiapine fumarate	Seroquel	Tablet	Peripheral edema, weight gain, postural hypotension, hyperglycemia, and increased risk of suicidal thoughts

TABLE 9–13 Examples of Narcotic Analgesics

Generic Name	Trade Name	Dosage Form	Major Adverse Effects
codeine	Codeine Sulfate	Injection, oral solution, tablet	Shortness of breath, anaphylactoid reaction, hypotension, circulatory collapse, sedation, convulsions, and respiratory depression
hydrocodone and homatropine	Hycodan	Syrup, tablet	Dry mouth, sedation, and respiratory depression
hydromorphone	Dilaudid	Injection, oral liquid, tablet	Dizziness, sedation, hypotension, and respiratory depression
meperidine	Demerol	Injection, syrup, tablet	Respiratory depression, convulsions, cardiovascular collapse, and bronchoconstriction
methadone	Dolophine, Methadose	Injection, oral solution, tablet	Drowsiness, dry mouth, and respiratory depression
pentazocine and naloxone	Talwin	Injection	Flushing, allergic reaction, sweating, and respiratory depression
propoxyphene	Darvon	Tablet	Confusion, sedation, toxic psychosis, coma, respiratory depression, and circulatory collapse

TABLE 9–14 Stages of General Anesthesia

Stages	Characterized By:
Stage I	Analgesia Euphoria Perceptual distortions Amnesia
Stage II	Delirium Hypertension Tachycardia
Stage III	Surgical anesthesia
Stage IV	Medullary depression begins with cessation of respiration and circulatory collapse

Table 9–15, and examples of general anesthetics that are currently used are shown in Table 9–16.

PHARMACOLOGY AND THE RESPIRATORY SYSTEM

Upper respiratory tract infections (URIs), more common than lower respiratory tract infections, may be caused by viruses, bacteria, or fungi. Upper respiratory tract infections can be treated by appropriate antibiotics, as discussed previously. Lower respiratory tract infections are less common, and the lungs are the primary site of tuberculosis and pneumonia.

TABLE 9–15 Examples of Local Anesthetics

Generic Name	Trade Name	Dosage Form	Major Adverse Effects
Amides			
bupivacaine	Sensorcaine, Marcaine	Injection	Syncope, hyperthermia, anxiety, convulsions, and respiratory arrest
bupivacaine and epinephrine		Injection	Syncope, hyperthermia, anxiety, convulsions, and respiratory arrest
lidocaine	Xylocaine	Cream, injection, jelly, ointment, patch	Difficulty breathing, tremors, psychosis, convulsions, and respiratory depression and arrest
Esters			
benzocaine	Americaine, Anbesol	Cream, gel, liquid, ointment, spray	Anaphylaxis
dibucaine	Nupercainal	Ointment	Irritation of skin
procaine	Novocain	Injection	Dizziness, sedation, convulsions, respiratory arrest, and urinary retention

TABLE 9–16 Examples of Currently Used General Anesthetics

Generic Name	Trade Name	Dosage Form	Major Adverse Effects
diazepam (a benzodiazepine)	Valium	Injection, rectal gel, tablet	Amnesia, vivid dreams, tremors, hypotension, and drowsiness
propofol (a sedative-hypnotic)	Diprivan	Injection	Dizziness, twitching, jerking, hypotension, and ventricular asystole (rare)
thiopental (a barbiturate)	Pentothal	Injection	Circulatory and respiratory depression, laryngospasm, amnesia, and skeletal muscle hyperactivity

Antihistamines

Counteracting the action of histamine, antihistamines are of two types. The conventional ones, those used in allergies, block H_1 histamine receptors. The second type, used for peptic ulcers and gastritis, block H_2 receptors. Antihistamines appear to compete with histamine for cell receptor sites on effector cells. Hence, histamine-related allergic reactions and tissue injury are blocked or diminished in intensity. Although there are newer products that are "nondrowsy," most antihistamines have a sedating effect and should be used carefully. Cetirizine, loratadine, and fexofenadine are among the newer products, with the latter two having the lower sedating effect. Table 9–17 shows some examples of antihistamines.

Antitussives

Agents that relieve or prevent coughing are called antitussives. The initial stimulus for cough probably arises in the bronchial mucosa, where irritation results in bronchoconstriction. Antitussives are classified into two major groups: opioid and nonopioid. Cough suppression agents are classified in Table 9–18.

Corticosteroids

The most potent and consistently effective anti-inflammatory agents currently available,

TABLE 9–17   Examples of Antihistamines

Generic Name	Trade Name	Dosage Form	Major Adverse Effects
First-Generation Drugs			
brompheniramine	Veltane	Elixir, injection, tablet	Increased sweating, sedation, drowsiness, disturbed coordination, and buzzing in ears
dexchlorpheniramine	Polaramine	Syrup, tablet	Drowsiness, excitation, insomnia, vertigo, blurred vision, dry mouth, and hypotension
dimenhydrinate	Dramamine	Injection, liquid, tablet	Dizziness, insomnia, hypotension, and dry mouth
diphenhydramine	Benadryl	Capsule, injection, tablet	Drowsiness, tremor, insomnia, tachycardia, and cardiovascular collapse
Second-Generation Drugs			
cetirizine	Zyrtec	Syrup, tablet	Dry mouth, sedation, drowsiness, and depression
fexofenadine	Allegra	Capsule, tablet	Fatigue and throat irritation
loratadine	Claritin	Syrup, tablet	Dizziness, dry mouth, flushing, depression, and syncope

TABLE 9–18   Examples of Antitussives

Generic Name	Trade Name	Dosage Form	Major Adverse Effects
Opioids			
chlorpheniramine	Chlor-Trimeton	Syrup, tablet	Drowsiness, sedation, vertigo, insomnia, and blurred vision
codeine	Various with codeine	Oral solution	Anaphylactoid reaction, hypotension, dizziness, sedation, and respiratory depression
Nonopioids			
benzonatate	Tessalon	Capsule	Drowsiness, sedation, and mild dizziness
dextromethorphan	Delsym	Syrup	Dizziness, anxiety, restlessness, nervousness, confusion, hallucinations, slow and shallow breathing, allergic symptoms, and nausea

corticosteroids come in three commonly-used devices for inhalation administration, including metered dose inhalers, dry powder inhalers, and nebulizers. Drug administration with a metered dose inhaler (MDI) is often accomplished with one or two puffs from a hand-held pressurized device (see Figure 9–1).

A dry powder inhaler (DPI) delivers medication in the form of micronized powder into the lungs. Medications such as fluticasone and salmeterol are available for use this way. Breath-activated, DPIs are easier to use than MDIs.

A nebulizer uses a small machine that converts a solution into a mist. The patient inhales the mist droplets either through a facemask or through a mouthpiece. Examples of inhaled and non-inhaled corticosteroids are seen in Table 9–19.

Bronchodilators

Bronchodilators are agents that widen the diameter of the bronchial tubes. Bronchodilators include beta-adrenergic agonists, theophylline, anticholinergic drugs, and xanthine derivatives. Table 9–20 shows examples of bronchodilators to treat asthma.

Antitubercular Agents

The primary lesion of tuberculosis is located in the lungs. The patient's resistance to secondary tuberculosis

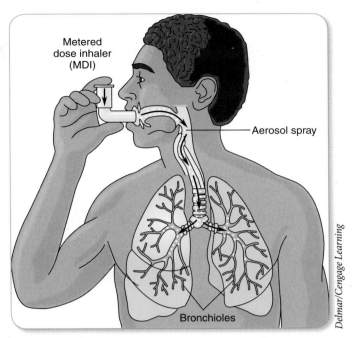

Figure 9–1 The metered dose inhaler aerosolizes medication for inhalation directly into the airways.

depends on general health and environment. In the United States, certain groups of the population are more prone to acquire active tuberculosis. These people include:

- Patients with AIDS
- Drug abusers
- Homeless shelter residents
- Nursing home residents

TABLE 9–19 Examples of Corticosteroids for Treating Asthma

Generic Name	Trade Name	Dosage Form	Major Adverse Effects
beclomethasone	Vancenase AQ	Tincture	Confusion, delirium, blurred vision, photophobia, and urinary retention
budesonide	Pulmicort, Pulmicort Turbohaler	Capsule, inhalation	Arthralgia, myalgia, dizziness, facial edema, agitation, insomnia, chest pain, and hypertension
fluticasone	Flovent	Inhalation	Acne, impaired wound healing, easy bruising, angioneurotic edema, and skin atrophy
prednisolone	Prelone	Tablet	Sensitivity to heat, hypotension, insomnia, and gastric irritation or ulceration
prednisone	Orasone	Oral solution, tablet	Insomnia, confusion, psychosis, edema, peptic ulcer, muscle weakness, and delayed wound healing

TABLE 9–20   Examples of Bronchodilators Used for Treating Asthma

Generic Name	Trade Name	Dosage Form	Major Adverse Effects
albuterol	Proventil, Ventolin	Inhalation, tablet	Tremor, anxiety, convulsions, hallucinations, and blurred vision
metaproterenol	Alupent, Metaprel	Inhalation, syrup, tablet	Tremor, tachycardia, cardiac arrest, hypertension, and palpitations.
salmeterol	Serevent	Inhalation	Dizziness, tremor, and tachycardia
terbutaline	Brethaire, Brethine	Inhalation, injection, tablet	Drowsiness, seizures, and tachycardia
Xanthenes			
aminophylline	Truphylline	Injection, oral liquid, suppository, tablet	Nervousness, restlessness, depression, insomnia, cardiac arrhythmias, severe hypotension, and cardiac arrest
dyphylline	Dilor, Lufyllin	Elixir, solution, tablet	Convulsions, tachycardia, nausea, palpitations, and vomiting
theophylline	Elixophyllin	Injection, tablet	Drug-induced seizures, marked hypotension, and circulatory failure

For treating tuberculosis, the primary antitubercular drugs include isoniazid, ethambutol, rifampin, pyrazinamide, and streptomycin.

PHARMACOLOGY AND THE ENDOCRINE SYSTEM

The endocrine system consists of specialized cell clusters, glands, hormones, and target tissues. Endocrine drugs are used to treat deficiencies or excesses of specific hormones, or nonendocrine diseases.

Selected Drugs for Thyroid Gland Conditions

Diseases of the thyroid gland include hypothyroidism and hyperthyroidism (overproduction of thyroid hormone). Selected medications used as drugs for the thyroid gland are shown in Table 9–21.

Selected Drugs for Diabetes Mellitus

The two general classifications for diabetes mellitus include:

- Type 1, or insulin-dependent diabetes mellitus (IDDM)
- Type 2, or non-insulin-dependent diabetes mellitus (NIDDM)

Characterized by a lack of insulin production from the pancreas, type 1 diabetes must be treated with insulin. Type 2 diabetes may be characterized by either decreased production of insulin or normal amounts of insulin with abnormal sensitivity of the tissues to the insulin that is present. Insulin can be given only by injection either subcutaneously or intravenously. Table 9–22 shows a list of different types of insulin.

Only regular insulin can be administered intravenously. Insulin doses are measured in units. Oral hypoglycemics are used to lower blood sugar in type 2 diabetes. Table 9–23 shows some examples of oral hypoglycemics.

Oral Contraceptives

The ovaries and placenta produce natural estrogenic hormones, and the ovarian cells secret progesterone. Both estrogen and progesterone control a female's menstrual cycle. Manipulating estrogen and

TABLE 9–21   Examples of Medications for Thyroid Gland Conditions

Generic Name	Trade Name	Dosage Form	Major Adverse Effects
Antithyroid Preparations			
potassium iodide	Pima, SSKI	Solution, syrup	Stomach pain, angioneurotic edema, mucosal hemorrhage, metallic taste, salivation, and pulmonary edema
methimazole	Tapazole	Tablet	Hepatotoxicity (rare), arthralgia, agranulocytosis, neuritis, and vertigo
Natural Thyroid Replacement			
(dessicated) thyroid (T_3 and T_4)	Armour Thyroid	Tablet	Hypermetabolic state may be caused only by overdosage
Synthetic Thyroid Replacement			
levothyroxine (thyroxine, T_4)	Levothroid, Synthroid	Injection, tablet	Nervousness, insomnia, arrhythmias, angina pectoris, and hypertension
liothyronine (triiodothyronine, T_3)	Cytomel, Triostat	Injection, tablet	Accelerated rate of bone maturation in children
liotrix (T_3, T_4)	Thyrolar	Tablet	Cardiac arrhythmias, abdominal cramps, weight loss, sweating, and insomnia

TABLE 9–22   Types of Insulin

Insulin Type	Onset of Action	Duration of Action
Rapid-Acting Insulin Analogs		
aspart (Novolog)	5–15 minutes	3–4 hours
glulisine (Apidra)		
lispro (Humalog)		
Longer-Acting Insulin Analog		
glargine (Lantus)	4 hours	24 hours (no peak)
Short-Acting Insulin		
regular insulin (Humulin R, Novolin R, etc.)	30–60 minutes	4–6 hours
Intermediate-Acting Insulins		
isophane insulin suspension (NPH, Humulin N, Novolin N, etc.)	2–4 hours	10–16 hours
insulin zinc suspension (Lente L, Humulin L, Novolin L, etc.)	3–4 hours	12–18 hours
Insulin Mixtures (Short- to Intermediate-Acting)		
NPH 70%/Regular 30% (Humulin 70/30, Novolin 70/30)	30–60 minutes	Up to 36 hours
NPH 50%/Regular 50% (Humulin 50/50)	30–60 minutes	Up to 24 hours

TABLE 9-23 Examples of Oral Hypoglycemic Drugs

Generic Name	Trade Name	Dosage Form	Major Adverse Effects
Sulfonylureas			
First Generation			
chlorpropamide	Diabinese	Tablet	Flushing, photosensitivity, alcohol intolerance, cholestatic jaundice, leucopenia, thrombocytopenia, and hypoglycemia
tolbutamide	Orinase	Tablet	Anorexia, agranulocytosis, aplastic anemia, seizures, and coma
Second Generation			
glimepiride	Amaryl	Tablet	Blurred vision, agranulocytosis, hypoglycemia, and urticaria
glipizide	Glucotrol, Glucotrol XL	Tablet	Hepatic porphyria, hypoglycemia, seizures, and coma
Meglitinides (secretogogues)			
nateglinide	Starlix	Tablet	Back pain, flu-like syndrome, dizziness, hypoglycemia, and upper respiratory infection
repaglinide	Prandin	Tablet	Hypoglycemia, upper respiratory infections, arthralgia, chest pain, and back pain
Biguanides			
metformin	Glucophage, Glucophage XR	Oral solution, tablet	Agitation, lactic acidosis, and bitter or metallic taste
Thiazolidinediones (Glitazones)			
pioglitazone	Actos	Tablet	Edema, exacerbation of heart failure, sinusitis, pharyngitis, and hypoglycemia
rosiglitazone	Avandia	Tablet	Edema, anemia, back pain, exacerbation of heart failure, and increased risk of heart attack
Alpha-Glucosidase Inhibitors			
miglitol	Glyset	Tablet	Abdominal pain, diarrhea, and hypoglycemia

progesterone levels can prevent pregnancy (a popular method of contraception). Oral contraceptives, the most commonly used drugs to prevent pregnancy, include:

1. Estrogen and progestin combinations

2. Progestin-only preparations

Table 9–24 shows some examples of the most commonly used contraceptive agents.

PHARMACOLOGY AND THE DIGESTIVE SYSTEM

The digestive tract is the organ system primarily responsible for food absorption and elimination of solid waste. Absorbed by movement across the lining of the digestive tract into the blood, digested food and its nutrients eventually reach every cell in the body. Many medications are used for different

TABLE 9–24   Examples of Contraceptive Agents

Generic Name	Trade Name	Dosage Form	Major Adverse Effects
Monophasic Agents			
ethinyl estradiol / desogestrel	Desogen, Ortho-Cept	Pill	Hives, stomach pain, symptoms of depression, difficulty breathing, and chest pain
ethinyl estradiol / levonorgestrel	Alesse, Levlen, Nordette	Pill	Hives, difficulty breathing, facial or oral swelling, chest pain, and symptoms of depression
ethinyl estradiol / drospirenone	Yasmin	Pill	Hives, difficulty breathing, facial or oral swelling, chest pain, and symptoms of depression
ethinyl estradiol / norelgestromin	Ortho Evra	Topical patch	Hives, difficulty breathing, facial or oral swelling, chest pain, and symptoms of depression
Biphasic Agents			
ethinyl estradiol / norethindrone	Ortho-Novum 10/11	Pill	Allergic reaction, sudden numbness or weakness, sudden headache, chest pain, and jaundice
Triphasic Agents			
ethinyl estradiol / levonorgestrel	Tri-Levlen, Triphasil	Pill	Allergic reaction, sudden numbness or weakness, sudden headache, chest pain, and symptoms of depression
ethinyl estradiol / norethindrone	Ortho-Novum 7/7/7, Tri-Norinyl	Tablet	Allergic reaction, bleeding, jaundice, symptoms of depression, and vaginal candidiasis
Estrophasic Agents			
ethinyl estradiol / norethindrone	Estrostep	Tablet	Thrombophlebitis, bleeding, jaundice, symptoms of depression, and vaginal candidiasis
Progestin Only Agents			
norethindrone	Micronor, Nor-Q.D.	Tablet	Menstrual irregularity, bleeding, headache, nausea, and hirsuitism
norgestrel	Ovrette	Tablet	Menstrual irregularity, symptoms of depression, skin rash, changes in flow of breast milk, and difficulty breathing
Long-acting Agents			
progesterone	Progestasert	IUD	Menstrual irregularity, infections, fainting, genital sores, and bloody or black stool
levonorgestrel	Mirena	IUD	Menstrual irregularity, pelvic or abdominal pain, ovarian cysts, symptoms of depression, and headache
medroxyprogesterone acetate	Depo-Provera	Injection, suspension	Menstrual irregularity, weakness or fatigue, abdominal pain, headache, and nervousness

disorders of the digestive system. In this chapter, we focus on treatment of peptic ulcer, diarrhea, and constipation.

In general, ulcers occur whenever there is an increase in acid secretion or a decrease in mucosal resistance. Mucosal injury in acid peptic diseases includes gastric ulcer, duodenal ulcer, and gastroesophageal reflux disease, which are mediated by gastric acid.

Antacids

The various types of antacids differ in **cation** content, neutralizing capacity, duration of action, side effects, and cost. When choosing an antacid for therapeutic use, these factors must be considered. Antacids are over-the-counter (OTC) drugs, and some of the common antacids are shown in Table 9–25. The most widely used

antacids are sodium bicarbonate, calcium carbonate, aluminum hydroxide, and magnesium hydroxide.

Histamine Receptor Antagonists

Three types of histamine receptors are available. One of these types mediates acid secretion by gastric parietal cells and is inhibited by the H_2-receptor-blocking drugs. Because of their convenience of use and lack of effect on GI motility, these drugs may be preferred to other antiulcer agents. H_2-receptor antagonists are listed in Table 9–26.

Proton Pump Inhibitors

The final common pathway in gastric acid secretion is the proton pump—an H1/K1-adenosine triphosphatase. The physiological essence of this enzyme is

TABLE 9–25 Examples of Common Antacids

Generic Name	Trade Name	Dosage Form	Major Adverse Effects
aluminum hydroxide	Amphojel	Capsule, suspension, tablet	Constipation, fecal impaction, and intestinal obstruction
calcium carbonate	Tums	Capsule, oral suspension, powder, tablet	Hives, difficulty breathing, facial or oral swelling, nausea, or vomiting
magaldrate	Riopan	Suspension	Hypermagnesemia (in patients with impaired kidney function)
magnesium hydroxide and aluminum hydroxide	Maalox Concentrate	Suspension	Diarrhea, constipation, hypermagnesemia, hypophosphatemia, and osteomalacia
sodium bicarbonate (baking soda)	Neut	IV, tablet	Gastric distention, flatulence, metabolic alkalosis, and electrolyte imbalance

TABLE 9–26 Examples of Histamine (H_2) Receptor Antagonists

Generic Name	Trade Name	Dosage Form	Major Adverse Effects
cimetidine	Tagamet	Injection, tablet	Cardiac arrhythmias and cardiac arrest after rapid IV bolus dose, aplastic anemia, and paranoid psychosis
famotidine	Pepcid	Injection, tablet	Constipation, diarrhea, dry skin, and thrombocytopenia
nizatidine	Axid	Capsule, oral solution, tablet	Sweating and hyperuricemia
ranitidine	Zantac	Capsule, injection, tablet	Mental confusion, insomnia, bradycardia, and thrombocytopenia

TABLE 9–27 Examples of Proton Pump Inhibitors

Generic Name	Trade Name	Dosage Form	Major Adverse Effects
esomeprazole	Nexium	Capsule, injection, powder for oral suspension	Diarrhea, nausea, vomiting, headache, rash, and dizziness
lansoprazole	Prevacid	Capsule, injection, tablet	Fatigue, dizziness, and anorexia
omeprazole	Prilosec	Capsule, powder for oral suspension	Headache, dizziness, hematuria, and proteinuria
rabeprazole	AcipHex	Tablet	Toxic epidermal necrolysis and erythema multiform

the exchange of hydrogen ions for potassium ions. Hence, the parietal cell secretes hydrogen into the gastric lumen in exchange for potassium. Patients should take the proton pump inhibitors before meals because these drugs are more potent when taken orally and before meals. They are also absorbed more effectively in the morning. Examples of proton pump inhibitors are shown in Table 9–27.

Antidiarrheal Agents

The manifestation of many illnesses, diarrhea has many causes, including infections (bacterial, viral, fungal, and parasitic), irritable bowel syndrome, inflammatory bowel disease (ulcerative colitis and Crohn's disease), toxins (food poisoning), drugs, and other causes. Treatment should be focused on the underlying cause.

The use of antidiarrheal agents is occasionally necessary for convenience or for conditions for which there is no primary treatment. The most commonly used antidiarrheals are anticholinergics, opioid narcotics, meperidine congeners (diphenoxylate), and loperamide. Opioid antidiarrheals are the most effective drugs for controlling diarrhea. Selected agents used to treat diarrhea are shown in Table 9–28.

Laxatives and Stool Softeners

Constipation is difficult or infrequent passage of stools. Normal stool frequency ranges from two or three times daily to two or three times per week. Because constipation is a symptom, rather than a disease, a medical evaluation should be undertaken in patients who develop constipation.

Laxatives are drugs that either accelerate fecal passage or decrease fecal consistency. They work by promoting one or more of the mechanisms that cause diarrhea. Because of the wide availability and marketing of OTC laxatives, many patients will probably not seek an appropriate diagnosis. Some examples of laxatives and stool softeners are shown in Table 9–29.

TABLE 9–28 Examples of Antidiarrheal Agents

Generic Name	Trade Name	Dosage Form	Major Adverse Effects
attapulgite	Donnagel	Liquid, tablet	Constipation
bismuth subsalicylate	Pepto-Bismol	Caplet, liquid, tablet	Constipation
diphenoxylate with atropine	Lomotil	Liquid, tablet	Constipation
loperamide	Imodium	Caplet, capsule, liquid	Constipation

TABLE 9–29   Examples of Laxatives and Stool Softeners

Generic Name	Trade Name	Dosage Form	Major Adverse Effects
Bulk-Forming Laxatives			
methylcellulose	Citrucel	Powder, tablet	Nausea, vomiting, and diarrhea
psyllium seed	Metamucil	Powder	Allergic reaction, chest pain, difficulty swallowing, difficulty breathing, and vomiting
Fecal Softener Laxatives			
docusate	Colace, Dialose, Surfak	Capsule, enema, liquid	Diarrhea
Saline and Osmotic Laxatives			
magnesium citrate	Citrate of Magnesia	Solution	Diarrhea
sorbitol	Generic only	Solution	Diarrhea
Stimulant Laxatives			
bisacodyl	Dulcolax	Suppository, tablet	Diarrhea and nausea
senna	Senokot	Granules, syrup, tablet	Allergic reaction, kidney inflammation, poor bowel function, rectal bleeding, and abdominal cramping
Oral Lubricant Laxatives			
mineral oil	Kondremul	Solution	None
Stool Softener			
lactulose	Cephulac	Solution	Diarrhea

ANTIMICROBIAL AGENTS

Pathogenic microorganisms produce infections of different organs or systems of the body. Invading microorganisms include viruses, bacteria, fungi, protozoa, and parasites. The emphasis of this section is on drugs used to treat bacteria, along with some antiviral and antifungal drugs.

Antibacterial Agents

Antibacterial agents are classified in two groups: bactericidal and bacteriostatic. Bactericidal refers to an agent that is capable of killing bacteria, whereas bacteriostatic means that an agent inhibits bacterial growth but does not necessarily kill bacteria. Examples of antibacterial agents are discussed in the following paragraphs.

Beta-Lactam Antibiotics

An antibiotic is one that is derived from a natural, rather than a synthetic, source. The most common sources of antibiotics are molds and other bacteria. Sulfa drugs, although effective for treating many bacterial infections, are not truly antibiotics because they are derived from synthetic sources. Broad-spectrum and having relatively few adverse effects, beta-lactam antibiotics include penicillins, cephalosporins, carbapenems, and monobactams.

Penicillins

One of the first antibiotics developed, penicillins are classified in three groups:

TABLE 9–30   Examples of Common Penicillins

Generic Name	Trade Name	Dosage Form	Major Adverse Effects
Natural Penicillins			
penicillin G potassium	Pfizerpen	Injection	Systemic anaphylaxis, laryngospasm, circulatory collapse, and cardiac arrest
penicillin G benzathine	Permapen	Injection	Anaphylaxis, nephrotoxicity, and hemolytic anemia
penicillin G procaine	Penicillin G Procaine	Injection	Procaine toxicity, unusual tastes, and palpitations
penicillin V potassium	Beepen VK	Oral suspension	Anaphylaxis, hemolytic anemia, and superinfections
Penicillinase-Resistant Penicillins			
cloxacillin	Cloxapen	Oral suspension	Anaphylaxis and superinfections
dicloxacillin	Dycill, Dynapen	Capsule, oral suspension	
nafcillin	Nafcil, Unipen	Injection	
Semisynthetic Penicillins			
amoxicillin	Amoxil, Trimox	Oral suspension, tablet	Hypersensitivity and agranulocytosis
amoxicillin/clavulanate potassium	Augmentin	Tablet (regular, chewable, and extended-release)	Rash, urticaria, and candidal vaginitis
ampicillin	Principen, Ampicillin Sodium	Capsule, injection, oral suspension	Anaphylactoid reaction, hemolytic anemia, and pseudomembranous colitis

1. Natural penicillins
2. Antistaphylococcal penicillins (Penicillinase-resistant)
3. Extended-spectrum penicillins (semisynthetic)

Penicillin allergies can be fatal. All patients should be carefully questioned about their allergy histories before they are administered any drug of this class. Table 9–30 shows examples of common penicillins.

Cephalosporins

Structurally and pharmacologically related to penicillins, cephalosporins are semisynthetic antibiotics and are classified into four different "generations." It is important to understand that a cross-sensitivity exists to cephalosporins for those allergic to penicillins. (Approximately 5% of people allergic to cephalosporins are also allergic to penicillins.) Table 9–31 shows some examples of cephalosporins.

Macrolides

Macrolides are especially useful against respiratory infections, and patients who are allergic to penicillins can usually take any of the macrolides. Table 9–32 shows common macrolides.

Sulfonamides

The first drugs to prevent and cure human bacterial infections successfully, sulfonamides are generally classified as short-acting, intermediate-acting, and long-acting. Hematuria (presence of blood in urine) and crystalluria are two of the major adverse effects of sulfonamide agents, and patients with kidney impairment should use them with caution. To prevent or minimize the risks of renal damage while taking sulfonamides, patients should be advised to take in adequate fluids. See Table 9–33 for examples of sulfonamides.

TABLE 9–31 Examples of Cephalosporins

Generic Name	Trade Name	Dosage Form	Major Adverse Effects
First Generation			
cefadroxil	Duricef	Capsule, oral suspension, tablet	Angioedema and superinfections
cefazolin	Ancef	Injection	Anaphylaxis
cephalexin	Keflex	Capsule, oral suspension, tablet	Anaphylaxis
Second Generation			
cefaclor	Ceclor	Capsule, oral suspension, tablet	Pseudomembranous colitis and superinfections
cefotetan	Cefotan	Injection	Pseudomembranous colitis and superinfections
cefoxitin	Mefoxin	Injection	Pseudomembranous colitis and superinfections
Third Generation			
cefdinir	Omnicef	Capsule, oral suspension	Hematuria and vaginitis
cefoperazone	Cefobid	Injection	Superinfections and pseudomembranous colitis
cefotaxime	Claforan	Injection	Superinfections and pseudomembranous colitis
cefprozil	Cefzil	Oral suspension, tablet	Superinfections and vaginal candidiasis
ceftriaxone	Rocephin	Injection	Superinfections and vaginal candidiasis
Fourth Generation			
cefepime	Maxipime	Injection	Oral moniliasis and vaginitis

TABLE 9–32 Examples of Common Macrolides

Generic Name	Trade Name	Dosage Form	Major Adverse Effects
azithromycin	Zithromax	Injection, oral suspension, tablet	Hepatotoxicity
clarithromycin	Biaxin	Oral suspension, tablet	Diarrhea and abnormal taste
erythromycin	Erythrocin, Ilotycin	Capsule, ointment, tablet, topical solution	Abdominal cramping, superinfections, and ototoxicity
erythromycin ethylsuccinate	E.E.S., EryPed	Oral suspension, tablet	Anorexia and hepatotoxicity

Tetracyclines

Broad-spectrum agents, tetracyclines are effective against certain bacterial strains that are resistant to other antibiotics. Because tetracyclines can combine with iron, calcium, aluminum, and magnesium, which alter the effectiveness of the drug, they should not be given with iron tablets, antacids, or dairy products. Tetracyclines should not be used in children younger than 8 years of age unless other appropriate drugs are ineffective or are contraindicated. When used in this age group, tetracyclines can be absorbed into the bones and teeth, resulting in "mottled" teeth

TABLE 9–33 Examples of Sulfonamides

Generic Name	Trade Name	Dosage Form	Major Adverse Effects
Short-Acting Sulfonamides			
sulfisoxazole	Gantrisin	Ophthalmic ointment, oral suspension, tablet	Allergic reaction, bloody stool, cyanosis, joint pain, and seizures
Intermediate-Acting Sulfonamides			
sulfadiazine	Microsulfon	Tablet	Aplastic anemia, anaphylactoid reactions, crystalluria, and toxic nephrosis
Long-Acting Sulfonamides			
sulfasalazine	Azulfidine	Oral suspension, tablet	Blood dyscrasias, liver injury, and allergic reactions
Combination Sulfonamides			
trimethoprim / sulfamethoxazole	Bactrim, Septra	IV, oral suspension, tablet	Toxic epidermal neurolysis, pseudomembranous enterocolitis, and allergic myocarditis

TABLE 9–34 Examples of Tetracyclines

Generic Name	Trade Name	Dosage Form	Major Adverse Effects
demeclocycline	Declomycin	Capsule, tablet	Pericarditis and anaphylaxis
doxycycline	Vibramycin	Capsule, IV, oral suspension, tablet	Interference with color vision, enterocolitis, and superinfections
minocycline	Minocin	Capsule, IV, oral suspension, tablet	Hepatotoxicity
oxytetracycline	Terramycin	Capsule	Allergic reaction, pericarditis, intracranial hypertension, hemolytic anemia, and inflammatory lesions
tetracycline	Achromycin, Sumycin	Capsule, oral suspension	Jaundice, hyperphosphatemia, acidosis, and irreversible shock

(meaning that they may become spotted or blotched with different colors). Examples of tetracyclines are shown in Table 9–34.

Aminoglycosides

Used primarily for infections caused by gram-negative enterobacteria, aminoglycosides have a toxic potential. They can cause serious adverse effects such as ototoxicity and nephrotoxicity; hence, their use is limited.

Neomycin is the most nephrotoxic aminoglycoside, and streptomycin is the least nephrotoxic. Examples of aminoglycosides are shown in Table 9–35.

Fluoroquinolones

Fluoroquinolones, related to nalidixic acid, may be useful in penicillin-allergic patients. Because of their potential chrondrotoxicity, which is defined as "toxicity of the articular cartilage," fluoroquinolones should

TABLE 9–35 Most Commonly Used Aminoglycosides

Generic Name	Trade Name	Dosage Form	Major Adverse Effects
gentamicin	Garamycin, Genoptic	Cream, IM, IV, ophthalmic	Ototoxicity, optic neuritis, and nephrotoxicity
kanamycin	Kantrex	Injection	Allergic reaction, seizures, hearing or balance changes, changes in urination, and numbness or tingling
neomycin	Mycifradin	Cream, ointment, solution, tablet	Respiratory paralysis, nephrotoxicity, and ototoxicity
streptomycin		Injection	Anaphylactic shock and respiratory depression
tobramycin	Nebcin	Injection, ophthalmic	Neurotoxicity, ototoxicity, and nephrotoxicity

not be taken by children of all ages, up to age 18, or pregnant women. Examples of fluoroquinolones are shown in Table 9–36.

Miscellaneous Antibacterial Agents

Some antibiotics such as chlorampenicol, clindamycin, metronidazole, and vancomycin are classified as miscellaneous antibacterial agents. To prevent a severe drug reaction, patients taking metronidazole must avoid alcohol.

- *Chloramphenicol:* Because of its potential toxicity, bacterial resistance, and the availability of other effective drugs (e.g., cephalosporins), chloramphenicol is not used as widely as it once was.

- *Clindamycin:* Clindamycin is effective against many organisms found on the skin and in the mouth. However, it has marked toxicity.

- *Metronidazole:* Metronidazole is the most effective antibiotic against anaerobic bacteria (bacteria that grow without oxygen) that cause infections primarily in the abdomen and vagina.

- *Vancomycin:* Vancomycin can destroy most gram-positive organisms and is also useful for treating infections in patients who are allergic to penicillin. Vancomycin is usually given intravenously. It should be well diluted and given slowly. A reaction, referred to as *red man syndrome*, may occur if the drug is given

TABLE 9–36 Examples of Fluoroquinolones

Generic Name	Trade Name	Dosage Form	Major Adverse Effects
cinoxacin	Cinobac	Capsule	Blood in urine or stool, unusual bleeding or bruising, seizures, bone pain, and joint pain
ciprofloxacin	Cipro	Injection, ophthalmic, oral suspension, tablet	Tendon rupture, cartilage erosion, and vertigo
gatifloxacin	Zymar	Ophthalmic solution, tablet	Abnormal dreams, insomnia, vaginitis, and abnormal vision
lomefloxacin	Maxaquin	Tablet	Peripheral neuropathy and risk of tendon rupture (rare)
norfloxacin	Noroxin	Tablet	Joint swelling, cartilage erosion, tendonitis, and leukopenia
ofloxacin	Floxin	IV, ophthalmic, and tablet	Allergic reaction, bloody diarrhea, seizures, hallucinations, and easy bruising or bleeding

too rapidly. Flushing and/or a rash affecting the face, neck, and upper torso characterize this syndrome. It may also cause hypotension and angioedema (rapid swelling of the skin, mucosa, and submucosal tissues).

Antiviral Agents

Influencing viral replication, antivirals are used to treat viral infections. The majority of antiviral drugs are active against only one type of virus, either the DNA or the RNA type. DNA viruses include:

- Herpes simplex virus (HSV) 1 and 2
- Varicella-zoster virus (VZV)
- Cytomegalovirus (CMV)
- Influenza A virus

Table 9–37 shows some examples of antiviral agents that are currently approved for the treatment of DNA viruses.

RNA viruses include:

- Picornavirus (polio)
- Rhabdovirus (rabies)
- Paramyxovirus (mumps and measles)
- Retrovirus (HIV)

Most patients with the HIV infection are receiving combination therapy with different antiviral agents.

Presently, four classes of antiretroviral agents effective against HIV-1 and HIV-2 have been approved. They include:

1. Nucleoside reverse transcriptase inhibitors (NRTIs)
2. Non-nucleoside reverse transcriptase inhibitors (NNRTIs)
3. Protease inhibitors (PIs)
4. Fusion inhibitors (FIs)

Table 9–38 shows examples of HIV antiviral agents.

Highly Active Antiretroviral Therapy (HAART)

Antiviral agents are being used currently either alone, or in combination, for the treatment of HIV infection. HAART has been shown to offer the following effects:

- Reducing viral load
- Increasing CD4 lymphocytes in persons infected with HIV
- Delaying the onset of AIDS
- Prolonging the survival of patients with AIDS

HAART involves the combination of three to four drugs that are effective against HIV. Two distinct categories of drugs are combined: nucleoside analogs and protease inhibitors.

TABLE 9–37   Antivirals for the Treatment of DNA Viruses

Generic Name	Trade Name	Dosage Form	Major Adverse Effects
acyclovir	Zovirax	Capsule, IV, ointment, oral suspension, tablet	Acute renal failure and thrombocytopenia
amantadine	Symmetrel	Capsule, syrup	Orthostatic hypotension, insomnia, confusion, and leukopenia
famciclovir	Famvir	Tablet	Somnolence and anorexia
ganciclovir	Cytovene	Capsule, powder for injection	Confusion, coma, and bone marrow suppression
rimantadine	Flumadine	Syrup, tablet	Dizziness, drowsiness, and dry mouth
valacyclovir	Valtrex	Tablet	Mood changes, lack of appetite, tiredness, difficulty in concentrating and/or sleeping
zanamivir	Relenza	Inhalant	Dizziness, bronchitis, and cough

TABLE 9–38   Examples of HIV Antiviral Agents

Generic Name	Trade Name	Dosage Form	Major Adverse Effects
NRTIs			
abacavir (ABC)	Ziagen	Solution, tablet	Malaise, myalgia, shortness of breath, hypotension, and hepatomegaly
didanosine (DDI)	Videx, Videx EC	Capsule, powder, tablet	Arrhythmias, insomnia, seizures, photophobia, and pancreatitis
lamivudine (3TC)	Epivir	Solution, tablet	Hepatomegaly, myalgia, and lactic acidosis
stavudine (d4T)	Zerit	Capsule, powder	Peripheral neuropathy, pancreatitis, and myalgia
zalcitabine (ddC)	Hivid	Tablet	Peripheral neuropathy, abnormal hepatic function, fatigue, skin rash, and nausea/vomiting
zidovudine (AZT)	Retrovir	Capsules, IV, syrup	Insomnia, agitation, bone marrow depression, granulocytopenia, and anemia
NNRTIs			
delavirdine (DLV)	Rescriptor	Capsule, tablet	Allergic reaction, arthralgia, neutropenia, and chest pain
efavirenz (EFZ)	Sustiva	Capsule	Insomnia, hypercholesterolemia, erythema multiforme, and toxic epidermal necrolysis
nevirapine (NVP)	Viramune	Capsule, tablet	Hepatotoxicity and myalgia
PIs			
amprenavir	Agenerase	Capsule, oral solution	Peripheral paresthesia, depression, taste disorders, and hyperglycemia
indinavir (IDV)	Crixivan	Capsule	Insomnia, fatigue, anxiety, splenomegaly, and anemia
nelfinavir (NFV)	Viracept	Powder, tablet	Anorexia, GI bleeding, pancreatitis, and anemia
ritonavir (RTV)	Norvir	Capsule, oral solution	Nausea/vomiting, diarrhea, asthenia, taste disorders, and peripheral paresthesia
FIs			
enfuvirtide	Fuzeon	Injection	Hypersensitivity reactions, depression, insomnia, and pancreatitis

Antifungal Agents

Antifungals are often used to treat systemic, local, and topical fungal infections. Some examples of antifungal drugs are listed in Table 9–39.

PHARMACOLOGY AND THE MUSCULOSKELETAL SYSTEM

Some of the most common disorders in humans at any age are those affecting the musculoskeletal system. Pain or inflammation of the muscles or joints is common. Acetylcholine can be released at the neuromuscular junction for contraction of skeletal muscles, and in some conditions, causes spasms and pain.

Muscle Relaxants

Skeletal muscle relaxants work by blocking somatic motor nerve impulses through depression of specific neurons within the CNS. These drugs are called **neuromuscular blocking agents**, which prevent muscles from moving. These drugs have no effect on pain or level of consciousness. Examples of these agents are listed in Table 9–40.

TABLE 9–39 Examples of Antifungal Agents

Generic Name	Trade Name	Dosage Form	Major Adverse Effects
amphotericin B	Amphocin, Fungizone	Cream, lotion, ointment, powder for injection, suspension	Anaphylaxis reaction, cardiac arrest, nephrotoxicity, hypokalemia, and hypotension
butenafine	Mentax	Cream	Contact dermatitis, erythema, and itching
ciclopirox	Loprox, Penlac Nail Lacquer	Cream, nail lacquer, ointment, shampoo	Irritation, pruritus, and burning
fluconazole	Diflucan	Injection, suspension, tablet	Headache, abdominal pain, and diarrhea
flucytosine	Ancobon	Capsule	Confusion, hallucinations, anemia, leucopenia, and agranulocytosis
griseofulvin	Fulvicin-U/F	Capsule, tablet	Hypersensitivity, severe headache, insomnia, confusion, decreased or unpleasant taste, nephrotoxicity, and hepatotoxicity
ketoconazole	Nizoral	Cream, gel, shampoo, tablet	Anaphylaxis, fatal hepatic necrosis (rare), gynecomastia, and renal hypofunction
nystatin	Mycostatin, Nilstat	Cream, ointment, oral suspension, powder, tablet	Nausea, vomiting, and epigastric distress

TABLE 9–40 Examples of Neuromuscular Blocking Agents

Generic Name	Trade Name	Dosage Form	Major Adverse Effects
Short Duration			
succinylcholine	Anectine, Quelicin, Sucostrin	Injection	Hypotension or hypertension, respiratory depression, apnea, and malignant hyperthermia
Intermediate Duration			
atracurium	Tracrium	Injection	Arrhythmia, respiratory depression, and increased salivation
cisatracurium	Nimbex	Injection	Bradycardia, hypotension, flushing, and bronchospasm
Extended Duration			
mivacurium	Mivacron	Injection	Hypotension, flushing of the face, neck, and chest

Another group of skeletal muscle relaxants is used orally for painful muscle conditions. These agents are called centrally acting skeletal muscle relaxants. Some examples of these drugs are listed in Table 9–41.

Analgesics, Antipyretics, and Anti-inflammatory Drugs

Some pain is relieved with opioid analgesics; other pain, with nonopioid analgesics. Many of the nonopioid analgesics affect pain, fever, and inflammation, depending on their properties (see Tables 9–42, 9–43, and 9–44). Fever-reducing medications, antipyretics, include acetaminophen, aspirin, and ibuprofen. They are designed to lower body temperature while treating the underlying cause of the fever. Available in various dosages and concentrations, some antipyretics, are specially designed for infants and children; others, designed more for adults.

TABLE 9–41   Examples of Centrally Acting Skeletal Muscle Relaxants

Generic Name	Trade Name	Dosage Form	Major Adverse Effects
baclofen	Kemstro, Lioresal	Injection, tablet	Vertigo, insomnia, tinnitus, blurred vision, diplopia, and nystagmus
carisoprodol	Rela, Soma	Tablet	Anaphylactic shock, postural hypotension, drowsiness, tremor, syncope, and insomnia
chlorzoxazone	Paraflex	Tablet	Drowsiness, malaise, rash, and pruritus
cyclobenzaprine	Cycloflex, Flexeril	Tablet	Edema of tongue, face sweating, hepatitis, alopecia, syncope, and orthostatic hypotension
diazepam	Valium	Injection, oral solution, rectal gel, tablet	Amnesia, slurred speech, hypotension, and cardiovascular collapse

TABLE 9–42   Examples of Anti-inflammatory and Analgesic Agent Salicylates

Generic Name	Trade Name	Dosage Form	Major Adverse Effects
aspirin	Bayer Aspirin, Ecotrin	Suppository, varied tablets	Bronchospasm, anaphylactic shock, drowsiness, hearing loss, occult bleeding, and hemolytic anemia
magnesium salicylate	Magan, Mobidin	Caplet, tablet	Dizziness, tinnitus, hearing loss, nausea, and vomiting
mesalamine	Asacol, Pentasa	Capsule, tablet	Weakness, dizziness, abdominal pain, pruritus, and alopecia
salsalate	Artha-G, Salsitab	Tablet	Heartburn, GI bleeding, tinnitus, hearing loss, hyperventilation, and sweating
sulfasalazine	Azulfidine	Tablet	Bloody diarrhea, anorexia, arthralgia, blood dyscrasias, and allergic reactions

TABLE 9–43   Examples of Nonsalicylate Anti-inflammatory and Analgesic Agents (NSAIDs)

Generic Name	Trade Name	Dosage Form	Major Adverse Effects
diclofenac	Cataflam, Solaraze, Voltaren	Tablet	Tinnitus, abdominal pain, peptic ulcer, hypertension, joint pain, hyperglycemia, and prolonged bleeding time
ibuprofen	Advil, Motrin, Rufen	Drops, oral suspension, tablet	Anxiety, emotional instability, drowsiness, hypertension, peripheral edema, blurred vision, gingival ulcerations, abdominal pain, and hemolytic or aplastic anemia
indomethacin	Indocin, Indocin SR	Capsule, injection, oral suspension, suppositories	Hypersensitivity, syncope, insomnia, nightmares, confusion, and coma
meclofenamate	Meclomen	Capsule	Dizziness, tinnitus, peptic ulceration, GI bleeding, blurred vision, and kidney failure
meloxicam	Mobic	Tablet	Ulceration, GI bleeding, dizziness, pharyngitis, and pruritus

TABLE 9–44   Examples of Second-Line Agents for Rheumatoid Arthritis

Generic Name	Trade Name	Dosage Form	Major Adverse Effects
auranofin	Ridaura	Capsule	Thrombocytopenia, leucopenia, agranulocytosis, aplastic anemia, and renal failure
gold sodium thiomalate	Myochrysine	Injection	Bradycardia, hepatitis, metallic taste, agranulocytosis, aplastic anemia, glomerulitis, and pulmonary fibrosis
methotrexate	Amethopterin, Rheumatrex	Injection, tablet	Hepatotoxicity, hepatic cirrhosis, glossitis, and GI ulcerations

Anti-inflammatory drugs are classified into two groups: corticosteroids and nonsteroidal anti-inflammatory drugs (NSAIDs). They include aspirin and ibuprofen, which are widely prescribed for mild to moderate inflammation. NSAIDs block inflammation by inhibiting cyclooxygenase (COX).

EXPLORING THE WEB

Visit http://www.familydoctor.org for information about antacids.

Visit http://www.cypharmacology.com for more information on antianginal drugs.

Visit http://allergyandasthmarelief.org to learn more about antihistamines.

Visit http://www.spinal-health.com for more information about muscle relaxants.

Visit http://www.pharmacology2000.com to learn more about pharmacology and the endocrine system.

Visit http://www.endocrineweb.com to learn more about the role of the thyroid gland.

Visit http://www.rxlist.com to learn which drugs made the Top 200 Drugs List.

REVIEW QUESTIONS

1. Which drug is used for the treatment of Parkinson's disease?

   A. phenytoin
   B. amantadine
   C. lithium
   D. morphine

2. What is the trade name of alprazolam?

   A. BuSpar
   B. Ativan
   C. Serax
   D. Xanax

3. Which agent is a loop diuretic?

   A. methimazole (Tapazole)
   B. diltiazem (Cardizem)
   C. nadolol (Corgard)
   D. furosemide (Lasix)

4. Which agent is an anticonvulsant?

   A. carbamazepine
   B. estazolam
   C. levodopa
   D. perphenazine

5. Conventional antipsychotics act by blocking the action of which of the following neurotransmitters?

   A. dopamine
   B. serotonin
   C. acetylcholine
   D. all of the above

6. The generic name of Demerol is:

   A. hydrocodone
   B. meperidine
   C. pentazocine
   D. propoxyphene

7. Which symptom signifies stage III of general anesthesia?

   A. euphoria
   B. delirium
   C. surgical anesthesia
   D. cessation of respiration

8. Which agent is used for the treatment of thyroid gland disorders?

   A. glipizide
   B. metformin
   C. norgestrel
   D. potassium iodide

9. Which agent is a beta-adrenergic blocker?

   A. nadolol
   B. nitroglycerin
   C. diltiazem
   D. nifedipine

10. The trade name of verapamil is:

    A. Edecrin
    B. Diachlor
    C. Calan
    D. Hygroton

11. All of these agents are examples of aminoglycosides, except:

    A. gentamicin
    B. nafcillin
    C. neomycin
    D. kamikacin

12. Which drug is an antiviral?

    A. ciclopirox
    B. mupirocin
    C. amphotericin B
    D. amantadine

13. Fluconazole is classified as an:

    A. antifungal
    B. antiviral
    C. antihypertensive
    D. immunosuppressant

14. Typical antipsychotics are thought to act by blocking the action of which neurotransmitter?

    A. dopamine
    B. acetylcholine
    C. serotonin
    D. A and C

15. What is the trade name of diazepam?

    A. Prosom
    B. Ativan
    C. Valium
    D. Xanax

Safety in the Workplace

OUTLINE

GLOSSARY

Barrier precautions – types of personal protective equipment (PPE) used to minimize risk of exposure

Biohazard symbol – an image or object that serves as an alert that there is a risk such as ionizing radiation or harmful bacteria or viruses to organisms

Exposure control plan – a written procedure for the treatment of persons exposed to biohazardous or similar chemically harmful materials

Fire safety plan – a written procedure that includes fire extinguisher locations, fire alarm pull-box locations, sprinkler system location, exit signs, and clear directions to the quickest and safest way to exit a building during an emergency

Hazard communication plan – a plan that informs employees about all hazardous materials found in the workplace; it should outline employee training and an exposure control plan, should list locations of any existing hazards, and should explain hazard signs and chemical labels, especially the use and location of personal protective equipment and how to handle various types of spills

Laminar airflow hood – a system of circulating filtered air in parallel-flowing planes in hospitals or other health-care facilities; reduces the risk of airborne contamination and exposure to chemical pollutants in surgical theaters, food preparation areas, hospital pharmacies, and laboratories

Personal protective equipment – gloves, gowns, face shields, goggles, laboratory coats, and masks used to protect against blood, bodily fluids, and microorganisms

Standard precautions – a set of guidelines for infection control

SAFETY

Safety issues are present in any place, and employees need to take practical precautions in the workplace, particularly in the pharmacy. The purpose of environmental protection measures is to minimize the risk of occupational injury by isolating or removing any physical or mechanical health hazards in any workplace. In 1970, the federal government passed the Occupational Safety and Health Act, the first national heath and safety law, with the goal of ensuring safe and healthful working conditions for all workers in the United States. The act established the Occupational Safety and Health Administration (OSHA) in the Department of Labor. OSHA establishes safety regulations for employers and monitors compliance.

Occupational Safety and Health Administration Standards

Part of the Department of Labor, OSHA establishes standards requiring employers to provide their workers with workplaces free from recognized hazards that could cause serious injury or death. In addition, employees must abide by all safety and health standards that apply to their jobs. OSHA regulates all workplace environments by enforcing protocols for the proper removal of hazards and for observance of fire safety and emergency plans. Table 10–1 outlines some of the safety practices pharmacy technicians must follow in the workplace.

Two specific functions related to the pharmacy, specifically the hospital pharmacy, are protection of employees from exposure to disease and protection of their exposure to chemicals. OSHA has the right to inspect private and public worksites to ensure that all protocols and guidelines are being followed. The employee's general health must be protected, and many standards require plans, training of employees, and monitoring of injuries with detailed records. In addition, the employer must provide general protective equipment (such as fire extinguishers and first-aid kits), as well as specialized protective equipment as needed. OSHA provides for research, information, education, and training in the field of occupational safety and health and authorized enforcement of OSHA standards.

TABLE 10–1 Safety Practices in the Workplace

Safety Concern	Instructions
Body surfaces	If exposed body surfaces come into contact with body fluids, scrub with soap and water as soon as possible.
Decontamination	Decontaminate test materials before reprocessing or place them in impervious bags and dispose of them according to policy.
Eyes	If the eyes are exposed to body fluids, flush them with water, preferably using an eyewash station.
Food and drinks	Do not keep food and drink inside refrigerators, freezers, shelves, or cabinets, on countertops where blood or other potentially hazardous chemical materials could be present.
Gloving	Bandage any breaks or lesions on the hands before gloving.
Hemostats	Use hemostats to attach and remove scalpel blades from handles.
Labeling	Observe warning labels on biohazard containers and equipment.
Sharps	Do not recap, bend, or break contaminated needles and other sharps.
Splashes	Minimize splashing, spraying, and splattering of potentially harmful chemicals or infectious materials. Splattering of blood onto skin or mucous membranes is a proven mode of transmission of hepatitis B virus.
Tubing	Do not use mouth pipetting or suck blood or other harmful chemicals through tubing.

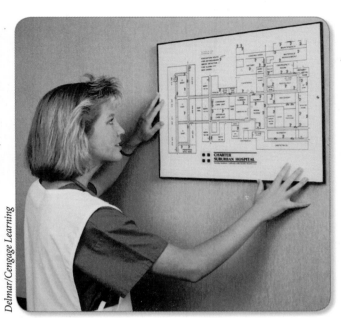

Delmar/Cengage Learning

Figure 10–1 Fire safety (emergency) plans should include clearly posted and marked escape routes.

Fire Safety Plan

An OSHA-compliant fire safety plan must include written procedures. Exits must be marked and escape routes published (see Figure 10–1). Fire safety plans, which are sometimes referred to as *Fire Safety Emergency Plans*, must include information about smoke detectors, fire alarms, pull boxes, fire doors, fire escapes, and sprinkler systems. Instructions for using all of these devices must be included as well. Employers must train employees on the correct procedures to take in case of a fire or other emergency.

Electrical Safety

If not handled correctly, electricity is capable of causing severe injury to employees and other people in the workplace. Electrical equipment must be properly grounded at all times. When being repaired, electrical equipment must be unplugged before work begins. Electrical cords and plugs must be checked for exposed wires or "frays" in cords. Because of the potential fire hazard, electrical circuits must never be overloaded. Extension cords should be avoided to reduce potential electrical safety hazards, as well as to prevent people from tripping over them.

Hazard Communication Standard

OSHA's *Hazard Communication Standard* ensures that employees and employers receive information on the hazardous chemicals they may encounter in the workplace. These chemicals may include chlorine bleach, cleaning supplies, disinfectants, and other products. Other hazards include electrical equipment, glassware, and pharmacy instruments. All hazards must be communicated in a hazard communication plan.

Hazard Communication Plan

A hazard communication plan protects the rights of employees by informing them about all hazardous materials found in the workplace. In addition to outlining employee training, as well as employees' responsibilities about working with hazardous materials, the plan should also outline an exposure control plan, including the posting of safety signs throughout the facility. The hazard communication plan should list locations of material safety data sheets, hazard-related information, and any existing hazards. Also, the plan should explain hazard signs and chemical labels, the use and location of personal protective equipment, and how to handle various types of spills.

Inventory of Products

An inventory of potentially hazardous materials must be included in a hazard communication plan. Every product identified on the list must have a material safety data sheet (MSDS). Common products that may be listed include inks, cleaners, glues, oil products, silicone lubricants, controlled substances, toner, alcohols, gases, chemotherapeutic agents and radio-pharmaceuticals. OSHA considers many drugs to be hazardous, including ethinyl estradiol, interferon-A, methotrexate, vinblastine, and others.

Labeling Hazardous Materials

Manufacturers are required to properly label all of their products, and these products must retain legible, intact labels while stored in the workplace (see Figure 10–2). Each label should identify the chemical, its hazard warnings, and the name and address

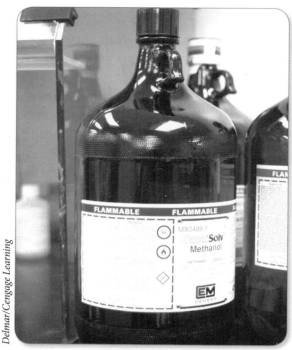

Delmar/Cengage Learning

Figure 10–2 Hazardous materials should bear labels indicating potential danger if they come into contact with personnel.

of the manufacturer. Hazardous products must be kept inside their original containers, and health-care facilities must store all chemicals in locked cupboards.

Material Safety Data Sheet

A *material safety data sheet (MSDS)* is a document outlining a chemical substance's structure. In identifying the potential hazards of the substance, the MSDS must include the chemical name, common name, chemical composition, substance characteristics, substance hazards, guidelines for safe handling and disposal, and guidelines for emergency procedures. Employers must maintain an accurate, up-to-date MSDS for each hazardous chemical in their facilities, and employees must have access to this information.

Bloodborne Pathogen Standard

The *Bloodborne Pathogen Standard* was designed to reduce occupational-related cases of HIV and HBV infections among health-care workers. All employees who can be "reasonably anticipated" to come into contact with blood, body fluids, and other potentially infectious materials are covered. The standard seeks to limit their exposure to these bloodborne pathogens.

Exposure Control Plan

Designed to minimize risk of exposure to infectious material and bloodborne disease, the exposure control plan must be written and updated as necessary. OSHA also has regulations for or provides information about hazards associated with radioactive materials, use of lasers, and latex allergies.

Exposure Determination

Exposure control plans must define employee risks in three levels, as follows:

- I – exposure anticipated when normally performing the job (such as by physicians or nurses)
- II – occasional exposure anticipated when normally performing the job (such as by pharmacists or pharmacy technicians)
- III – no exposure anticipated when normally performing the job

Standard Precautions

A set of guidelines for infection control, standard precautions require employers and employees to assume that all human blood and specified human body fluids are infectious for human immunodeficiency virus (HIV), hepatitis B virus, and other bloodborne pathogens (Figure 10–3). Employees must use standard precautions for blood, other body fluids containing visible blood, semen, vaginal secretions, cerebrospinal fluid, pleural fluid, synovial fluid, and any other body fluids. A health-care worker must undertake proper disposal of hazardous waste containers, which are marked. OSHA regulations require that all health-care workers be immunized against hepatitis B because they are at risk for infection from bloodborne pathogens.

Personal Protective Equipment

Many medical employees use personal protective equipment (PPE) as a barrier between them and

STANDARD PRECAUTIONS

Assume that every person is potentially infected or colonized with an organism that could be transmitted in the healthcare setting.

Hand Hygiene

Avoid unnecessary touching of surfaces in close proximity to the patient.

When hands are visibly dirty, contaminated with proteinaceous material, or visibly soiled with blood or body fluids, wash hands with soap and water.

If hands are not visibly soiled, or after removing visible material with soap and water, decontaminate hands with an alcohol-based hand rub. Alternatively, hands may be washed with an antimicrobial soap and water.

Perform hand hygiene:
  Before having direct contact with patients.
  After contact with blood, body fluids or excretions, mucous membranes, nonintact skin, or wound dressings.
  After contact with a patient's intact skin (e.g., when taking a pulse or blood pressure or lifting a patient).
  If hands will be moving from a contaminated-body site to a clean-body site during patient care.
  After contact with inanimate objects (including medical equipment) in the immediate vicinity of the patient.
  After removing gloves.

Personal protective equipment (PPE)

Wear PPE when the nature of the anticipated patient interaction indicates that contact with blood or body fluids may occur.

Before leaving the patient's room or cubicle, remove and discard PPE.

Gloves

Wear gloves when contact with blood or other potentially infectious materials, mucous membranes, nonintact skin, or potentially contaminated intact skin (e.g., of a patient incontinent of stool or urine) could occur.

Remove gloves after contact with a patient and/or the surrounding environment using proper technique to prevent hand contamination. Do not wear the same pair of gloves for the care of more than one patient.

Change gloves during patient care if the hands will move from a contaminated body-site (e.g., perineal area) to a clean body-site (e.g., face).

Gowns

Wear a gown to protect skin and prevent soiling or contamination of clothing during procedures and patient-care activities when contact with blood, body fluids, secretions, or excretions is anticipated.

Wear a gown for direct patient contact if the patient has uncontained secretions or excretions.

Remove gown and perform hand hygiene before leaving the patient's environment.

Mouth, nose, eye protection

Use PPE to protect the mucous membranes of the eyes, nose and mouth during procedures and patient-care activities that are likely to generate splashes or sprays of blood, body fluids, secretions and excretions.

During aerosol-generating procedures wear one of the following: a face shield that fully covers the front and sides of the face, a mask with attached shield, or a mask and goggles.

Respiratory Hygiene/Cough Etiquette

Educate healthcare personnel to contain respiratory secretions to prevent droplet and fomite transmission of respiratory pathogens, especially during seasonal outbreaks of viral respiratory tract infections.

Offer masks to coughing patients and other symptomatic persons (e.g., persons who accompany ill patients) upon entry into the facility.

Patient-care equipment and instruments/devices

Wear PPE (e.g., gloves, gown), according to the level of anticipated contamination, when handling patient-care equipment and instruments/devices that are visibly soiled or may have been in contact with blood or body fluids.

Care of the environment

Include multi-use electronic equipment in policies and procedures for preventing contamination and for cleaning and disinfection, especially those items that are used by patients, those used during delivery of patient care, and mobile devices that are moved in and out of patient rooms frequently (e.g., daily).

Textiles and laundry

Handle used textiles and fabrics with minimum agitation to avoid contamination of air, surfaces and persons.

SPR   ©2007 Brevis Corporation www.brevis.com

Figure 10–3 Standard Precautions. *(Courtesy of BREVIS Corporation)*

blood or bodily fluids, while pharmacy technicians use PPE to protect the sterile environment during IV compounding from sloughing skin, hair, or other type of contamination. **Barrier precautions**, such as gloves, gowns, face shields, goggles, laboratory coats, shoe covers, and masks help to protect sterile IV medications against contamination from dangerous microorganisms (see Figure 10-4). In addition, eye wash stations are required in workplaces for emergency situations. Using these stations, employees can flush out their eyes or mucous membranes with water immediately after exposure to blood, bodily fluids, or chemicals (see Figure 10–5). Eye wash stations are designed to allow the rinsing of the eye for a minimum of 15 minutes after contact with a potentially harmful substance.

Latex Allergy

Made from Brazilian rubber trees, latex may cause some people to experience an allergic response to the proteins it contains. These reactions consist of allergic or irritant contact dermatitis and, in rare cases, immediate systemic hypersensitivity. Approximately 8% to 12% of health-care workers have a latex allergy; so nonlatex gloves have been created. Also available are powder-free, low-allergen latex gloves that are less likely to produce allergic responses.

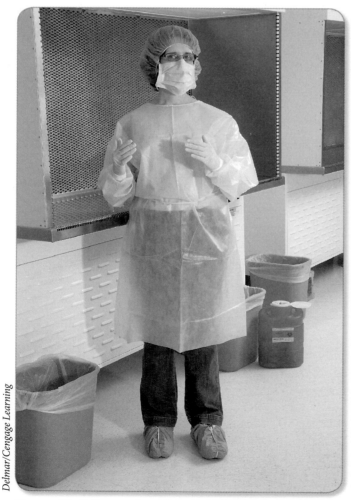

Delmar/Cengage Learning

Figure 10–4 Personal protective equipment is used to protect the sterile environment during IV compounding.

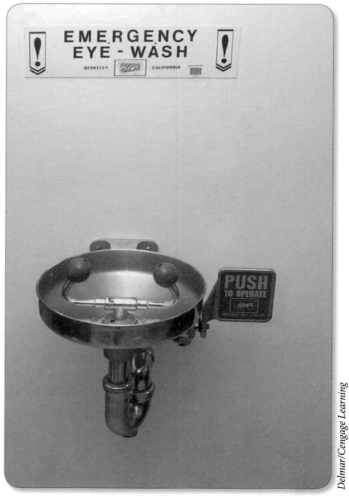

Delmar/Cengage Learning

Figure 10–5 Eye wash stations should be located in any workplace where potentially harmful chemicals and substances are used.

Safe Handling of Cytotoxic and Hazardous Medications

The exposure hazard for nuclear pharmacy technicians or pharmacy technicians that prepare chemotherapeutic medications can be very dangerous. Exposure to radiation can be minimized by increasing distances between radiopharmaceuticals and personnel, decreasing contact times, using film badges to monitor exposure, following proper labeling of radioactive materials, and using appropriate radiation shields. Figure 10–6 shows a film badge used to monitor radiation levels.

When working with chemotherapeutic medications, proper PPE should be worn to not only protect the sterility of the IV drug, but to protect the pharmacy technician from these hazardous agents. The compounding of IV chemotherapeutic medication is similar to the compounding of non-chemotherapeutic medication, but must always be performed in a vertical laminar airflow hood instead of a horizontal airflow hood. A technician should always have proper, thorough training before working with cytotoxic and hazardous medications.

Cleaning Up a Spill

Spill cleanup kits are available for all pharmacies and health-care facilities where potentially harmful substances are used (see Figure 10–7). Ordinary paper

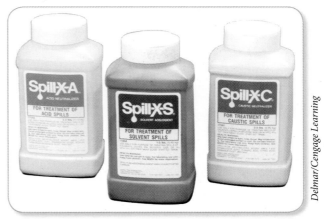

Figure 10–7 Spill cleanup kits are used for various types of spills, and contain special formulations of substances designed for specific types of cleanups.

towels should not be used to clean up potentially harmful substance spills. Spill cleanup kits have specifically designed substances that absorb and neutralize dangerous substances of varying types. For blood spills, bleach is recommended to kill any pathogens that may be present. For extremely toxic spills, a specially trained hazardous cleanup team should handle them.

Disposing of Hazardous Waste

Any materials that have come into contact with blood or body fluids are treated as hazardous waste. For collection of hazardous materials, waste containers are labeled with the biohazard symbol to ensure that all employees are aware of the contents (see Figure 10–8). Plastic bags are used for gloves,

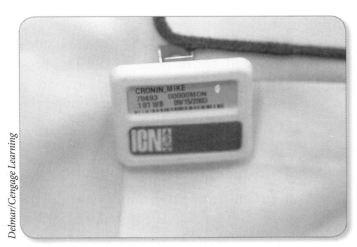

Figure 10–6 A film badge used to monitor radiation exposure.

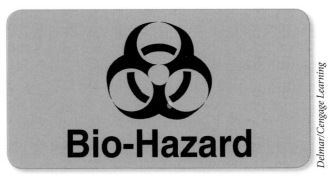

Figure 10–8 Biohazard symbols will appear on containers used to dispose of contaminated waste.

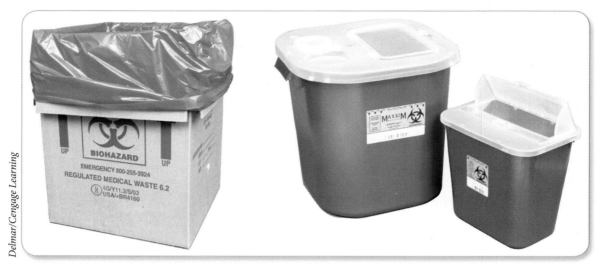

Delmar/Cengage Learning

Figure 10–9 Red plastic biohazard bags are used to dispose of gloves, contaminated gowns, and bedding; hard plastic sharps containers are used to dispose of needles, glass slides, and scalpel blades.

paper towels, dressings, and other soft material; rigid containers, for sharps such as needles, glass slides, scalpel blades, or disposable syringes (see Figure 10–9). Most facilities contract with a company that specializes in removal and disposal of hazardous waste. Cleaning staff should be instructed not to empty hazardous waste containers. When changing hazardous waste bags, health-care workers must wear gloves, masks, and protective eyewear; close the bags securely; and put the bag inside a second hazardous waste bag (double bag) if there is any chance of leakage.

Any expired, unused, spilled, or contaminated pharmaceutical product is pharmaceutical waste. Among these products are drugs, vaccines, and other substances that are no longer required. Additional pharmaceutical waste products include bottles and boxes with residues, gloves, masks, tubing, and vials. According to each state's hazardous waste disposal guidelines, pharmaceutical waste must be disposed of properly. The U.S. Environmental Protection Agency has published guidelines for pharmaceutical waste. They can be found at: http://edocket.access.gpo.gov/2008/pdf/E8-28161.pdf.

CLEAN AIR ENVIRONMENTS

A *clean room* is defined as a specific area that allows no more than 3,500 airborne particles, of no larger than 0.5 microns each, per square meter of air. "Clean" or "critical" room environments are commonly classified as "Class 100" or "Grade A." Parenteral products are regularly prepared in clean air environments, where the air is rapidly cycled through at between 90 and 100 feet per minute. The air first passes through a pre-filter and then is electrostatically charged. After this step, it goes through a high-efficiency particulate air (HEPA) filter. Strict control is maintained of air conditioning and humidity, and a positive air pressure is maintained, meaning that air outside the clean room is of lower pressure and, therefore, kept out by the higher pressure within the clean room.

Clean Rooms

In a clean room, air quality, humidity, and temperature are highly regulated to reduce risks of cross-contamination. The air in a clean room is repeatedly filtered to remove impurities such as dust and other particulates. Clean rooms, discussed in more detail in Chapter 15, provide safe areas for sterile compounding.

Laminar Airflow Hoods

A laminar airflow hood is a piece of equipment designed for the handling of materials whenever a sterile working environment is required. This device uses a system of circulating filtered air in parallel flow planes. This flowing air, called *laminar*, allows for safe and sterile compounding in a controlled work area. Various types of laminar airflow hoods will be discussed in detail in Chapter 15.

ASEPTIC TECHNIQUE

The most effective way to eliminate transmission of disease from one host to another is through asepsis, which means "sterile" (free from microorganisms). There are two types of asepsis: medical asepsis and surgical asepsis, which will be discussed in detail in Chapter 15.

EMPLOYEE RESPONSIBILITIES

Employee responsibilities concerning safety in the workplace include:

- Reading the OSHA poster at the job site

- Complying with all applicable OSHA standards
- Following all employer safety and health rules and regulations and wearing or using required protective equipment while working
- Reporting hazardous conditions to the supervisor
- Reporting any job-related injury or illness to the employer and seeking prompt treatment
- Cooperating with OSHA compliance officers conducting an inspection if they inquire about safety and health conditions in the workplace
- Exercising rights under the OSHA act in a responsible manner

EXPLORING THE WEB

Visit http://www.cdc.gov; the Centers for Disease Control and Prevention (CDC) features a link on "Workplace Safety & Health."

Visit http://www.dol.gov; the U.S. Department of Labor (DOL) also has a link on "Workplace Safety & Health."

Visit http://www.epa.gov; you can learn more about current environmental issues and concerns on the Environmental Protection Agency's (EPA) site.

Visit http://www.osha.gov; among other topics, the Occupational Safety and Health Administration (OSHA) site has information about job hazard analyses, bloodborne pathogens, and hazard communications.

REVIEW QUESTIONS

1. Which form is used to identify the potential hazards of a substance?

    A. MSDS
    B. OSHA
    C. HIPAA
    D. PPE

2. Clean room environments are commonly classified as:

    A. Grade A
    B. Grade B
    C. Grade C
    D. Grade D

3. Which statement is false about workplace safety?

    A. Employers must train employees on the correct procedures to take in case of a fire or other emergency.
    B. Unplug electrical equipment before working on it.
    C. Many drugs are considered hazardous materials.
    D. Use extension cords to plug in equipment.

4. Standard Precautions are issued by the:

    A. Food and Drug Administration
    B. Occupational Safety and Health Administration
    C. Health and Human Services Department
    D. Centers for Disease Control and Prevention

5. Which product is used to destroy bloodborne pathogens in the hospital pharmacy?

    A. phenol
    B. alcohol
    C. ammonium hydroxide
    D. bleach

6. OSHA requires all health-care workers who may be at risk to be vaccinated against which disease?

    A. tuberculosis
    B. acquired immunodeficiency syndrome (AIDS)
    C. hepatitis B
    D. hepatitis C

7. Pharmacy technicians who deal with radiopharmaceutical substances can reduce radiation exposure by which of these methods?

    A. using appropriate gowns
    B. labeling all radiation exposure sites in their body
    C. monitoring radiation exposure with film badges
    D. maximizing time in contact with radiation sources

8. Hazardous wastes should only be disposed of by which of these methods?

    A. flushing them down a toilet
    B. throwing them into the facility's trash containers
    C. burning them in an approved container
    D. using a licensed disposal service

9. If sensitive to latex gloves, pharmacy technicians:

    A. should put powder in the gloves
    B. should ask for nonlatex gloves
    C. should wear the latex gloves anyway
    D. need not wear gloves

10. Standard precautions are focused on:

    A. avoiding contact with and touching patients with AIDS
    B. avoiding contact with the body of a patient suspected of having hepatitis B
    C. avoiding contact with terminally ill patients
    D. avoiding contact with blood and body fluids

Hospital Pharmacy Practice

OUTLINE

GLOSSARY

Automation – the automatic control or operation of equipment, processes, or systems that often involves robotic machinery controlled by computers

Centers for Medicare and Medicaid (CMS) – a government agency that inspects and approves institutions to provide Medicaid and Medicare services

Computerized physician order entry system (CPOE) – a computerized system in which the physician inputs the medication order directly for electronic receipt in the pharmacy

Controlled substance medication order – an order for medication (generally narcotics) that requires monitored documentation of procurement, dispensation, and administration

Demand/stat medication order – an order for medication to be given in rapid response to a specific medical condition

Department of health (DOH) – an organization that oversees hospitals, including the pharmacy department

Emergency medication order – an order for a medication to be given in response to a medical emergency

Floor stock system – a system of drug distribution in which drugs are issued in bulk form and stored in medication rooms on patient care units

Group purchasing – many hospitals working together to negotiate with pharmaceutical manufacturers to get better prices and benefits based on the ability to promise high-committed volumes

Hospital pharmacy – the provision of pharmaceutical services within an institutional or hospital setting

Independent purchasing – the director of the pharmacy or buyer directly contacts and negotiates pricing with pharmaceutical manufacturers

Investigational medication order – an order for a medication given under direction of research protocols that also require strict documentation of procurement, dispensing, and administration

The Joint Commission – an organization that surveys and accredits health-care organizations

Just-in-time (JIT) inventory system – an inventory control system in which stock arrives just before it is needed

Medication order – the written order for particular medications and services to be provided to a patient within an institutional setting; physicians, nurse practitioners, or physician's assistants write medication orders

Patient prescription system – a system of drug distribution in which a nurse supplies the pharmacy with a transcribed medication order for a particular patient and the pharmacy prepares a 3-day supply of the medication

Policy – statement of the definite course or method of action selected to support goals of the overall organization

Policies and procedures manual – a formal document specifying guidelines for operations of an institution

PRN (as needed) medication order – an order for medication to be given in response to a specific defined parameter or condition

Procedure – statement of a series of steps to implement the policies of the department or organization

Scheduled intravenous (IV)/total parenteral nutrition (TPN) solution order – an order for medication given via an injection; these medications are to be prepared in a controlled (sterile) environment

Scheduled medication order – an order for medication that is to be given on a continuous schedule

State board of pharmacy (BOP) – an agency that registers pharmacists and pharmacy technicians

Sterile product – a substance that contains no living microorganisms

Unit-dose drug distribution system – a system for distributing medication in which the pharmacy prepares single doses of medications for a patient for a 24-hour period

WHAT IS HOSPITAL PHARMACY?

In the simplest terms and in today's practice setting, hospital pharmacy, can be defined as the provision of pharmaceutical services within an institutional or hospital setting. The practice of pharmacy within an institution comprises several types of services:

- **Support services:** Ordering and properly storing medications and maintaining an inventory of pharmaceuticals and associated medical supplies, billing for services, and installing and maintaining computer systems

- **Product services:** Dispensing, preparing, and processing medication orders for inpatients and maintaining required patient records and drug control records

- **Clinical services:** Managing the formulary system, evaluating drug use, and reviewing drug orders for appropriateness

- **Educational services:** Providing education about medications to pharmacy staff, other health-care professionals, the public, and patients and their caregivers

Hospital pharmacy practice now encompasses all aspects of drug therapy through the total continuum of medical care.

ORGANIZATION OF THE HOSPITAL

The structure of a hospital or a health-care system varies greatly from organization to organization. The basic structure includes a board of directors, who are responsible for the overall governance of the organization. Answering to the board are several layers of management. The primary leadership position is chief executive officer (CEO), also called hospital director or hospital president. Depending upon the size of the hospital, a senior vice president or chief operating officer (COO) who answers to the CEO may be present. The CEO usually works with the medical staff leadership; the COO, the operating staff leadership. Both staffs consist of vice presidents, functional department heads, assistant department heads, and supervisors. A sample organizational chart for an institutional setting is shown in Figure 11–1.

ORGANIZATION OF THE HOSPITAL PHARMACY

The pharmacy department within an institution is responsible for all aspects of drug use, including product-related services, clinical services, support services, and educational services. The personnel in a hospital pharmacy are classified into three categories:

- **Professional:** All pharmacists and management

- **Technical:** Pharmacy technicians involved in the drug-related processes

- **Support:** Nonlicensed personnel involved in providing services that support the drug-related processes and/or management functions

All hospital pharmacies have a leadership position in the department, usually titled director of pharmacy. The aforementioned individual is responsible for all the pharmacy services provided in or by the organization. The rest of the department's structure depends on the size of the organization. Smaller hospitals may have a small staff, consisting of a pharmacy director and a staff pharmacist. As the institution grows, additional pharmacists may be added, along with pharmacy technicians. Larger hospital systems will have many different positions categorized by functions:

1. Management—almost always pharmacists
   A. Director
   B. Manager
   C. Supervisor—may have a technician supervisor supervising technicians

2. Dispensing and preparation
   A. Pharmacist—unit dose, satellite
   B. Technician—unit dose, cart fill, medication and supply delivery
   C. Central intravenous (IV) admixture and sterile processing
   D. Controlled drug storage and distribution

3. Support—generally nonpharmacists
   A. Department secretary
   B. Buyer
   C. Biller
   D. Systems analyst

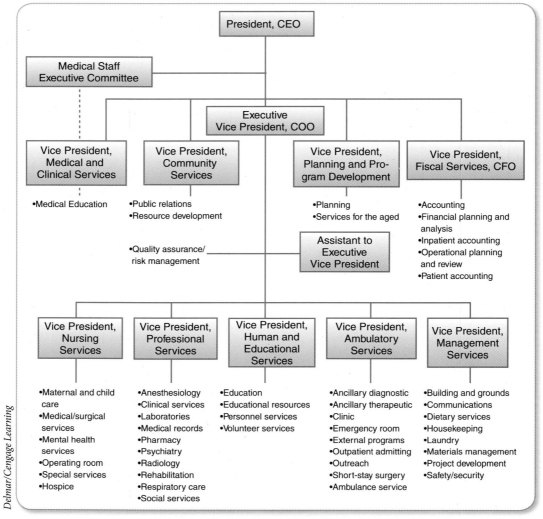

Figure 11–1 Hospital organizational chart according to traditional divisions of responsibility.

4. Clinical

   A. Clinical coordinator

   B. Clinical pharmacist

   C. Clinical specialist

5. Education and research

   A. Drug information specialist

   B. Research coordinator

As the pharmacy department becomes more involved in providing direct patient care, many departments are beginning to redesign their organizational structure to support the practices of the future. Figure 11–2 shows an example of one possible structure and organization of a pharmacy department within a hospital organization.

MEDICATION ORDERS

When the physician generates a medication order, the practice of hospital pharmacy begins. In the hospital pharmacy, the medication order is the equivalent to the prescription in the retail pharmacy. All medications, including prescription and over-the-counter (OTC), ordered in a hospital require a medication order. When the pharmacy department receives a

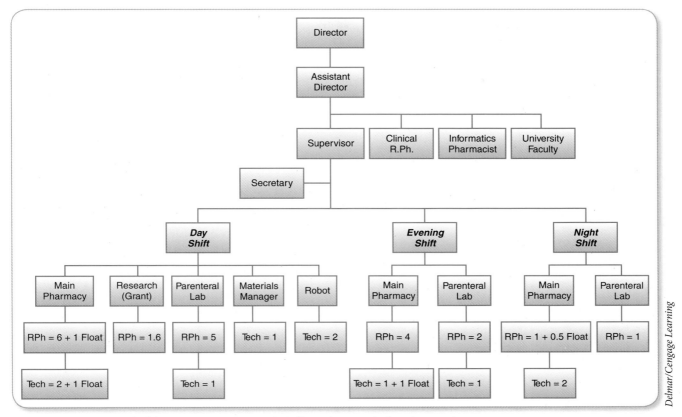

Figure 11–2 Hospital pharmacy organizational staffing chart with the pharmacist and technician teams.

copy of the original medication order, the medication fulfillment process begins. The original physician's order can be a carbon copy or an electronically scanned copy.

The medication order must contain the following information (see Figure 11–3):

- Patient's name, height, weight, date of birth, medical record number, medical condition, and known allergies
- Patient's room and bed number
- Dosage schedule
- Instructions for preparing the drugs
- The exact dosage form of the drug
- The dosage strength
- Directions for use
- Route of administration

Pharmacists and technicians must be able to distinguish between various types of orders that are written on the medication order. Many nonmedication orders, not pertaining to the pharmacy, can also exist on this document, including diet, laboratory, radiology, and physical activity orders. Also, pharmacists and pharmacist technicans may encounter a variety of types of medication orders, as listed below:

- **Scheduled medication order**: A medication that is given on a continuous schedule according to the medication order.

- **Scheduled intravenous (IV)/total parenteral nutrition (TPN) solution order**: A medication that is given by the injectable route and must be prepared in a controlled environment.

- **PRN (as needed) medication order**: A medication that may be given in response to

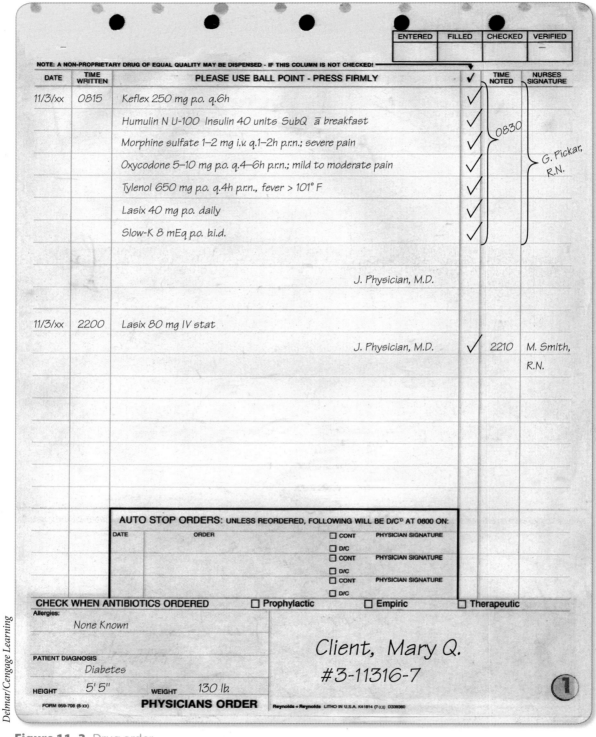

		ENTERED	FILLED	CHECKED	VERIFIED

NOTE: A NON-PROPRIETARY DRUG OF EQUAL QUALITY MAY BE DISPENSED - IF THIS COLUMN IS NOT CHECKED!

DATE	TIME WRITTEN	PLEASE USE BALL POINT - PRESS FIRMLY	✓	TIME NOTED	NURSES SIGNATURE
11/3/xx	0815	Keflex 250 mg p.o. q.6h	✓		
		Humulin N U-100 Insulin 40 units SubQ ā breakfast	✓	0830	
		Morphine sulfate 1–2 mg i.v. q.1–2h p.r.n.; severe pain	✓		
		Oxycodone 5–10 mg p.o. q.4–6h p.r.n.; mild to moderate pain	✓		G. Pickar, R.N.
		Tylenol 650 mg p.o. q.4h p.r.n., fever > 101° F	✓		
		Lasix 40 mg p.o. daily	✓		
		Slow-K 8 mEq p.o. b.i.d.	✓		
		J. Physician, M.D.			
11/3/xx	2200	Lasix 80 mg IV stat			
		J. Physician, M.D.	✓	2210	M. Smith, R.N.

AUTO STOP ORDERS: UNLESS REORDERED, FOLLOWING WILL BE D/Cᴰ AT 0800 ON:

DATE	ORDER		
		☐ CONT	PHYSICIAN SIGNATURE
		☐ D/C	
		☐ CONT	PHYSICIAN SIGNATURE
		☐ D/C	
		☐ CONT	PHYSICIAN SIGNATURE
		☐ D/C	

CHECK WHEN ANTIBIOTICS ORDERED ☐ Prophylactic ☐ Empiric ☐ Therapeutic

Allergies:
None Known

PATIENT DIAGNOSIS
Diabetes

HEIGHT 5' 5"   WEIGHT 130 lb.

Client, Mary Q.
#3-11316-7

FORM 959-708 (8-XX)   **PHYSICIANS ORDER**   Reynolds + Reynolds LITHO IN U.S.A. K41814 (7-XX) D330080

①

Delmar/Cengage Learning

Figure 11–3 Drug order.

a given parameter or condition defined in the medication order. If the defined situation does not occur, the medication is not given.

- **Controlled substance medication order:** A narcotic that requires controlled documentation of procurement, dispensing, and administration. Storage is usually in a secured environment.

- **Demand/stat medication order:** A medication that is needed for a rapid response to a given medical condition.

- **Emergency medication order:** A medication that is needed in response to a medical emergency, e.g., cardiac arrest.

- **Investigational medication order:** A medication that is given under the direction of research protocols. Strict documentation of the procurement, dispensing, and administration of the medication is required.

MEDICATION DISPENSING SYSTEMS

Because the pharmacist's role has changed from being a product dispenser to having expanding responsibility for the entire medication process, the medication dispensing systems have changed to support this increasing responsibility. In the past, medications were stored in the pharmacy in bulk quantities and then dispensed in bulk quantities and multidose containers to "mini" pharmacies located on the patient care units. Nurses prepared doses for administration to patients. This system has evolved into sophisticated unit-dose and automated dispensing processes to allow pharmacists and their support staff to concentrate on the final preparation of the medications for administration to the patient and the monitoring of the proper use of medications.

Commonly used inpatient dispensing systems include:

- **AcuDose-Rx (by McKesson Corporation):** This decentralized mediciation distribution system uses physician orders being entered into patient profiles, allowing authorized users to choose the desired profile and select the appropriate drug.

- **Baxter ATC 212:** This system uses microcomputers to package unit doses in the pharmacy for oral administration. Drugs are stored in specially designed, calibrated canisters that are assigned a specific numbered location. Each packaged dose is ejected into a strip-packing device that labels and hermetically seals it.

- **MedCarousel (by McKesson Corporation):** This storage and retrieval system is designed for hospital pharmacies and offers vertically rotating shelves and bar code scanning.

- **McLaughlin Dispensing System:** This system offers bedside dispensing and programmable magnetic cards linked into the pharmacy computer system. This locked system handles individual patient medications that the patient can remove from a bedside drawer device when it is time for medications to be administered. The dosing time is signified by a light that illuminates, notifying the patient to take his or her medication.

Floor Stock System

In the floor stock system, the pharmacy's role in the medication process is only product related. Drugs are purchased in bulk and multidose dosage forms. The drugs are issued to patient care units via a bulk drug order form and are stored in medication rooms. Once the drugs are placed in the medication room, a nurse prepares them for administration to patients. A medication could be used for more than one patient. In this system, the nurse is responsible for most of the steps in the medication process.

The disadvantages of this system include the following:

- Potential for medication errors

- Potential for drug diversion and misappropriation resulting in economic loss

- Increased inventory needs

- Inadequate space for medication storage on the patient care unit

Patient Prescription System

To improve on the floor stock system, the patient prescription system was developed. In this system, the nurse orders medications on a specific patient form. Transcribing information from the physician-prepared medication order, the nurse prepares the patient form. The pharmacy then dispenses a 3-day supply of medication.

Unit-Dose Drug Distribution System

In response to the increasing availability of new and more complex medications, pharmacists are expected to play an expanded role in the medication process. The distribution system that evolved as a result is the unit-dose drug distribution system, considered to be the safest, most-efficient, and most-effective medication system for distributing medications. The features of the unit-dose system include:

- The pharmacy receives a copy of the original physician's order and uses it as the dispensing document.

- Medications, including liquid and injectable medications, are prepared in ready-to-use forms and are dispensed per individual patient.

- Individual doses of medications are labeled (see Figure 11–4).

- The pharmacy receives more patient information, including drug allergies, weight, and possibly a medication history.

- No more than a 24-hour supply of medication is dispensed.

In the unit-dose drug distribution system, each patient has two medication drawers designated. While one drawer is in the pharmacy being filled, the other is on the patient care unit; and the nursing staff uses this drawer to give medication to the patient (see Figure 11–5).

The advantages of using the unit-dose drug distribution system include:

- Reduction in medication errors

- Improved medication control

- Decreased overall cost of medication distribution

- More precise medication billing

- Reduction in medication credits (medications returned unused)

- Reduced drug inventories

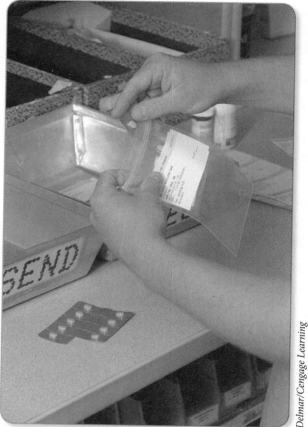

Delmar/Cengage Learning

Figure 11–4 Following the unit-dose system, the pharmacy technician prepares a single dose of medication for the hospital patient.

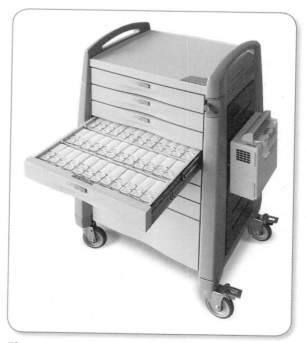

Figure 11–5 Unit-dose system. *(Courtsey of Artromick International, Inc).*

STERILE PRODUCTS

A **sterile product**, one that contains no living micro-organisms, is usually associated with drugs that are administered by injection or via the ophthalmic route. When a sterile product is not available commercially, the responsibility for preparing the medication resides in the pharmacy department. The pharmacy department will do the following:

- Ensure that the person preparing these products is properly and carefully trained in the use of aseptic technique.

- Prepare the product in an environment (clean room and laminar flow hood) that will prevent contamination (see Figure 11–6).

- Prepare the product using aseptic technique to prevent contamination.

- Ensure that all contents of the preparation are chemically, physically, and therapeutically compatible.

- Ensure that the product is stable over the time it is to be used.

- Ensure that the prepared product is stored under proper conditions.

- Ensure that the product is labeled properly.

- Keep records of preparation.

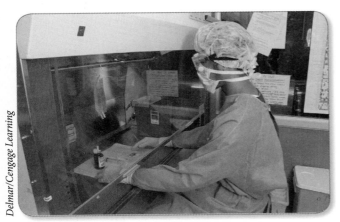

Delmar/Cengage Learning

Figure 11–6 Sterile products must be prepared in an aseptic environment.

- Use proper quality control processes to ensure that a proper preparation has been produced.

INVENTORY CONTROL

The director of pharmacy is responsible for maintaining an adequate medication inventory and establishing specifications for the procurement of all drugs, chemicals, and biologic agents related to the practice of pharmacy. The director usually delegates this duty to a pharmacy buyer or a pharmacy technician. Customers of pharmacy services expect to have high-quality drugs quickly and cheaply and those that have been stored properly. In the hospital pharmacy, the pharmacy and therapeutics committee determine which medications will be purchased and maintained in stock. Inventory control is discussed in detail in Chapter 20.

Purchasing Systems

The hospital must then decide on the system of purchasing the medications. The two types of systems are as follows:

1. **Independent purchasing**: The director of pharmacy or pharmacy buyer contracts directly with pharmaceutical manufacturers to negotiate prices and other conditions affecting purchases from that manufacturer. Larger institutions are more likely to use the independent purchasing system because they can offer larger committed volumes independent of other institutions. Smaller hospitals will form coalitions to achieve the larger committed volumes needed to obtain competitive prices.

2. **Group purchasing** (**group purchasing organization [GPO]**): This type of purchasing involves the collaboration of many hospitals in negotiations with pharmaceutical manufacturers to achieve advantageous pricing and other benefits. The main advantage of this process is that the manufacturer offers more competitive pricing because of the promise of high-committed volumes.

Modes of Purchasing

The next consideration is to determine the method of acquisition of the pharmaceuticals. There are three modes of purchasing:

1. Direct purchasing from the pharmaceutical manufacturer

2. Purchase from a wholesaler

3. Purchase from a prime vendor

Direct Purchasing

Although direct purchasing eliminates the middleman and handling fees, it requires a significant commitment of time, larger inventories, and more storage space. Purchases must be made from many vendors.

Wholesaler Purchasing

Purchasing from a wholesaler means that a hospital purchases many items from one source. The wholesaler is usually located close to the institution, can provide next-day delivery, and will maintain the larger portion of the inventory. This enables the hospital to reduce inventory costs. Wholesaler purchasing also reduces the need for a large commitment of personnel to support the purchasing process. The primary disadvantage is the higher costs of pharmaceuticals.

Prime Vendor Purchasing

The prime vendor system of purchasing is a relationship the hospital establishes with a single wholesaler. The hosptial establishes a contract, stipulating a committed volume of purchases. In return, the vendor charges a highly competitive service fee and provides a guaranteed service level, guaranteed delivery schedule, and a guarantee that individual or group contract prices will be the base price. A contract with a prime vendor may be an independent agreement with the hospital or an agreement that the GPO makes. Generally, the GPO is better able to negotiate a competitive contract.

The prime vendor system has the advantages of both the direct and wholesaler purchasing processes without the disadvantages. To reduce inventory costs, most pharmacy departments will attempt to have a just-in-time (JIT) inventory system. Under this system, the pharmacy maintains sufficient inventory to function until the next reorder period. With the prime vendor system, the reorder period could be as little as 24 hours.

AUTOMATION

The automatic control or operation of equipment, processes, or systems, automation often involves robotic machinery controlled by computers. The advent of automation (pharmacy information systems) has improved the efficiencies of the pharmacy. One of the innovators in the use of automation for cart filling, McKesson has developed the Robot-Rx® for this purpose (see Figure 11–7). Automation provides the ability to rapidly process large volumes of medication orders accurately and quickly. From the automated processing of medication orders, patient profiles are generated; medication labels, medication fill lists, and medication administration records are produced; and medication charges are processed. Some disadvantages of the pharmacy's increased involvement in the medication process are the need for massive amounts of information and the need to process many transactions quickly.

Clinical screening can occur to check for drug interactions, drug allergies, and dosage ranges. Reports can also be generated to produce data to monitor appropriate drug utilization. Utilization and usage data from the pharmacy information system can be used to order and maintain a medication inventory. One of the problems identified with this process is the medication order. A handwritten document from a physician, nurse practitioner, or physician's assistant, the medication order is prone to error because the handwriting may be illegible. Currently, in many facilities, the physician, rather than the pharmacy staff, is responsible for entering medication orders into the hospital information system. This type of system is generically called a computerized physician order entry system (CPOE).

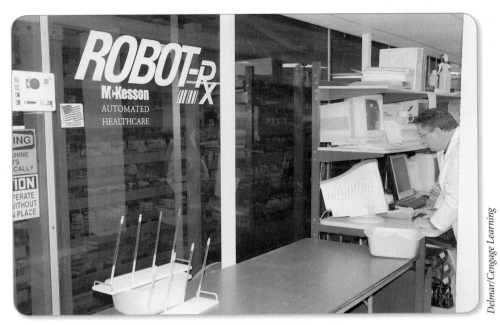

Figure 11–7 Robot-Rx.

Delmar/Cengage Learning

Popular physician order entry systems include:

- **MedDirect:** This system uses automation to communicate medication ordering information and manage documents.

- **Medstation and Medstation Rx (by Pyxis):** Used on nursing units for automated dispensing, this system interfaces with pharmacy computer systems. Physicians enter their orders into the pharmacy computers, and the orders are transferred, along with patient profiles, to the nurses who use passwords for easy access of verified medications. Charges are calculated automatically, by the unit, for dispensed drugs.

- **OmniLinkRx (by Omnicell):** This system manages handwritten physician orders and simplifies communication between the pharmacy and remote nursing stations.

- **Robot-Rx (by McKesson Corporation):** A centralized robotic drug distribution system, Robot-Rx automates storage, dispensing, returning, restocking, and crediting.

- **Saf-T-Pak:** An automated bar code packaging system, Saf-T-Pak is used for unit doses

and multidoses; it automatically replenishes decentralized cabinets and fills individual patient medication bins.

Many unit-dose systems use the 24-hour medication cart exchange process. These carts contain a 24-hour supply of medication for each patient on a patient care unit. A pharmacy technician usually fills the carts, and a pharmacist checks them. A robotic device interfaced with the pharmacy information system will fill each patient medication tray in the cart. This robotic device is also capable of returning credited medication to proper stock locations.

Automation is also used to create point-of-service storage cabinets that are interfaced with the pharmacy information system. Use of these cabinets eliminates the medication cart-filling process. An example of this type of automation is the automated dispensing cabinet. Many fear that automation will decrease the need for pharmacy personnel. However, these devices require human intervention for appropriate use. The pharmacy technician of the future will be controlling these machines and providing proper maintenance, repair, and quality assurance processes. If mechanical failure occurs, manual backup processes must be in place; and human intervention will be needed to repair failed mechanical systems. Human intervention can never be replaced.

RESPONSIBILITIES OF PHARMACISTS IN HOPSITALS

Hospital pharmacists have two major areas of responsibilities—dispensing medications and performing general operations responsibilities. A pharmacist's dispensing responsiblities include checking for accuracy of dispensed medications, ensuring medication control, ensuring proper compounding techniques, reviewing medication orders, supervising medication administration, and monitoring medication use. General responsibilities include documentation, training, education, establishment of policies and procedures, and evaluations of medical use.

ROLES AND DUTIES OF PHARMACY TECHNICIANS IN HOSPITALS

The increasing complexity of health care in the modern hospital is creating ever-greater demands for the hospital pharmacy to broaden its scope of services. New health-care legislation and rapid changes in health-care technology are imposing new demands on hospital pharmacies, and meeting these demands result in a need for increased staffing. Personnel shortages limit the scope of pharmaceutical services being provided in most hospitals. By delegating routine tasks to pharmacy technicians under their supervision, hospital pharmacists can free much of their time. Supportive hospital pharmacy personnel are used in most hospitals today. Therefore, it is essential to understand the roles and duties of pharmacy technicians in the hospital setting, as listed in the following:

- Maintaining medication records
- Preparing unit doses
- Compounding medications
- Packaging

- Preparing and delivering prescriptions to nursing homes, hospice, and rehabilitation facilities
- Inputting data into the computer
- Inspecting nursing unit drug stocks
- Maintaining inventory
- Preparing labels
- Maintaining privacy
- Communicating effectively
- Working safely

Following Policies and Procedures

Pharmacy technicians must follow the policies and procedures of the hospital in which they work. Policy and procedure manuals focus on general responsibilities, technical resopnsibilities, documentation, and reporting duties of pharmacy technicians and other pharmacy personnel. Because they are accountable for all outcomes, including those that result from the failure to follow procedures, pharmacy technicians must understand and follow these standards.

Maintaining Medication Records

An important part of the pharmacy technician's job is to accurately maintain the patient records on the pharmacy information system. Records should include the patient's weight, as well as the care and counseling of the patient.

Maintaining Competence

Pharmacy technicians must improve their skills and knowledge because the practice of pharmacy is growing and evolving more quickly than ever. To keep up with changing demands, pharmacy technicians must attend continuing education lectures, courses, and seminars. In fact, if a pharmacy technician is nationally certified, their recertification requires 20 continuing education credits (with 1 hour being focused on pharmacy law) every two years.

Preparing Unit Doses

Pharmacy technicians are responsible for preparing the unit doses for individual patients each day, placing the medications by the patient's weight, diagnosis, treatment, therapy, diet plans, blood and laboratory test results, and the name of the primary physician. Maintaining up-to-date records allows the pharmacist to provide updated unit-dose carts that are delivered to the patient care areas of the hospital. The pharmacist must check these carts before they can be delivered to the patient care floors.

Compounding Medications

In some circumstances, a drug may need to be created from a prepared recipe (see Figure 11–8). If a written procedure exists for preparation of the drug, pharmacy technicians can prepare it. This process is called *compounding*. To create a compounded drug, technicians must be able to clearly understand the formula and be able to adjust it to increase or decrease amounts as necessary. A sound understanding of mathematical principles is required.

Packaging

Many drugs have to be placed in proper containers to remain active and potent. Pharmacy technicians must be aware of these characteristics of drugs to choose the appropriate containers for dispensing and storing them.

Using Aseptic Technique to Prepare Admixtures

Contamination of various types of admixtures by microorganisms may harm, permanently damage, or even cause the death of patients. As a result, pharmacy technicians must always use aseptic technique when preparing these products. Aseptic technique and admixtures are discussed in detail in Chapter 15.

Preparing and Delivering Outpatient Prescriptions

Some hospitals are affiliated with off-site facilities such as nursing homes and rehabilitation centers. Pharmacy technicians are responsible for preparing the medications these facilities need and for delivering them to the facilities in a timely manner.

Inputting Data into the Computer

Data entry is an important part of the pharmacy technician's job. Accurate entry of new data into the computer system and maintenance of records within the system are important. The pharmacy then can be run efficiently because patient records are accurate,

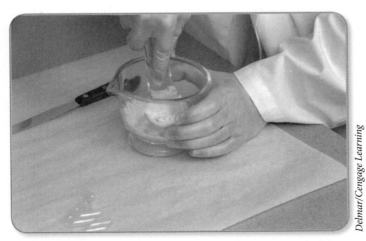

Delmar/Cengage Learning

Figure 11–8 To compound a drug, the pharmacy technician must be able to accurately follow written procedures and formulas.

inventory is maintained at appropriate levels, and billing can be done in an accurate and timely manner.

Ensuring Billing Accuracy

During the billing process, inaccuracies can occur. This is a result of the involved process of insurance claims, coding, and related forms. Failure to understand how this process works will cause errors in payments, reimbursements, and coverage. Pharmacy technicians should understand how Medicare, Medicaid, and other common insurance providers are correctly billed for the coverage of their patients. See Chapter 18 for detailed information on health insurance and billing.

Inspecting Nursing Unit Drug Stocks

The pharmacy must maintain nursing unit drug stocks, and pharmacy technicians are responsible for inspecting unit drug stocks for proper storage conditions, appropriate inventory, and replacement of expired or damaged stock.

Following Medication Control, Security, and Controlled Substance Accountability

The DEA monitors the use of scheduled drugs and those who prescribe them. Because of increasing crime involving controlled substances and prescription medications, proper security measures are vital. Medication controls should be in place so that any misappropriation of these substances may be discovered and dealt with as quickly as possible. This topic is one of the most important responsibilites of pharmacy technicians and pharmacy personnel, in general, because their ability to practice may be threatened by inefficient medication control policies. For detailed information on security procedures involving all types of medications, see Chapter 2.

Maintaining Inventory and Reorders

Pharmacy technicians often have the responsibilities of ordering stock and maintaining stock levels. As discussed earlier, many inventory systems are available for use within the pharmacy. Regardless of the system used, technicians must ensure that stock levels are appropriate to allow the pharmacy to operate efficiently without having to borrow stock or order stock at higher prices. When stock is delivered, pharmacy technicians generally check and verify the stock against the order and clearly mark receipt of the order on the invoice. All orders must be appropriately stored within the pharmacy (see Figure 11–9). Any damaged goods or expired drugs must be returned or properly disposed.

During inventory control processes, the pharmacy computer system should prompt the pharmacy staff when it is time to reorder specific medications and supplies. Therefore, pharmacy technicians must follow their organization's policies and procedures for reordering. They must know when to notify their pharmacist or pharmacy supervisor when specific drugs need to be reordered that they are not allowed (by law) to order themselves.

Preparing Labels

Each filled medication order must be appropriately labeled. The label should contain the name of the patient the drug is prescribed for, the patient's medical record number, the patient's room number, the name of the prescriber, the date of dispensing, the name of the drug, the strength of the drug, the quantity of the drug dispensed, the dosage directions, and the

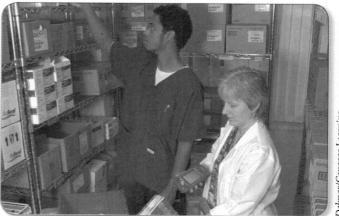

Figure 11–9 Proper maintenance of inventory levels is necessary to allow the pharmacy to run efficiently.

Delmar/Cengage Learning

expiration date. The label should also contain the initials of the person dispensing the drug. Proper labeling on medications is critically important, and a great deal of care should be taken in this task. The label should be checked and rechecked against the medication order. The pharmacist must check and initial all labels before the medications leave the pharmacy.

Maintaining Privacy

Pharmacy technicians are legally bound to uphold the privacy of all patients. New standards for maintaining a patient's privacy have been implemented with regulations in the Health Insurance Portability and Accountability Act (HIPAA). Please review Chapter 2 for more information.

Auditing and Reporting of Medication Processes

Pharmacy technicians must keep complete records of orders, reorders, and dispensations of all drugs (with scheduled drugs being most important) in their hospital pharmacy. For scheduled drugs, federal law requires records be kept on file for two years, and many state laws may require them to be kept for up to five years. Different federal and state agencies, as well as insurance companies, may audit medication records.

Communicating Effectively

Communication skills are very important in the field of pharmacy. Pharmacy technicians will need to communicate effectively and accurately with patients, as well as with other health-care workers.

Working Safely

For the health and safety of pharmacy personnel, a safe working environment must be maintained. Work areas should be clean, and accidental exposures to harmful substances should be avoided. Emergency and exposure treatment plans should be in place. Pharmacy technicians should be aware of and quickly be able to respond to any unsafe condition. Workplace safety is discussed in more detail in Chapter 10.

POLICIES AND PROCEDURES MANUAL

Hospitals today are very complex organizations. In addition, the hospital may be a member of an integrated health-care delivery system. This complexity dictates that the hospital and all its departments must have a set of standard operating statements to operate effectively and efficiently. The regulatory and quasi-legal organizations that oversee hospitals require a manual to fulfill this need. In support of the hospital and health-care delivery system, the pharmacy department must develop guidelines for operations. This document is formally called the policies and procedures manual, and it should answer the following questions:

- What action must be undertaken?
- What is its purpose (why must it be done)?
- When must it be done?
- Where must it be done?
- Who should do it?
- How must it be done?

The policies and procedures manual provides a standard direction for operating and functioning within an organization and its specific departments. All pharmacy personnel should be familiar with the contents of the manual. The minimum standards for pharmacies in the hospital include the following:

1. Preparing a comprehensive operations manual
2. Clearly defining lines of authority and areas of responsibility
3. Having written job descriptions that are developed and revised as needed
4. Updating the manual with revisions that include continuing changes
5. Familiarizing all personnel with the contents of the manual
6. Obtaining input from other disciplines

Policies and procedures should relate to the selection, distribution, and safe and effective use of drugs in the facility. The director of pharmaceutical services, the medical staff, the nursing service, and the administration should conjointly establish policies and procedures. Organizations that require polices and procedures include:

- **Food and Drug Administration:** Investigation of drug policies and procedures in hospital pharmacies and drug recall policies and procedures.

- **Drug Enforcement Administration:** Policies and procedures to show proper handling of controlled substances.

- **Occupational Safety and Health Administration:** Policies and procedures that ensure the health and safety of people in the workplace.

- **The Joint Commission:** Policies and procedures that guide the pharmacy department in providing safe, effective, and cost-effective drug therapy.

- **American Society of Health-System Pharmacists:** Policies and procedures showing implementation of its guidelines and standards of practice.

Benefits of a Policies and Procedures Manual

The primary benefit of having a policies and procedures manual is to document compliance with accrediting, certifying, and regulatory bodies. The second most beneficial effect of having a policies and procedures manual is to create a more effective departmental management program. Other benefits include:

- Establishing standards of practice for delivering pharmaceutical services

- Coordinating use of resources

- Improving intradepartmental relationships

- Providing consistency in orientation and training of personnel

- Providing a reference guide to all personnel in the performance of daily activities

- Creating a positive work environment, including increased job satisfaction and productivity

A department with a well-developed and enforced policies and procedures manual will function more efficiently and effectively.

Contents of a Policies and Procedures Manual

The purpose of a policies and procedures manual is to provide an authoritative source for organizational and departmental policies and procedures. In it, standards of operation are identified; and it is a guide and reference for personnel in the performance of their daily duties. The pharmacy director is responsible for creating the manual, and each employee is responsible for becoming familiar with its content. It is beyond the scope of this chapter to give examples of specific policies and procedures.

Policies and procedures will be either administrative or professional. Administrative policies and procedures are related to the control of resources (human resources, financial resources, supplies and equipment, job descriptions, and the physical plant) and relationships with other departments and administration. Professional policies and procedures pertain either directly or indirectly to patient care services. Representing the major portion of the manual, this section should include all dispensing and clinical functions.

To make the policies and procedures manual available to any department employee, a copy of the document needs to be located in each area of the pharmacy department. The document should start with a policy title followed by a **policy** statement. The next section of the document should contain the step-by-step **procedure** for placing the policy into operation. A section should be devoted to references to source material used in the creation of the policies and procedures manual. After the policies and procedures have been defined, signatures indicating proper approvals should be obtained.

REGULATORY AGENCIES THAT OVERSEE HOSPITAL PHARMACY

The agencies that oversee all aspects of hospital operations, including the pharmacy department, are as follows:

- **Joint Commission:** This organization surveys and accredits health-care services. All health-care organizations must undergo this accreditation process every three years. The Joint Commission identifies specific guidelines for every department within the hospital.

- **State Board of Pharmacy (BOP):** This agency licenses pharmacists and pharmacy technicians. Each state board of pharmacy has its own specific requirements concerning licensing, certification, and registration.

- **Centers for Medicare and Medicaid (CMS):** The CMS inspects and approves hospitals to provide care for Medicaid patients. Approval by this organization is required to receive reimbursement for any patients covered by Medicaid and Medicare.

- **Department of Health (DOH):** This organization oversees hospitals, including the pharmacy department. Hospitals undergo inspections by the DOH to assure compliance with laws concerning hospital practice.

FUTURE OF HOSPITAL PHARMACY

With the aging population and the increasing number of medications being produced by research, an increasing need for pharmacy services in all settings will be seen. Trends for the future include the following:

1. Continuing expansion of the responsibilities of pharmacy technicians to allow pharmacists to concentrate on direct patient care activities

2. Increasing need for education of both pharmacists and pharmacy technicians

3. Increasing need for pharmacists and pharmacy technicians to obtain the skills necessary to work directly with patients

4. Increasing multiprofessional approach to providing patient care, hence requiring better communication skills

5. Increasing use of automation to perform routine tasks and to handle the massive amounts of information and documentation that must occur as a result of providing patient care. Automation will also be used to make patient information available in the multiple settings in which patient care will be delivered

For those who choose pharmacy as a profession, the future is bright. Those in the field now have the responsibility to prepare for the requirements of the future directions of pharmacy.

EXPLORING THE WEB

Visit http://www.ahrq.gov; the Agency for Health Care Research and Quality (AHRQ) is the lead federal agency charged with improving the quality, safety, efficiency, and effectiveness of health care for all Americans.

Visit http://www.aha.org; the American Hospital Association's (AHA) mission is to advance the health of individuals and communities. The AHA leads, represents and serves hospitals, health systems and other related organizations that are accountable to the community and committed to health improvement.

Visit http://www.cms.hhs.gov; the Centers for Medicare and Medicaid Services (CMS) has as its mission to ensure effective, up-to-date health-care coverage and to promote quality care for beneficiaries.

Visit http://www.fip.org; the International Pharmaceutical Federation (FIP) is the global federation of national associations representing two million pharmacists and pharmaceutical scientists around the world.

Visit http://www.jointcommission.org; The Joint Commission, an independent, not-for-profit organization, accredits and certifies more than 17,000 healthcare organizations and programs in the United States.

Visit http://www.nabp.net; the National Association of Boards of Pharmacy (NABP) is the independent, international, and impartial association that assists its member boards and jurisdictions in developing, implementing, and enforcing uniform standards for the purpose of protecting the public health.

Visit http://www.nlm.nih.gov; the National Library of Medicine (NLM), the world's largest medical library, collects materials and provides information and research services in all areas of biomedicine and health care.

Visit http://pharmacytechnician.org; the National Pharmacy Technician Association (NPTA), the world's largest professional organization established specifically for pharmacy technicians, is dedicated to advancing the value of pharmacy technicians and the vital roles they play in pharmaceutical care.

Visit http://www.hhs.gov; the U.S. Department of Health and Human Services (HHS) is the government's principal agency for protecting the health of all Americans and providing essential human services, especially for those who are least able to help themselves.

REVIEW QUESTIONS

1. Who determines which medications are purchased and stocked in the hospital pharmacy?

   A. pharmacy buyer and the pharmacy technician
   B. pharmacy supervisors
   C. pharmacists on staff
   D. pharmacy and therapeutics committee

2. In preparing sterile products, the primary concern must be:

   A. safety and accuracy
   B. saving time and speeding
   C. availability and productivity
   D. cost

3. The disadvantages of the floor stock system include all of the following, except:

   A. potential for drug diversion and misappropriation resulting in economic loss
   B. decreased inventory needs
   C. inadequate space for medication storage on the patient care unit
   D. potential for scheduling errors

4. The Centers for Medicare and Medicaid Services (CMS) inspects and approves hospitals to provide care for:

   A. only young patients
   B. Medicaid patients
   C. only inpatients
   D. only pregnant patients

5. Who has the responsibility of setting up unit doses?

   A. pharmacy technician
   B. nurse
   C. pharmacy director
   D. support staff

6. Which of the following is not a mode of purchasing?

   A. purchase from a wholesaler
   B. purchase from a second vendor
   C. purchase from a prime vendor
   D. purchase from the pharmaceutical manufacturer

7. The provision of pharmaceutical services in the institutional setting is known as:

   A. nuclear pharmacy
   B. hospital pharmacy
   C. retail pharmacy
   D. mail-order pharmacy

8. Who generates the medication order?

   A. pharmacy technician
   B. nurse
   C. pharmacist
   D. physician

9. A medication needed in response to a cardiac arrest is which type of medication order?

   A. controlled substance
   B. demand or stat
   C. emergency
   D. investigational

10. The roles and duties of the technician in the hospital do not include:

   A. providing policies and procedures
   B. inputting data into the computer
   C. packaging
   D. maintaining inventory

Community Pharmacy

OUTLINE

GLOSSARY

Auxiliary labels – extra labels applied to products in the pharmacy that may contain warnings, cautions, directions for use, and dietary or other information

Drive-through – an external site at a pharmacy that can be accessed by driving up in a vehicle

Inscription – the main part of a prescription, which indicates the drugs and quantities of each to be used in the mixture

Legend drug – a medication that may be dispensed only with a prescription; also known as prescription drug

Over-the-counter (OTC) – a medication that may be purchased without a prescription directly from the pharmacy

Pharmacy compounding – the preparation, mixing, assembling, packaging, or labeling of a drug or device

Signa – a Latin term meaning "mark" or "label"; abbreviated as "Sig," the signa is the part of a prescription where the prescriber writes the directions for use

Subscription – the part of a prescription that includes directions for compounding; physicians seldom include it today, leaving product preparation to the pharmacist's discretion

Superscription – the part of a prescription below the patient's name and address that begins the body of the actual prescription; it is usually designated by the symbol "℞"

COMMUNITY PHARMACY

According to the National Association of Chain Drug Stores (NACDS), more than 56,000 community pharmacies exist across the United States. According to the Bureau of Labor Statistics, the number of pharmacy technicians, the primary providers of pharmaceuticals and pharmaceutical care services to patients, working in community pharmacies throughout the United States totals more than 264,000. In comparison, more than 54,000 pharmacy technicians work in institutional (hospital) pharmacy. Community pharmacies are found in a variety of locations such as shopping centers, grocery stores, department stores, and medical office buildings. These are classified into two main categories: independent pharmacies and chain pharmacies.

Local individuals own independent pharmacies. On the contrary, chain pharmacies such as Walgreens, CVS, and Rite Aid are usually regionally or nationally based. Giant regional or national mass merchandisers such as Walmart or Kmart also have pharmacies inside most of their stores. Pharmacists in the community pharmacy provide several important functions:

1. They provide distribution of prescribed drug products.

2. They are caretakers of the nation's drug supply.

3. They compound prescriptions to meet the specific needs of individual patients.

4. They educate the public to maximize the intended benefits of drug therapy and, at the same time, try to minimize the unintended side effects and adverse reactions patients may have to that therapy.

THE PRESCRIPTION

Issued by a physician, dentist, or other licensed medical practitioner, an order for medication is called a *prescription*. In certain states, nurse practitioners and even pharmacists can issue prescriptions with certain restrictions. The prescription order is a part of the professional relationship among the prescriber, the pharmacist, and the patient. It is the pharmacist's responsibility in this relationship to provide quality pharmaceutical care that meets the patient's medication needs. The pharmacist or pharmacy technicians not only must be precise in the manual aspects of filling the medication order, but they also must provide the patient with the necessary information and guidance to ensure the patient's compliance in taking the medication properly.

There are two broad legal classifications of medications: those that can be obtained only by prescription and those that may be purchased without a prescription. The latter are termed *nonprescription drugs* or over-the-counter (OTC) drugs. Medications that may be dispensed legally only by prescription are referred to as prescription drugs or legend drugs. The prescriber may write the prescription and give it to the patient for presentation at the pharmacy, may telephone or send the prescription directly to the pharmacist by fax, or send the prescription electronically from a physician's computer to a pharmacist's computer. The component parts of a prescription include the following:

- Information about the prescriber's office

- Information about the patient

- Date

- Medication prescribed (inscription), which states the name and quantities of ingredients

- Rx symbol (superscription), which gives directions to the pharmacist

- Dispensing directions to the pharmacist (subscription)

- Directions for patient (signa)

- Refill and special labeling

- Prescriber's signature and license or Drug Enforcement Agency (DEA) number

An example of a physician's prescription is shown in Figure 12–1.

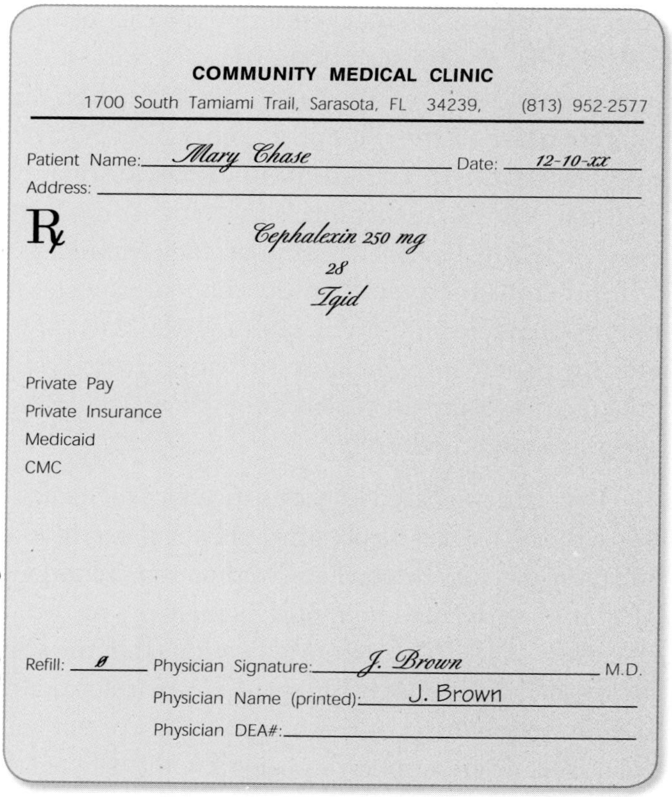

COMMUNITY MEDICAL CLINIC

1700 South Tamiami Trail, Sarasota, FL 34239, (813) 952-2577

Patient Name: _Mary Chase_ Date: _12-10-xx_

Address: _____

R℞   _Cephalexin 250 mg_
             _28_
             Iqid

Private Pay
Private Insurance
Medicaid
CMC

Refill: _0_ Physician Signature: _J. Brown_ M.D.

Physician Name (printed): _J. Brown_

Physician DEA#: _____

Delmar/Cengage Learning

Figure 12–1 A prescription.

Processing Prescriptions— Dispensing

Proper procedures and correct steps for processing prescriptions and dispensing drugs include receiving, reading and checking, numbering and dating, labeling, preparing, packaging, rechecking, delivering and patient counseling, recording and filing, pricing, and refilling.

Receiving

The pharmacy technician receives the prescription order directly from patients. This is a good opportunity to enhance the pharmacist- or the technician-patient relationship and to facilitate the gathering of essential information from patients, such as their history of diseases and a list of other drugs they may be taking. This information is critical for providing quality pharmaceutical care. The technician can also obtain the correct name, address, and other necessary information from patients and determine whether their medications are provided through insurance coverage.

Pharmacy technicians should ask patients whether they wish to wait, call back, or have the medication delivered. Many pharmacists try to price prescriptions before dispensing, especially for unusually expensive medication, to avoid subsequent questions concerning the charge.

Reading and Checking

After reading the prescription completely and carefully to be sure the ingredients or quantities prescribed are clear, pharmacy technicians should take the time to update the patient's profile. From the computer, technicians should determine the compatibility of the newly prescribed medication with other drugs that the patient is taking and should determine whether any drug-food or drug-disease interactions are possible. If some part of the information is illegible on the prescription or if it appears that the prescriber has made an error, technicians should notify the pharmacist who should then consult another pharmacist or the prescriber. Unfamiliar or unclear abbreviations represent a source of errors in interpreting and filling prescriptions.

Pharmacists must take great care and use their broad knowledge of drug products to prevent dispensing errors. The amount and frequency of a dose must be noted carefully and checked. In determining the safety of the dose of a medicinal agent, pharmacists must consider the age, weight, and condition of the patient; dosage form prescribed; possible influence of other drugs being taken; and the frequency of administration.

Numbering and Dating

As a legal requirement, the prescription order must be numbered and that same number must be placed on the label. The numbering helps to identify the bottle or package. Prescription computers assign consecutive numbers, or the numbers are provided manually by using numbering machines. Including the date the prescription was filled on the label is also a legal requirement. The information is important in determining the appropriate refill frequency and patient compliance and can be used as an alternate means of locating the prescription order if the patient loses the prescription number.

Labeling

Using the information that the pharmacist or pharmacy technician enters, the prescription label may be typewritten or prepared by computer. Figure 12–2 shows a computer-prepared prescription, including the label.

A prescription should have a professional-appearing label. With its size appropriate to the prescription container's size, the label should contain the following information:

- Pharmacy name, address, and telephone number
- Prescription number
- Prescriber's name
- Patient's name
- Directions for use
- Date of dispensing

The patient's address and strength of the medication are also commonly included.

Some state laws require that the dispensing pharmacist's name or initials appear on the label. Used to emphasize important aspects of the dispensed medication, including its proper use, handling, storage, refill status, and necessary warnings or precautions,

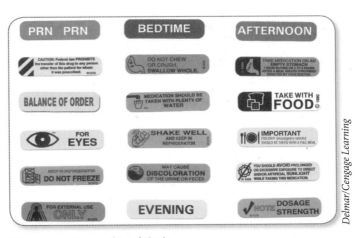

Figure 12–3 Auxiliary labels.

auxiliary labels are available in various colors to give them special prominence. Figure 12–3 shows some examples of pharmacy auxiliary labels.

Preparing

Most prescriptions call for dispensing of medications that pharmaceutical manufacturers have already prefabricated into dosage forms. In filling prescriptions with prefabricated products, the pharmacist should compare the manufacturer's label with the prescription to be certain it is the correct medication. Medications that show signs of poor manufacture or deterioration or for which the stated expiration date on the label has passed should never be dispensed.

Tablets, capsules, and some other solid, prefabricated dosage forms usually are counted in the pharmacy using a *counting tray*, which is shown in Figure 12–4. This device facilitates the rapid and sanitary counting and transferring of medication from

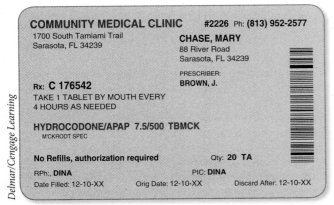

Figure 12–2 Computer-prepared prescription and label.

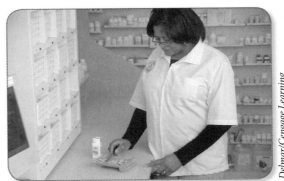

Figure 12–4 A counting tray.

the stock packages to the prescription container. To prevent contamination of capsules and tablets, the pharmacist or technician should wipe the counting tray with an alcohol wipe and/or a dry cloth after each use because powder, especially from uncoated tablets, tends to remain on the tray.

Although they represent a small percentage of the total, some prescriptions may require compounding. The pharmacist must have the knowledge and skills needed to prepare them accurately. **Pharmacy compounding** is defined as the preparation, mixing, assembling, packaging, or labeling of a drug or device. Extemporaneous compounding is essential in the course of professional practice to prepare drug formulations in dosage forms or strengths that are not otherwise commercially available.

Packaging

When in the process of filling a prescription, pharmacy technicians may select a container from among various types with different shapes, sizes, mouth openings, colors, and compositions. The type and quantity of medication to be dispensed and the method of its use generally determine this selection. Figure 12–5 shows some types of medication containers.

Pharmacists or pharmacy technicians must dispense all legend drugs intended for oral use to the patient in containers having child-resistant safety closures, unless the prescriber or the patient specifically requests otherwise. Drugs that are used by

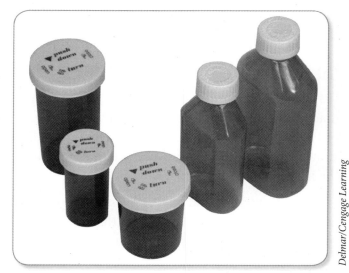

Figure 12–6 Various child-resistant caps.

or given to patients in hospitals, nursing homes, and extended-care facilities need not be dispensed in containers with safety closures unless they are intended for patients who are leaving the institution's confines. Examples of child-resistant caps are shown in Figure 12–6.

Rechecking

For verification, pharmacists must recheck every prescription that has been dispensed. All details of the label should be rechecked against the prescription order to verify directions, patient's name, prescription number, date, and prescriber's name. A repackaged medication must contain the generic name of the medication, lot number, manufacturer's name, and the expiration date after packaging. The repackaging date can be either six months from the date the medication is repackaged, or one quarter of the original length of time that the manufacture stated the drug was good for (whichever is less). Rechecking is especially important for those drug products available in multiple strengths. The maximum amount of time that can be assigned to a repackaged medication is six months.

Delivering and Patient Counseling

Unless patients specify that medications should be delivered to their homes or workplaces, pharmacists should personally present prescription medications

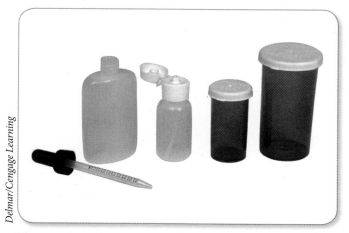

Figure 12–5 Various types of medication containers.

to the patients or to their family members. Because labeling instructions are often inadequate to ensure the patients' understanding of their medications, prescribers and pharmacists share the responsibility for ensuring that the patient receives specific instructions, precautions, and warnings for safe and effective use of the prescribed drugs.

Recording and Filing

Using computers and hard-copy prescription files, pharmacies maintain a record of the prescriptions dispensed. Today, many chain drugstores have central computers, which allow pharmacists from any location in the system to access a patient's record and refill a prescription previously dispensed at another store. Various types of units are available to keep original prescription orders. Most pharmacies use metal or cardboard units, which conveniently store approximately 1000 prescriptions, and some may use partitioned drawers for filing (Figure 12–7). The least common method of filing is microfilming of prescriptions.

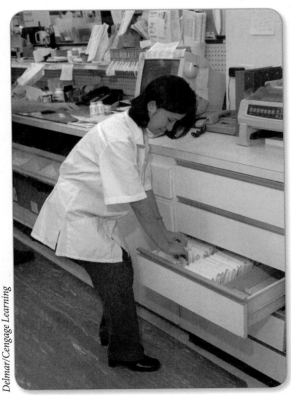

Delmar/Cengage Learning

Figure 12–7 Partitioned drawers may be used for filing prescription orders.

Pricing

Because the pharmacy is a business practice, pharmacy technicians must assist in the financial aspects of the business so that the pharmacy is maintained and makes a fair profit. A method of pricing prescriptions should be established to ensure the profitable operation of the prescription section. The charge applied to a prescription should cover the costs of the ingredients, which include the container and label, the time of the pharmacist or pharmacy technician and auxiliary personnel involved, the cost of inventory maintenance, and the pharmacy's operational costs. Obviously, pricing the prescription must provide a reasonable margin of profit on investment.

Refilling

In providing instructions for refilling a prescription, the prescriber indicates on the original prescription the number of appropriate refills. Although state laws may impose such limits, federal law does not limit the number of prescription refills for noncontrolled medications. On the other hand, refilling prescriptions for controlled agents is strictly regulated. A prescriber should not indefinitely renew any prescription without reevaluating the patient to ensure that the medication as originally prescribed remains the drug of choice. Maintaining accurate records of refills is important not only for complying with federal and state laws, but also for providing information on the patient's medication history.

FLOOR PLAN OF THE RETAIL PHARMACY

Having similar floor plans, almost all community pharmacies are generally organized into two areas: the front area and the prescription processing area. OTC drugs, cosmetics, and other merchandise items are located in the front area. Dispensing of legend drugs, which are regulated under federal law, always requires a prescription because these drugs are off-limits to customers. Only authorized individuals can enter the prescription processing areas. By state regulations, a description of the space and equipment is required. Figures 12–8 and 12–9 show the front and prescription dispensing areas of community pharmacies.

Drop-off Window

The drop-off window allows customers to drop off prescriptions, new hard copies (or Rx) or refills, as well as to verbally request a refill. Via the drop-off window, technicians obtain all personal information that is required for a hard-copy prescription.

Input Terminals

Before they can start the order, technicians must input the information into the computer. After entering the information for the prescription, technicians then route the order for filling.

Prescription Counter

The prescription counter is an area that pharmacists or technicians can use to prepare prescriptions.

Drive-Through

Some community pharmacies have drive-through windows that allow customers or patients to drop off prescriptions or to purchase their medications (Figure 12–10). Pharmacy technicians need to make sure that the correct people receive their orders, not another person's order, and they must ask if patients have any questions for the pharmacist about the prescriptions. The pharmacist should be available for consultation with patients.

Consultation Area

The consultation area is strictly for the pharmacist to counsel patients privately. Technicians must always remember that they are not legally permitted to counsel patients about medications. Consulting is the pharmacist's role and responsibility.

Customer Service Area

The community pharmacy is different from the hospital pharmacy. Technicians in the community pharmacy interact with patients as customers (Figure 12–11). Therefore, customer service is one of the most important aspects of the community pharmacy, and

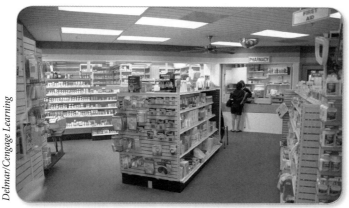

Figure 12–8 The front area of the retail pharmacy.

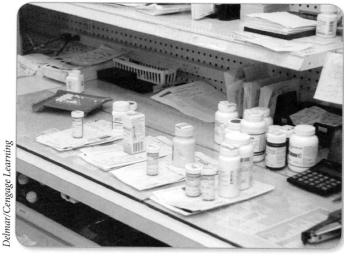

Figure 12–9 The dispensing area of the retail pharmacy.

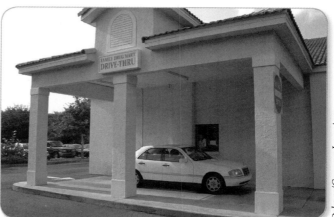

Figure 12–10 Drive-through windows allow patients to drop off prescriptions or to purchase their medications.

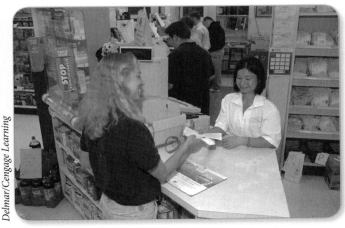

Figure 12–11 Technicians in the community pharmacy interact with patients as customers.

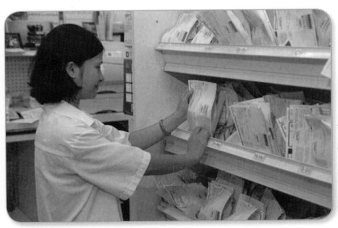

Figure 12–12 Shelves are used to store completed prescriptions that customers are not going to pick up right away.

technicians must have strong interpersonal skills. Customers inside the pharmacy can also pick up their prescriptions in this area.

Refrigerator

Each pharmacy must have a refrigerator to store drugs that are required to be kept at temperatures between 2°C and 8°C. The refrigerator must be used exclusively for medications. No food or beverages can be stored in any refrigerator designated for medications.

Prescription Shelves

When customers do not pick them up right away, completed prescriptions should be placed in a specific area or on shelves (Figure 12–12). For storage, prescriptions should be alphabetized by patient name.

Cash Register Area

Technicians may ring up prescriptions and other items, such as OTC products, into the cash register and accept payment for their purchase. Cash register machines are connected into the pharmacy's computer and can provide prices automatically by using barcode scanners. In handling cash payments properly, technicians must count the payment in the customer's presence, confirming the amount verbally.

PHARMACY COMPUTER SYSTEM

Because of pharmacists' expanded informational needs and because of the increased amount of paperwork required in practice, computers are now standard in pharmacy practice. Computer systems are essential for promoting efficiency by offering improving technology and expanding databases that provide needed support. Most chain pharmacies are linked together by dedicated telephone lines or satellites, hence facilitating the sharing of information between pharmacies.

Computerized systems can be used in the pharmacy in three areas:

1. Prescription dispensing and associated record maintenance

2. Clinical support and accounting

3. Business management

Many insurance and prescription plans now require online verification and authorization before medications can be dispensed. Pharmacists and pharmacy technicians can now use the Internet to obtain and download information about disease states and drug therapy for their patients.

COMPOUNDING

The vast majority of prescriptions dispensed are for dosage forms that are produced by manufacturers approved by the Food and Drug Administration (FDA). These standardized dosages meet the needs for most patients. Many patients, however, need custom-made dosages to treat specific problems. Many community pharmacists offer specialized compounding services. Extremely small doses for pediatric or geriatric use may be needed. Always a skill unique to pharmacists, compounding continues to be a part of contemporary pharmacy practice.

EXPLORING THE WEB

Visit http://www.cvs.com; this link opens the window into CVS/pharmacy's online pharmacy, where customers can not only request refills, but also learn about the drugs they take.

Visit http://www.riteaid.com; the Rite Aid Pharmacy site has a specialty link to "Pharmacy," where customers can request refills or courtesy refills of their prescriptions online and can learn more about the medications they take.

Visit http://www.walgreens.com; similar to Rite Aid, Walgreens has a specialty link to its "Pharmacy," where customers can request refills or express refills online and can learn about the medications they take.

REVIEW QUESTIONS

1. Prescribed medication is also called:

   A. superscription
   B. subscription
   C. inscription
   D. legend drug

2. Auxiliary labels are used to emphasize:

   A. important aspects of aseptic technique
   B. important characteristics of the dispensed medication
   C. that technicians complete the dispensed medication
   D. that technicians satisfy the customers

3. Child-resistant containers are used in which situation?

   A. dispensed medications for patients in the hospital
   B. dispensed medications for patients in nursing homes
   C. dispensed legend drugs—any of them
   D. dispensed drugs for extended-care facilities

4. Which area in the community pharmacy is the most important?

   A. customer service area
   B. consultation area
   C. drive-through area
   D. all of the above

5. The pharmacy technician may do which duty?

   A. count or pour medications
   B. empty returned medications to stock containers
   C. take new prescriptions over the phone
   D. counsel a patient

6. Refills for a prescription may be completed when the:

   A. patient loses the prescription
   B. prescriber fills in the refill blank
   C. prescriber leaves the refill blank
   D. patient tells the technician to refill the prescription

7. Which statement is correct in regard to a prescription?

   A. It must include the patient's full first and last names.
   B. It must include the patient's social security number.
   C. It must include the pharmacy technician's signature.
   D. It must include the pharmacist's signature.

8. Why do some pharmacists try to price prescriptions before dispensing them?

   A. The medication is close to being expired.
   B. The medication is manufactured in another country.
   C. Some medications are unusually expensive.
   D. They wish to keep a good relationship with the patients.

9. The prescription label's size should be appropriate for the:

   A. amount of medication prescribed
   B. prescription container's size
   C. patient's age
   D. patient's wishes

10. To prevent contamination of capsules and tablets, pharmacists or pharmacy technicians should wipe the counting tray after each use with:

    A. cold water
    B. their fingers
    C. bleach
    D. an alcohol wipe and/or a dry cloth

CHAPTER 13

Advanced Pharmacy

OUTLINE

GLOSSARY

Ambulatory care – medical care given on an outpatient basis where patients can come and go to an office or clinic for diagnostic tests or treatments

Enteral nutrition – feedings, other than normal eating, given into the gastrointestinal system; usually applied to specially prepared liquid feedings

Hospice – originally a facility, usually within a hospital, intended to care for the terminally ill, in particular, by providing physical comfort to the patient and emotional support and counseling to the patient and the family

Long-term care – a wide range of health and health-related support services

Long-term care pharmacy organization - an organization involving a licensed professional pharmacy or practice that provides medications and clinical services to long-term care facilities and their residents

Mail-order pharmacy – a licensed pharmacy that uses the mail or other carriers (e.g., overnight carriers or parcel services) to deliver prescriptions to patients

Nuclear pharmacy – a pharmacy that is specially licensed to work with radioactive materials; previously called radiopharmacy

Parenteral nutrition – a combination of amino acids, dextrose, fats, vitamins, minerals, electrolytes, and water administered intravenously that is capable of providing all the nutrients needed to sustain life

Radiopharmaceutical – a drug that is or has been made radioactive to treat diseases (e.g., radioactive iodine) but most commonly used as diagnostic agents

Starter kit – a group of medicines provided to a hospice patient to treat urgent problems that develop in the last days or weeks of life

Total parenteral nutrition (TPN) – an intravenous feeding that supplies all the nutrients necessary to sustain life

EXPANDING ROLE OF THE PHARMACIST

Today, the role of the pharmacist is expanding, and this evolution has guided the differentiation of pharmacy practice in various subspecialties. The rapid development of new drugs and drug delivery systems, changes in the health-care delivery system, an increase in the acuity of illness of institutionalized patients, and increased emphasis on patient outcomes and quality of health care are very important factors in this evolution.

The primary goals of changes in the health-care system are to reduce health-care costs and to increase the overall quality of life for the patient. To be effective in assisting pharmacists in the advancement of pharmacy practice, pharmacy technicians must be trained, skillful, and knowledgeable in these areas.

Long-Term Care Pharmacy Services

Long-term care is defined as a wide range of health and health-related support services. Recipients may be people of any age, ranging from children with congenital anomalies to elderly persons with chronic diseases and the multifaceted changes associated with aging (mental or physical impairment). The goal of long-term care is to enable a person to maintain the maximum possible level of functional independence.

Because of limited resources, most long-term care facilities contract dispensing and clinical pharmacy services and pay other companies to take care of the majority of patient medications. The licensed professional pharmacy or practice that provides medications and clinical services to long-term care facilities and their residents is called a long-term care pharmacy organization. Although a pharmacist or pharmacy technician does not have to be physically present at the facility during all hours, services must be made available 24 hours a day.

Pharmacists perform two types of functions for long-term care: distributive and consultant. The distributive pharmacist is responsible for making sure patients receive the correct medicines that were ordered. This job is mainly done outside of the long-term care facility itself. The impact and cost savings of consultant pharmacist services in long-term care have been documented.

The role of the consultant pharmacist has been shown to decrease overall medication costs, the occurrence of medication errors and adverse drug reactions and interactions, the length of hospitalization, and mortality rates of long-term care patients. Consultant pharmacists in long-term care are, in many ways, like hospital pharmacy directors in that they must supervise all aspects of the comprehensive pharmaceutical services delivered to patients. Interacting with doctors, nurses, and other health professionals, consultant pharmacists are responsible for several different nursing homes or other facilities and may only visit each at certain weekly or monthly intervals.

Home Health-Care Pharmacy

Home health-care pharmacy is one of the fastest growing segments of the health-care market. Today, most serious medical conditions and problems are treated outside of the hospital setting, many times at home. Home health care is an important part of the continuum of care.

Growth of this system is related to several factors, such as the increase in the number of elderly persons, patient preference, lower costs, improvement of technology, managed care, and physician acceptance. Several types of home health-care services are available, including:

• Pharmaceutical services

• Nursing services

• Personal care services

• Rehabilitation services

• Home medical supply services

Pharmacies today provide many home health-care products and services, including durable medical supplies, orthopedic supplies, oxygen therapy, wound care, artificial limbs, medical devices, prescription medications, infusion therapy (intravenous [IV]), and nutritional therapy. The patient may have multiple conditions that require monitoring of treatment beyond high-tech therapy for which other home care providers and the patient's regular physician continue to be involved.

The most common high-tech therapies include:

- IV antibiotic therapy
- Chemotherapy
- Pain medication
- Total parenteral nutrition (TPN)
- Enteral nutrition
- Renal dialysis
- Respiratory and ventilation therapy

High-tech home care requires close collaboration of the physician, the pharmacist, the registered nurse, and, depending on the type of therapy, the medical supply company.

Home Infusion Pharmacy

A unique area for pharmacists and pharmacy technicians where infusion therapies are prepared and dispensed to patients in the home. Home infusion pharmacy includes IV solutions, other injectable drugs, and enteral nutrition therapy. This type of service involves safe compounding of an IV solution and its delivery to the patient. Equipment and supplies needed to infuse the solution are also provided.

Home infusion pharmacies may be established in different areas, such as community pharmacies, long-term care pharmacies, and hospital pharmacies. Several types of infusion therapies are prescribed for home infusion, depending on the patient's condition. These therapies include antibiotic therapy, pain management therapy, hydration therapy, nutrition therapy, and chemotherapy.

A wide variety of equipment is used in the home infusion pharmacy including automated compounding and dispensing devices, horizontal and vertical laminar flow hoods, refrigerators with locked compartments for storage of drugs, computer hardware,

and printers. Supplies found in the home infusion pharmacy include syringes, needles, dispensing pins, IV solution containers, filters, transfer sets, IV tubing, alcohol preparation pads, gloves, masks, gowns, beard and shoe covers, and others.

In the home infusion pharmacy, one of the main duties of pharmacy technicians is the processing of equipment and supply orders. Pharmacy technicians must be familiar with vascular access and vascular access devices, infusion devices, and other IV delivery systems. In addition to compounding sterile products (Figure 13–1), pharmacy technicians handle home infusion equipment and supplies and must understand the three risk levels for contamination of sterile products under the USP Chapter 797. Chapters 10 and 15 discuss USP 797 and clean rooms in detail.

Pharmacy technicians must have knowledge and skills specific to home infusion therapies and nutritional products, sterile compounding, aseptic technique, pharmaceutical calculations, and computer skills; in addition, they must understand the laws and regulations pertaining to home infusion pharmacy. In the home infusion pharmacy, pharmacy technicians may be responsible for compounding, equipment and supplies, and computer functions.

Pharmacy technicians must also be familiar with the two types of nutrition therapy: parenteral and enteral. In **parenteral nutrition** therapy, nutrients

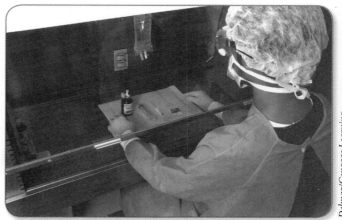

Figure 13–1 The technician is ready to perform the compounding of sterile products.

Delmar/Cengage Learning

are delivered directly into the bloodstream. Total parenteral nutrition (TPN) consists of amino acids (protein), dextrose (carbohydrates), lipids (fats), water, electrolytes, vitamins, trace elements, and medication (insulin and heparin). The base solutions of TPN (hyperalimentation) are made up of amino acids, dextrose, lipids, and water. TPN formulations are highly complex, and proper mixing is important. In preparing the formulations, pharmacists and technicians should follow a safe and effective order of mixing the ingredients. TPN formulations for home infusion are usually prepared several days before they are administered. When TPN solutions are mixed, the last base components added are lipids.

In the second type of nutritional therapy, enteral nutrition, foods and nutrients are delivered into the gastrointestinal (GI) tract through a feeding tube. This process, called *tube feeding*, is the most common home infusion nutritional therapy. For short-term therapy of up to three to four weeks, feeding tubes are placed into the stomach through the nose; for long-term therapy, into the stomach or small intestine through the skin. Used to supplement oral or parenteral nutrition, enteral nutrition can also be used to meet the patient's entire nutritional needs. Patients with swallowing problems resulting from conditions such as stroke, dementia, trauma, cancer, or acquired immunodeficiency syndrome (AIDS) are candidates for home enteral nutrition.

Hospice Pharmacy

An organized program of services to meet a terminally ill patient's physical, emotional, spiritual, and social needs, hospice care focuses on the patient's comfort, rather than on a cure for the disease. Hospice care allows patients to live the remainder of their lives as free from pain and other symptoms as possible. Hospice serves all types and ages of patients and is provided in a variety of settings. The preferred setting is in the home. An inpatient hospice facility may provide a safe and comfortable alternative. Medicare, Medicaid, and private insurance provide funding for hospice programs. For a patient to be eligible for hospice care under Medicare, a physician must certify that death is expected within six months.

Pharmacists have become involved in hospice by providing needed medications and pharmaceutical care services to patients who are terminally ill or nearing the end of life. A pharmacy must prepare and dispense medications, medication-related equipment and supplies, and pharmaceutical care services to hospice patients at home or in a facility. A hospice pharmacy can be part of a traditional community pharmacy, in which hospice is a part of its business, or it can be a pharmacy that services only hospice patients.

Hospice pharmacy services can be divided into two areas: clinical and dispensing. Clinical services include pain management, symptom management, medication monitoring, drug regimen review, drug information services, and formulary development and management. Dispensing services include medications and related equipment and supplies, sterile IV compounding (pain, hydration, and chemotherapy), starter kits, and 24-hour on-call coverage. A starter kit is a group of medications that the hospice pharmacy gives to a hospice patient to provide a "start" in treatment for the majority of urgent problems that can develop during the last days or weeks of life. Patients may suffer from pain, fever, nausea, vomiting, anxiety, agitation, increased secretions, and constipation.

Ambulatory Care Pharmacy

A significant trend in health care has been the emphasis on shorter hospital stays and on outpatient care. Now a standard for health-care delivery, ambulatory care includes a wide range of services such as outpatient pharmacies, emergency department, primary care clinics, specialty clinics, ambulatory care centers, and family practice groups.

The increase in ambulatory care services has greatly expanded the opportunities for ambulatory care pharmacy practitioners. Many outpatient pharmacies provide only traditional pharmaceutical services. Ambulatory care pharmacy practitioners, more commonly referred to as *clinical pharmacists*, practice in a wide variety of primary care clinics. The clinical pharmacist improves drug therapy documentation, improves patient compliance, decreases duplicate prescriptions, and prevents the risk of overdosage.

The pharmacy clinic provides refills to drop-in patients. Physicians refer patients to clinical pharmacists, who provide physical assessment, order laboratory tests, alter dosages, and change medications. One of the most successful pharmacist-managed ambulatory clinics has been the anticoagulation clinic. The value of clinical pharmacists in the chronic management of patients with hypertension, diabetes, or allergies and of patients receiving anticoagulation therapy is obvious.

An important aspect of ambulatory care practice is the clinical pharmacist's involvement in drug therapy decisions. The pharmacist must be available and accessible when the patient is being seen. Successful ambulatory care pharmacy services must be comprehensive and continual, and clinical pharmacy services must be provided 80% to 90% of the time.

Mail-Order Pharmacy

One of the fastest growing areas in pharmacy practice, a mail-order pharmacy is one that dispenses *maintenance medications* (those required on a continual basis for the treatment of a chronic condition) to patients through mail delivery. Offered by the majority of health plans today, mail-order pharmacy is an option to the traditional retail pharmacy for obtaining prescriptions. In most cases, mail-order pharmacies contract with health insurers and fill prescriptions at discounted rates for members of those plans. Patients receive their medications through mail or delivery services. As a unique practice setting for pharmacists and pharmacy technicians, the mail-order pharmacy staff consists of licensed pharmacists, registered nurses, and technicians.

Providing services to all 50 states, mail-order pharmacies operate at a high volume (which results in discounts) and are generally more economical for

patients. Mail-order pharmacies can also serve more patients, particularly those who have chronic illnesses such as diabetes, high blood pressure, depression, heart disease, arthritis, or gastrointestinal disorders. Because they can predict the need for medication, mail-order pharmacies can more easily maintain supply by mail delivery.

Telepharmacy

Integrating pharmacy software, remotely controlled dispensing cabinetry, and telecommunications technologies, *telepharmacy* provides pharmaceutical services from a distance. Telepharmacy, commonly used in rural areas to provide pharmacy services that otherwise do not exist, extends pharmaceutical services to multiple points of care. Through telepharmacy, pharmacists can reach new patients and markets, improve patient care, and enhance medication safety, all while controlling prescription costs. Using automated drug dispensing systems to integrate remote or local pharmacist-controlled dispensing, telepharmacy brings real-time medication dispensing and pharmacist counseling directly to the point-of-care.

Nuclear Pharmacy

A branch of the pharmacy profession, nuclear pharmacy deals with the provision of services related to radiopharmaceuticals, radioactive drugs used in the diagnosis and treatment of disease. Radioactive drugs contain radioactive elements. A radionuclide can release three types of radiation, including alpha, beta, and gamma radiation. Gamma radiation is the most penetrating. Pharmacy technicians working in the nuclear pharmacy must wear special badges that monitor radiation levels. These badges are checked monthly to determine amounts of radiation exposure.

The nuclear pharmacy consists of several areas, as follows:

- Compounding or dispensing areas
- Storage of finished radiopharmaceuticals in the packaging area

- A breakdown room (to store empty or used radiopharmaceuticals before they are returned or dismantled for reuse)

- A storage room for radioactive waste

Nuclear medicine uses very small quantities of radio-nuclides for the diagnosis and treatment of disease. Used as tracers for assessing the structure, function, secretion, excretion, and volume of a particular organ or tissue, radiopharmaceuticals are also used to analyze biological specimens, to treat specific diseases such as hyperthyroidism, thyroid cancer, and polycythemia vera, and to alleviate bone pain.

Most radiopharmaceuticals are prepared as sterile, pyrogen-free intravenous solutions or suspensions to be administered directly to the patient. An important component of nuclear medicine is imaging, which involves administering radiopharmaceuticals to a patient orally, intravenously, or by inhalation to localize a specific organ or system and its structure and function. Essentially a sterile compounding practice, nuclear pharmacy involves the procuring, storage, compounding, dispensing, and provision of information about radiopharmaceuticals and is one possible area of specialization for both pharmacists and pharmacy technicians (Figure 13–2).

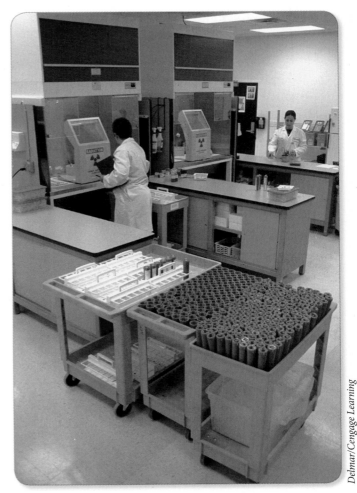

Figure 13–2 The pharmacist and the technician are working in the nuclear pharmacy dealing with radiopharmaceuticals.

Delmar/Cengage Learning

EXPLORING THE WEB

Visit http://www.ascp.com/members; the American Society of Consultant Pharmacists (ASCP) empowers pharmacists to enhance quality of care for all older persons through the appropriate use of medication and the promotion of healthy aging.

Visit http://www.hospicepharmacia.com; Hospice Pharmacia deals with the management of end-of-life medication and helps hospice nurses, physicians, and administrators to focus on caring for patients and their families.

Visit http://www.ltcpa.org; the Long Term Care Pharmacy Alliance (LTCPA) provides medications to millions of the nation's long-term care residents.

Visit http://www.nutritioncare.org; the American Society for Parenteral and Enteral Nutrition (A.S.P.E.N.) seeks to improve patient care by advancing the science and practice of nutrition support therapy.

Visit http://www.uspharmd.com; US PharmD includes much information about pharmacy degrees, pharmacy schools, and the role of the pharmacist.

REVIEW QUESTIONS

1. What is one of the fastest growing areas in pharmacy?

   A. mail-order pharmacy
   B. ambulatory care pharmacy
   C. nuclear pharmacy
   D. home infusion therapy

2. The most common high-tech therapies include:

   A. chemotherapy
   B. pain medication
   C. IV antibiotic therapy
   D. all of the above

3. What is the one main duty of pharmacy technicians in the home infusion pharmacy?

   A. ordering Schedule II drugs
   B. attending professional development seminars
   C. processing equipment and supply orders
   D. counseling patients

4. In long-term care pharmacy, using a consultant pharmacist has been shown to:

   A. increase the length of hospitalization
   B. increase overall medication costs
   C. decrease overall medication costs
   D. decrease occurrence of communicable diseases

5. The growth of home health-care pharmacy is related to all of the following factors, except:

   A. lower costs
   B. improvement of technology
   C. erection of more hospitals
   D. increased numbers of elderly patients

6. What is a starter kit?

   A. medications from an organization that provides day-care services
   B. a group of medications that a hospice pharmacy provides for a hospice patient to treat most of the urgent problems that develop in the last days or weeks or life
   C. medications for a hospital patient who is discharged right away
   D. medications for a hospice patient who is discharged

7. Home infusion pharmacy includes all of the following, except:

   A. IV solutions
   B. radiation therapy
   C. other injectable drugs
   D. enteral nutrition therapy

8. For whom has the increase in ambulatory care services greatly expanded opportunities?

   A. physicians who seek positions in a hospital
   B. pharmacy technicians to get a license
   C. hospital pharmacy technicians
   D. ambulatory pharmacy practitioners

9. Which is not a duty of pharmacy technicians in home infusion pharmacy?

   A. ordering medications
   B. counseling patients
   C. managing inventory
   D. compounding total parenteral nutrition formulations

10. Which of the following base components must be mixed last into a TPN bag?

    A. amino acids
    B. dextrose
    C. lipids
    D. sterile water

The Role and Duties of Pharmacy Technicians

OUTLINE

GLOSSARY

Compounding – mixing drugs or other substances specifically for a certain patient

Drug Enforcement Agency (DEA) – the government agency responsible for enforcing the controlled substance laws and regulations of the United States

Extemporaneous – a medication that is made based upon a particular set of circumstances or criteria

Professionalism – the conduct or qualities characterized by or conforming to the technical or ethical standards of a profession; exhibiting a courteous, conscientious, and generally businesslike manner in the workplace

Role of the Pharmacy Technician in Community Pharmacies

As the practice of pharmacy develops, so does the role of pharmacy technicians. The number of prescriptions dispensed in the United States has rapidly increased, as has the number of settings in which pharmacists practice. To keep up with the rising demand for pharmaceutical products and services, pharmacy technicians will play a greater role in support of pharmaceutical care in their communities. Having an important role in every pharmacy setting, pharmacy technicians have the primary goal of assisting the pharmacist in serving patients.

Job Responsibilities

Recent studies indicate that pharmacy technicians are now involved in more areas of pharmacy practice. In addition to assisting with outpatient prescription dispensing, many community pharmacy technicians participate in purchasing, controlling inventory, billing, and repackaging products.

Receiving and Reviewing Prescriptions

Prescriptions come to the pharmacy in three main ways: by person, fax, or telephone. In the community setting, the prescriber typically writes the prescription and the patient delivers it to the pharmacy. Rules govern special prescriptions such as those for controlled substances or narcotics and those that need special compounding.

Many states require that only licensed professionals can call in prescriptions. Another requirement is that a pharmacist must receive telephone prescriptions, although some states do allow pharmacy technicians to receive called-in prescriptions. In states that allow only pharmacists to receive original called-in prescriptions, technicians are often allowed to receive called-in requests for refills. Technicians should consult their pharmacy's policies and procedures manual about how to handle called-in prescriptions.

Technicians should screen prescriptions for anything that looks unusual, such as a dispense quantity in excess of normal quantities or an unrecognizable signature. If something looks suspicious, technicians should present the prescription to the pharmacist for more evaluation. Also, technicians must recognize and verify the practitioner's **Drug Enforcement Agency (DEA)** number. By following the steps in the example below, technicians can verify DEA numbers.

Example:

A technician receives a prescription from a practitioner, say, Andrea Smith, who has the DEA number CS-1424326.

Step 1:

Verify the first two letters in the DEA number. The first letter, *C*, is a standard letter that the DEA assigns. In this case, *C* signifies the registrant as a "practitioner." The first letter may be a variety of different letters based on the type of practice holding the DEA registration. The second letter, *S*, is the first letter of the registrant's last name, which is "Smith."

Step 2:

Now, check the number portion as follows:

- Add the first, third, and fifth digits:

$$1 + 2 + 3 = 6$$

- Add the second, fourth, and sixth digits:

$$4 + 4 + 2 = 10$$

- Now, multiply the second sum by 2:

$$10 \times 2 = 20$$

- Add this product to the first sum:

$$20 + 6 = 26$$

- Note that "26" ends in a "6." The rule here is that the final digit in the complete DEA number must be identical to the final digit in this sum in order to be valid. Therefore, because "6" matches the final DEA number digit, this number is a valid DEA number.

When dispensing a prescription, pharmacy technicians must enter the following information into the computer:

- Patient information

- Patient profile

- Correct drug and dosage

- Correct physician's name

- DEA number of physician for controlled substances

- Directions for use

- Quantity of medication

- Refill number

- Brand name or a generic product

- Patient counseling provided

- Dispensing pharmacist's initials

One major duty of pharmacy technicians is processing new and refill prescriptions. Depending on the community pharmacy, this process may differ. Because most pharmacies use computers, technicians must process the prescription accurately and efficiently on the system.

Most pharmacy computers allow pharmacists or technicians to look up a refill through the patient profile for the medication. Technicians must be sure that a refill is available. Although they may use many different mechanisms to request refills without involving the pharmacist, technicians should consult the pharmacist if they are confused about how to handle refills.

Dispensing Prescriptions

The last step in the prescription-processing function is dispensing. To prepare a medication for the patient, technicians print a prescription label that has all the patient and prescription information they entered into the system. When the label is ready, technicians then prepare the medication. A large and important component of the dispensing function is patient counseling, which only the pharmacist can perform.

Prescription dispensing is becoming more automated as a result of rapid advances in robotics and other technology. Many of the processes that pharmacists and pharmacy technicians previously handled may now be done automatically, including the "picking" of medications for prescriptions, counting, pouring, sealing, labeling, and other functions. Automated dispensing systems integrated with pharmacy computers are becoming more commonplace every day. The most commonly recognized names in this area of pharmacy include Pyxis, Baxter, and ScriptPro. See "Exploring the Web" section for Web sites that offer more detail about automation.

Labeling Prescriptions

In addition to listing the name of the patient, the pharmacy, and the prescriber, the prescription label should accurately identify the medication and provide directions for its use. The prescription label for a controlled substance must contain the following information:

1. Name and address of the pharmacy

2. Serial number assigned to the prescription by the pharmacy

3. Name of the medication being dispensed

4. Strength of the medication

5. Dosage form

6. Date of the initial filling

7. Name of the patient

8. Name of the prescriber

9. Directions for use

10. Cautionary statements as required by law

11. Refill information

The patient needs to be informed of some specific properties of the medication. For example, the medication may make the patient sensitive to sunlight; a drug may change the color of urine or must be taken with food. In preparing the medication,

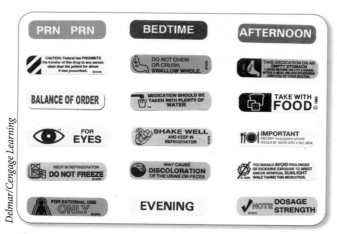

Figure 14–1 Auxiliary labels.

technicians or pharmacists attach *auxiliary labeling*, also referred to as *strip labels*, to the container to warn the patient of these properties (see Figure 14–1).

Keeping Records

A medication order or prescription becomes part of the patient's medical record (see Figure 14–2A and B). Pharmacies keep this information in the patient's computer record, and third-party payers such as insurance companies rely on this correct patient-identifying information to properly process and pay submitted claims for drugs.

Pricing

A pharmacy, similar to any other business, deals with expenses and receipts and must make a profit. Hence, pharmacy technicians have the additional responsibility to help ensure that receipts are greater than expenses so that the pharmacy can continue to operate. If assigned pricing, pharmacy technicians often follow directions to mark products up a certain percentage over their cost, or their average wholesale price, or mark products down by a certain percentage for discounts.

Insurance companies often use either a percentage-based payment for prescription products or a capitation fee. Pharmacy technicians also have responsibility for monitoring and correcting insurance billing for prescription products.

Maintaining Patient Profiles and Billing Records

Usually organized by medication type or by order of input, patient medication profiles include all of the patient's prescription information such as original date, refill dates, and prescribing physician. Active medication orders should be listed first, and they should be separated from the discontinued medications, which should be available only for review after entering an appropriate command at the end of the profile.

Third-party payer information such as medical insurance information, including any copayment amount, is entered in patient profiles. After filling the prescription and preparing the label, technicians or pharmacists can complete the billing. Many pharmacy customers have prescription drug insurance, and their insurance carriers, the third party, must be billed. The patient's prescription card contains information such as the name of the insured person, the insurance carrier, a group number, a cardholder identification number, information on dependents covered, an

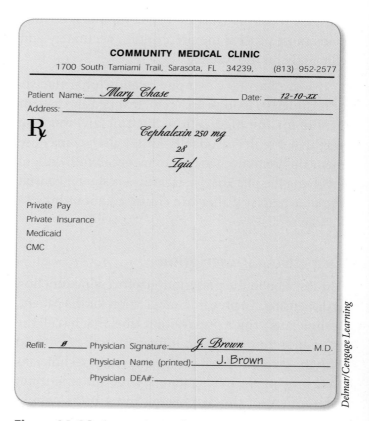

Figure 14–2A A prescription form.

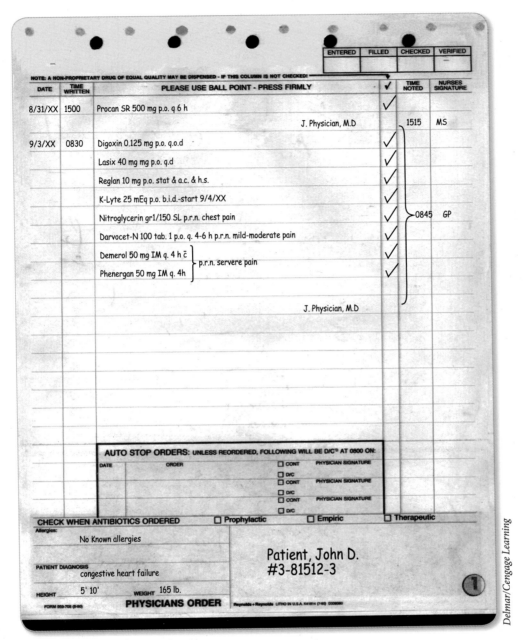

Figure 14–2B A physician's order.

expiration date, and the amount of the copayment (see Figure 14–3). Technicians must enter all of this information into the computer system.

Answering Telephone Calls

Fielding phone calls for the pharmacist from patients, customers, or health-care professionals falls to technicians. They must answer the phone in a pleasant and courteous manner, referring any questions they cannot answer to the pharmacist (e.g., when a call requires the pharmacist's judgment or questions are about medications or general health).

Operating the Cash Register

Pharmacy technicians also handle the pharmacy cash register. Operating a cash register successfully requires taking care of payments properly. The cash register is connected to the pharmacy's computer. If

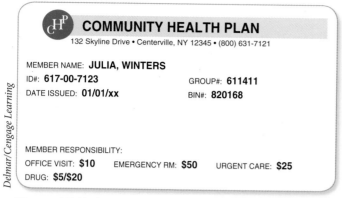

Figure 14–3 A prescription card.

a bar code scanner is available, technicians can automatically enter prices for any product. If the scanner is not available, however, pharmacy technicians must manually enter, or ring in, the prescription.

Purchasing

Pharmacy technicians often order products for use or sale. They may work alone with a purchasing agent and deal directly with pharmaceutical or medical supply companies on matters such as price. After completing a purchase order that includes the product name, amount, and price, technicians then transmit the order directly to manufacturers or wholesalers. Although the pharmacist always has responsibility for selection of drugs, technicians may prepare purchase orders (see Figure 14–4).

Checking Deliveries and Controlling Inventory

When pharmaceutical products arrive, technicians must carefully check the products against the purchase order and report damaged products without delay

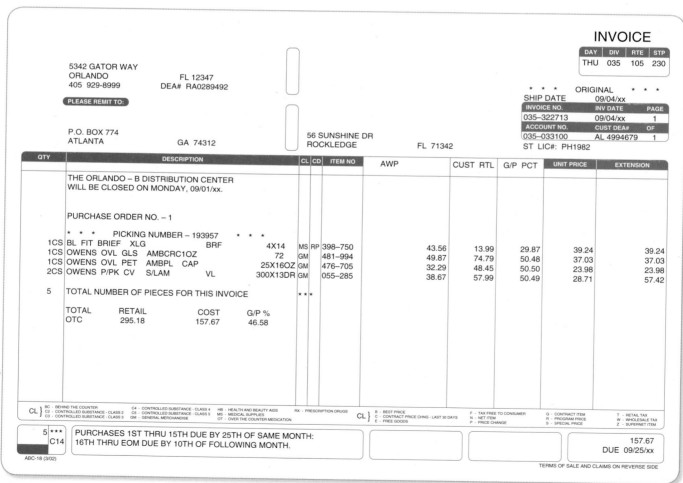

Figure 14–4 A purchase order.

and return them to the manufacturer or wholesaler. Also, pharmacy technicians must check all products for expiration dates.

Working with Computer Applications

After the telephone, the computer is probably the most frequently used and possibly the most important piece of equipment in the modern pharmacy. Pharmacy technicians must be familiar with the computer equipment used in the pharmacy and with all different programs that they will be asked to use. All patient information for pharmacy record keeping, such as insurance carriers and diagnostic codes, can be computerized. Other information entered into the computer may include payroll and bills the pharmacy pays.

ROLE OF THE PHARMACY TECHNICIAN IN INSTITUTIONAL PHARMACIES

Institutional pharmacies have ever-greater demands requiring them to broaden their scope of services. Because these pharmacies are open 24 hours a day, 7 days a week, pharmacy technicians must understand all the facility's various departments and how they interact with the pharmacy.

As they assist the pharmacist, technicians have a variety of roles and duties in institutional settings. Under the pharmacist's supervision, pharmacy technicians can handle many routine tasks that they have been trained to do. It is essential to understand the roles and duties of technicians in the hospital setting.

Following Policies and Procedures

Pharmacy technicians must follow the policies and procedures of the hospital in which they work. Policy and procedure manuals focus on general responsibilities, technical responsibilities, documentation, and reporting duties of pharmacy technicians and other pharmacy personnel. Because they are accountable for all outcomes, including those that result from the failure to follow procedures, pharmacy technicians must understand and follow these standards.

Maintaining Medication Records

An important part of the pharmacy technician's job is to accurately maintain the patient records on the pharmacy information system. Records should include the patient's weight, as well as the care and counseling of the patient. Patient medication profiles are usually organized by medication type.

Preparing Unit Doses

Pharmacy technicians are responsible for preparing the unit doses for individual patients each day, placing a 24-hour supply of the medications that have been ordered by the physicians into medication bins. Maintaining up-to-date records allows the pharmacist to provide the most correct unit doses for patients. The pharmacist must check each patient drawer in a drug cart before the carts are delivered to patient care floors.

Compounding Medications

In some circumstances, a drug may need to be created from a prepared recipe. If a written procedure exists for preparation of a drug, pharmacy technicians can prepare it. This process is called compounding. Pharmacy technicians can handle the majority of compounding activities, such as intravenous admixtures and total parenteral nutrition. However, unless pharmacy technicians have been specially trained to handle these agents, the pharmacist commonly handles certain types of compounding, such as chemotherapy drugs. The pharmacist must always directly supervise pharmacy technicians who handle these types of drugs.

To create a compound drug, technicians must be able to clearly understand the formula and be able to adjust it to increase or decrease amounts as necessary. A sound understanding of mathematical principles is required. Extemporaneous prescription compounding will be discussed in detail in Chapter 15.

Packaging

Many drugs have to be placed in proper containers to remain active and potent. Pharmacy technicians must be aware of these characteristics of drugs to choose the appropriate containers for dispensing and storing them.

Using Aseptic Technique to Prepare Admixtures

Contamination of various types of admixtures by microorganisms may harm, permanently damage, or even cause the death of patients. As a result, pharmacy technicians must always use aseptic technique when preparing these products. Aseptic technique and admixtures are discussed in detail in Chapter 15.

Preparing and Delivering Outpatient Prescriptions

Some hospitals are affiliated with off-site facilities such as nursing homes and rehabilitation centers. Pharmacy technicians are responsible for preparing the medications these facilities need and for delivering them to the facilities in a timely manner.

Inputting Data into the Computer

Data entry is an important part of the pharmacy technician's job. Accurate entry of new data into the computer system and maintenance of records within the system are important. The pharmacy then can be run efficiently because patient records are accurate, inventory is maintained at appropriate levels, and billing can be done in an accurate and timely manner.

Pharmacy technicians need basic skills in computer use. These skills include:

- **Keying:** The standard speed is approximately 35 words per minute. Fast and accurate keying helps to increase the number of prescriptions that a pharmacy can process each day.

- **Familiarity with hardware and software:** Learning about the pharmacy computer system will help pharmacy technicians perform the

computer activities of their jobs with skill, confidence, and speed. Pharmacy technicians must study and understand the basic programs used for word processing and spreadsheets, as well as specialized pharmacy programs. Also, to keep the workflow progressing smoothly, pharmacy technicians should be familiar with operating all types of hardware (such as scanners, printers, etc.).

Ensuring Billing Accuracy

During the billing process, inaccuracies can occur. This is a result of the complicated process of insurance claims, coding, and related forms. Failure to understand how this process works will cause errors in payments, reimbursements, and coverage. Pharmacy technicians should understand how Medicare, Medicaid, and other common insurance providers are correctly billed for the coverage of their patients. See Chapter 18 for detailed information on health insurance and billing.

Inspecting Nursing Unit Drug Stocks

The pharmacy must maintain nursing unit drug stocks, and pharmacy technicians are responsible for inspection of unit drug stocks for proper storage conditions, appropriate inventory, and replacement of expired or damaged stock.

Following Medication Control, Security, and Controlled Substance Accountability

The DEA monitors the use of scheduled drugs and those who prescribe them. Because of increasing crime involving controlled substances and prescription medication, proper security measures are vital. Medication controls should be in place so that any misappropriation of these substances may be discovered and dealt with as quickly as possible. This topic is one of the most important responsibilities of pharmacy technicians and pharmacy personnel, in general, because their ability to practice may be threatened by inefficient medication control policies.

Maintaining Inventory and Reorders

Pharmacy technicians often have the responsibilities of ordering stock and maintaining stock levels. As discussed earlier, many inventory systems are available for use within the pharmacy. Regardless of the system used, technicians must ensure that stock levels are appropriate to allow the pharmacy to operate efficiently without having to borrow stock or order stock at higher prices. When stock is delivered, pharmacy technicians generally check and verify it against the order and clearly mark receipt of the order on the invoice. All orders must be appropriately stored within the pharmacy. Any damaged goods or expired drugs must be returned or properly disposed.

During inventory control processes, the pharmacy computer system should prompt the pharmacy staff when it is time to reorder specific medications and supplies. Therefore, pharmacy technicians must follow their organization's policies and procedures for reordering. They must know when to notify their pharmacist or pharmacy supervisor when specific drugs need to be reordered that they are not allowed (by law) to order themselves. If drugs are close to expiring, pharmacists or pharmacy technicians must remove them from inventory.

Preparing Labels

Each filled medication order must be appropriately labeled. The label should contain the name of the patient the drug is prescribed for, the patient's medical record number, the patient's room number, the name of the prescriber, the date of dispensing, the name of the drug, the strength of the drug, the quantity of the drug dispensed, the dosage directions, and the expiration date. The label should also contain the initials of the person dispensing the drug. Proper labeling on medications is critically important, and a great deal of care should be taken in this task. The label should be checked and rechecked against the medication order. The pharmacist must check and initial all labels before the medications leave the pharmacy.

Maintaining Patient Privacy

Pharmacy technicians are legally bound to uphold the privacy of all patients. New standards for maintaining a patient's privacy have been implemented with regulations in the Health Insurance Portability and Accountability Act (HIPAA). Please review Chapter 2 for more information.

Auditing and Reporting of Medication Processes

Pharmacy technicians must keep complete records of orders, reorders, and dispensations of all drugs (with scheduled drugs being most important) in their hospital pharmacy. For scheduled drugs, federal law requires records be kept on file for two years, and many state laws may require them to be kept for up to five years. When state and federal laws differ, the stricter law should take precedence. Different federal and state agencies, as well as insurance companies, may audit medication records.

Working Safely

For the health and safety of pharmacy personnel, a safe working environment must be maintained. Work areas should be clean, and accidental exposures to harmful substances should be avoided. Emergency and exposure treatment plans should be in place. Pharmacy technicians should be aware of and quickly be able to respond to any unsafe condition. Workplace safety is discussed in more detail in Chapter 10.

ACCOUNTABILITY

Pharmacy technicians must understand the boundaries of what they can and cannot do legally and must be accountable for their performance and also for their mistakes. An error, even a small one, can have disastrous consequences for a patient, a customer, or the pharmacy itself. Pharmacy technicians must develop work habits to ensure accuracy and expect to be held responsible for what they do on the job.

To avoid mistakes, technicians must always double-check everything.

ETHICAL STANDARDS AND PROFESSIONAL BEHAVIOR

Ethics is the study of moral values or principles, and a *professional* is an individual qualified to perform the activities of a specific occupation. Professionalism goes beyond the knowledge, skills, and abilities required to perform those activities.

As professionals, pharmacy technicians represent the profession of pharmacy. Always being courteous and listening with focus, technicians must respect the privacy of patients and keep all information confidential. The most important character traits of good pharmacy technicians are honesty, organization, reliability, and dependability. The pharmacist must be able to count on technicians to maintain confidentiality and privacy of patients and behave ethically, even when not under direct supervision, because of the higher level of trust needed to provide excellent patient care.

Technicians are accountable for the laws and regulations dictated by the Health Insurance Portability and Accountability Act of 1996 (HIPAA). The HIPAA privacy rule became effective on April 14, 2001, and *compliance was required by April 14, 2003*. This rule sets national standards for the protection of health information of patients. To be in compliance, covered entities must implement standards to protect individually identifiable health information and guard against the misuse of that information. The privacy rule does not replace federal, state, or other laws that grant individuals even greater privacy protection. Therefore, pharmacy technicians must always keep in mind that they must maintain confidentiality and privacy of patients.

Each covered entity must have a privacy officer, an individual responsible for all activities related to an organization's policies and procedures covering the privacy of, and access to, patient health information.

The privacy officer ensures compliance with federal and state laws as related to issues about private health information. Overseeing all security systems that are in place to protect patient health information, the privacy officer also interacts as needed with legal counsel and governmental bodies.

Both federal and state laws regulate the disposal of patient information, with each state having varying degrees of regulation. A covered entity should make and retain a record of all disposed patient health information and keep this record permanently. With such record, the covered entity can legally demonstrate that the patient information records were destroyed or disposed of in the regular course of business. This record should include:

- Date of destruction or disposal
- Method of destruction or disposal
- Description of the actual type of information destroyed or disposed of
- The time period covered by the information destroyed or disposed of
- A statement that the patient information records were destroyed or disposed of in the normal course of business
- The signatures of the individuals supervising and witnessing the destruction or disposal

Communication Skills

To be efficient, pharmacy technicians must have effective verbal communication, both oral (spoken) and written. Written communication has traditionally been thought of as being more formal than oral conversation. Today, however, with the increasing use of e-mail, written communication is often as informal as oral communication.

Nonverbal communication is easy to understand, and one needs only to pay attention to the other party to interpret what is being conveyed. Facial expression, eye contact, and body position are all methods of communicating without using words. Listening to the words and the tone of voice is important. Pharmacy technicians must always use a nonjudgmental expression and tone of voice.

Teamwork

Pharmacy technicians need to be genuinely interested in helping people, be warm and caring, and be able to put the needs of others first. An effective health-care team working together does not just happen. To be effective, team members work together to provide appropriate care for each patient. Each member of the team must be committed to solving problems, focusing on the patient, and communicating.

A team approach to patient care ensures comprehensive service without expensive duplication of effort. Because technicians work closely with others to perform their duties, teamwork is also necessary for the smooth operation of the entire pharmacy.

Ability to Handle a Fast Pace and Stress

Learning new ideas, modifying thinking, adapting to new situations, and handling stress—pharmacy technicians will find all these as increasingly important skills in today's evolving and complex health-care delivery system. Most difficult problems can be solved if an individual simply looks at the situation from the other person's point of view. Team members should try to see what obstacles are present and then work together to move past the problem.

A team member in the pharmacy should expect to deal with a high stress environment. Examples of common stressors in the pharmacy setting include interacting with angry customers, needing to multitask, and solving or resolving difficult insurance issues. Pharmacy technicians must handle any workload and other specific situations in a professional manner.

EXPLORING THE WEB

Visit http://www.healthcareitnews.com to learn more about auditing and reporting of medication processes.

Visit http://www.baxter.nl to learn more about the Baxter automated dispensing systems.

Visit http://www.bls.gov for information about pharmacy technicians and assistants and their career opportunities.

Visit http://www.pharmacoethics.com to learn more about pharmacy ethics.

Visit http://www.healthcareerweb.com to find more job information about pharmacy technicians.

Visit http://www.carefusion.com to learn about the Pyxis Dispensing Systems.

Visit http://www.rxamerica.com to review a sample pharmacy policies and procedures manual.

Visit http://www.scriptpro.com for more information about the ScriptPro Dispensing Systems.

REVIEW QUESTIONS

1. By what criterion are patient medication profiles usually organized?

   A. medication type
   B. discontinued medications
   C. physician's specialty
   D. patient's condition

2. To avoid mistakes, what must pharmacy technicians do?

   A. refer all questions to the pharmacist
   B. reenter all patient insurance information
   C. initial medication orders
   D. double-check everything

3. What is the last step in the prescription-processing function?

   A. entering all the patient information into the computer system
   B. counseling with the pharmacist
   C. dispensing the medication
   D. purchasing supplies

4. The prescription label for a controlled substance must contain all of the following information, except:

   A. serial number that the pharmacy assigns to the prescription
   B. patient's social security number
   C. prescriber's name
   D. pharmacy's name and address

5. Which component of the dispensing function can only the pharmacist perform?

   A. counseling patients
   B. accessing the computer system
   C. labeling medications
   D. pricing medications

6. If drugs are close to expiration, what action must be taken?

   A. They must be dispensed quickly, at discounted prices to the patients.
   B. They must be removed from inventory.
   C. They must be tested to see if they are still potent.
   D. The pharmacy technician must return them to the manufacturer.

7. The term *extemporaneous* refers to:

   A. destroying a single-unit package that is not immediately used
   B. destroying medication at the time of expiration
   C. preparing medication that is made based on a particular set of circumstances or criteria
   D. preparing labels for all medications

8. Mixing drugs or other substances specifically for certain patients is called:

   A. unit dosing
   B. dispensing
   C. calculating
   D. compounding

9. What information does not need to be entered into the computer when dispensing a prescription?

   A. correct drug and dosage
   B. technician's initials
   C. refill number
   D. correct physician's name

10. Which laws regulate the disposal of patient information?

    A. state
    B. federal
    C. both
    D. neither

Sterile and Nonsterile Compounding

OUTLINE

Elixirs

Emulsions

Compounding Semisolid Drugs

Ointments

Creams

Pastes

Gels

Compounding Suppositories

Compounding Solid Drugs

Capsules

Tablets

Powders

GLOSSARY

Aseptic technique – preparing and handling sterile products in a manner that prevents microbial contamination

Autoclave – a sterilizing machine that uses a combination of heat, steam, and pressure to sterilize equipment

Beyond-use date – a date after which a product is no longer effective and should not be used

Chemical sterilization – a method of cleaning equipment used for instruments that cannot be exposed to the high temperatures of steam sterilization

Class A prescription balance (electronic balance) –a two-pan device that may be used for weighing small amounts of drugs (not more than 120 g)

Compounding slab – made of ground glass, a plate with a hard, flat, and nonabsorbent surface for mixing compounds

Conical graduates – used for measuring liquids, devices that have wide tops and wide bases and taper from the top to the bottom

Conjunctiva – mucous membrane of the eyes

Counter balance – a device, a double-pan balance, capable of weighing much larger quantities, up to about 5 kg

Cylindrical graduates – used for measuring liquids, devices that have narrow diameters that are the same from top to base

Disinfection – ability to kill microorganisms on the surfaces of various items

Dry heat sterilization – a method of sterilization that uses heated dry air at a temperature of 320°F to 365°F (160°C to 180°C) for 90 minutes to 3 hours

Elixir – a sweetened liquid containing alcohol and water

Emulsion – a suspension containing two different liquids and an agent that holds them together

Extemporaneous compounding – the preparation, mixing, assembling, packaging, and labeling of a drug product based on a prescription order from a licensed practitioner for the individual patient

Gas sterilization – the use of a gas such as ethylene oxide to sterilize medical equipment

Geometric dilution – when mixing agents, the medicament is first mixed with an equal weight of diluent; a further quantity of diluent equal in weight to the mixture is then incorporated; this process is repeated until all the diluent has been mixed in

Levigate – to grind into a smooth substance with moisture

Medical asepsis – complete destruction of organisms after they leave the body

Meniscus – meaning "moon-shaped body"; indicates that the level of the liquid will be slightly higher at the edges

Mortar – a cup-shaped vessel in which materials are ground or crushed

Pestle – a solid device that is used to crush or grind materials in a mortar

Piggyback – a medication, many times an antibiotic, that is added into an IV bag of medication

Pipette – a long, thin, calibrated hollow tube, which is made of glass and used for measuring liquids

Sanitization – a process of cleansing to remove undesirable debris

Solvent – a liquid vehicle in which active ingredients are dissolved

Solution – a liquid drug that does not require shaking before use

Spores – forms that some bacteria assume to increase their chances of surviving heat, dehydration, and antiseptics or antibiotics

Sterilization – complete destruction of all forms of microbial life

Surgical asepsis – the complete destruction of organisms before they enter the body

Suspension – a liquid dosage form that contains solid drug particles floating in a liquid medium

Tablet triturate – solid, small, and usually cylindrically molded or compressed tablets

Tare – the weight of an empty capsule used to compare with the full capsule

Triturate – to reduce to a fine powder by friction

PARENTERAL PREPARATIONS

Only properly educated and fully trained pharmacy technicians should be involved in pharmaceutical compounding. In the pharmacy, all of the ingredients needed to compound a specific formulation are listed on a master formula sheet, also referred to as a *bulk compounding formula record*, which lists the amounts of each ingredient to be used, as well as the manufacturer, lot number, and expiration date. It also has a section where the compounding activities can be documented with the preparer's initials.

Parenteral preparations are given when a medication is rendered inactive in the gastrointestinal tract or when a patient is unable to take medication by mouth (due to vomiting or unconsciousness). Fluids, electrolytes, and nutrients are often administered parenterally. Irrigations used in surgery and ophthalmics are also examples of parenteral preparations.

Parenteral products must have the following unique qualities:

- They must be sterile

- They must be free from contamination by endotoxins

- They must be free from visible particles, which include reconstituted sterile powders

- They should be isotonic; the correct level of isotonicity depends on the route of administration

- They must be chemically, physically, and microbiologically stable

- They must be compatible with IV delivery systems, diluents, and other drug products to be co-administered

For administration, injections may be classified in these six categories:

1. Solutions ready for injection

2. Dry and soluble products ready for combination with a solvent just prior to use

3. Suspensions ready for injection

4. Dry, insoluble products ready for combination with a vehicle just prior to use

5. Emulsions

6. Liquid concentrates ready to be diluted prior to administration

Formulation modifications, or different routes of injection, can be used to slow a drug's onset, hence prolonging its action. Because intestinal absorption is bypassed, parenteral administration more readily controls the therapeutic response of a drug. Disadvantages of parenteral administration, however, include the following:

- Asepsis required at administration

- Risk of tissue toxicity from local irritation

- Pain

- Difficulty in correcting errors

Pharmacy technicians must follow the pharmacy's policies and procedures concerning sterile compounding. The goal is to handle and prepare parenteral preparations in a manner that is as free from biological, chemical, and physical contaminants as possible. This requires proper aseptic technique because parenteral preparations are often unstable and highly potent, yet their characteristics must be preserved without contaminating them.

ASEPTIC TECHNIQUE

Microorganisms include bacteria, fungi, viruses, protozoa, spirochetes, and rickettsia. *Microbiology* is defined as the study of microorganisms, which are organisms that cannot be seen without a microscope. In the pharmacy setting, bacteria, fungi, and viruses most often cause contamination. The most effective way to eliminate transmission of disease from one host to another is through asepsis, which means "being completely sterile (free from microorganisms)." There are two types of asepsis: medical and surgical.

Medical Asepsis

Medical asepsis, also called *clean technique*, is the removal of pathogens to reduce transfer of microorganisms by cleaning any body part or surface that has been exposed to them. Clean technique is used in pharmacy during IV compounding to prevent exposure of pathogens into the sterile parenteral product.

Hand Hygiene

The single most important means of preventing the spread of infection is frequent and effective hand hygiene by all health-care workers. Hands must be washed using the correct technique. Although an extended scrub is not needed each time health-care workers wash their hands, the first scrub in the morning should be extensive, lasting two to four minutes, unless the hands are excessively contaminated. A good antimicrobial soap with chlorhexidine, such as Hibiclens®, which has antiseptic residual action that will last several hours, should be used. Proper hand washing depends on two factors: running water and friction. The water should be warm because water that is too cold or too hot will cause the skin to chap. Friction involves the firm rubbing of all surfaces of the hands and wrists.

Cleaning and Sanitizing

Sanitization, the cleansing process that decreases the number of microorganisms to a safe level, as dictated in public health guidelines, removes debris such as blood and other body fluids from instruments or equipment. Blood and debris must be removed so that when instruments are later disinfected or sterilized, chemicals (disinfection) or steam, heat, or gases (sterilization) can penetrate to all surfaces of the instruments. Items that cannot be cleaned at once are usually rinsed with cold water and placed in a soaking solution to prevent anyone from touching them and to prevent the residue from hardening. When instruments are sanitized, the soaking solution is drained off, and each instrument is rinsed in cold, running water.

Disinfection

Disinfection, the ability to kill microorganisms on the surface of various items, can be accomplished by using a chemical disinfectant or by boiling. Disinfection is also used for items that are sensitive to heat such as glass thermometers or rubber materials. Large equipment and counter surfaces that cannot fit into an autoclave for sterilization should be disinfected by use of chemical disinfectants. Although it kills many microorganisms, boiling does not kill bacterial spores.

Labels of disinfectant solutions provide directions for proper use, including the proper length of time to soak items. Many pharmacies use commercial solutions or prepare solutions containing household bleach. A 1:10 solution of household bleach (1 part bleach to 10 parts water) provides disinfection. Pharmacy staff can clean small spills of blood or body fluids on counter surfaces with bleach solution and paper towels (see Figure 15–1).

Surgical Asepsis

Surgical asepsis is the destruction of all microorganisms, pathogenic and nonpathogenic, on an object or instrument. Therefore, all equipment used is sterile. The goal of surgical asepsis is to prevent

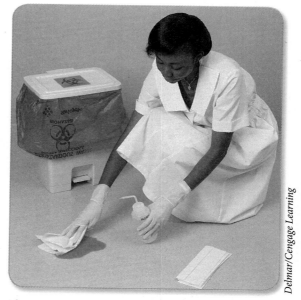

Figure 15–1 Blood spills can be cleaned with a bleach solution.

Delmar/Cengage Learning

any microorganisms from entering the patient's body through an open wound, especially during surgery.

Sterilization

Sterilization, the process of killing or destroying all microorganisms and their pathogenic products, includes the application of steam under pressure, dry heat, gas, chemicals, and radiation. Sterilization can be achieved through the use of an autoclave, which generates steam under pressure (see Figure 15–2). When moist heat of 270°F (or 132°C) under pressure of 30 pounds is applied to instruments, all organisms will be killed in 20 minutes. As one of the most effective methods for destruction of all types of microorganisms, the autoclave must be cleaned after each load.

Dry heat sterilization is another method of sterilization that uses heated dry air at a temperature of 320°F to 356°F (160°C to 180°C) for 90 minutes to 3 hours. When the gas ethylene oxide is used to sterilize items that are sensitive to heat, this method of sterilization is called gas sterilization. Because it is highly flammable and toxic, gas sterilization requires special equipment and aeration of materials. Many prepackaged products for intravenous infusion and bandages are sterilized using this method. **Chemical sterilization** is used for instruments; and chemicals such as iodine, household bleach, and alcohol can be applied topically to the body for disinfection.

EQUIPMENT AND SUPPLIES

Parenteral products must be prepared in a manner that avoids contamination. The following equipment and supplies are used in sterile compounding and IV administration:

- **Administration sets:** Disposable tubing that connects IVs to injection sites (see Figure 15–3).

- **Ambulatory pumps:** Small pumps that patients wear.

- **Ampule breakers:** Used to break necks of ampules.

- **Ampules:** Long glass containers with breakable necks.

- **Catheters:** Inserted into veins for direct vascular system access.

- **Clamps:** Adjust flow rates of solutions.

- **Drip chambers:** Hollow areas where IV solutions drip without allowing air bubbles to enter IV tubing (see Figure 15–4).

- **Filters:** Used to remove particulates and microorganisms from solutions.

- **Filter needles:** Used to prevent glass from ampule breakage from entering final solution withdrawn from the ampule.

- **Filter straws:** Used to pull medication out of ampules.

- **Flexible bags:** Plastic containers that hold 50 mL to 3000 mL of solution.

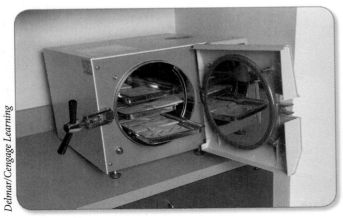

Delmar/Cengage Learning

Figure 15–2 An autoclave is used to sterilize equipment.

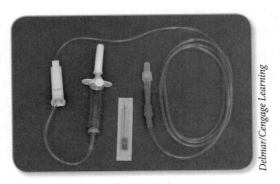

Delmar/Cengage Learning

Figure 15–3 IV administration set.

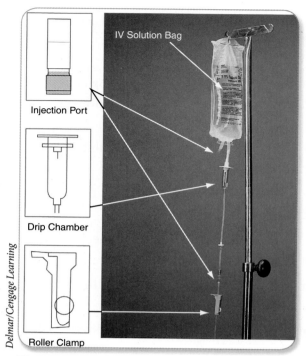

Delmar/Cengage Learning

Figure 15–4 Parts of an IV administration set.

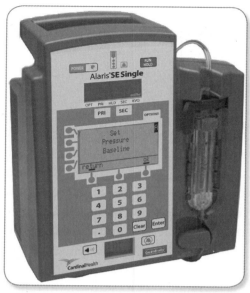

Figure 15–5 An infusion pump. *(Courtesy of Cardinal Health [Alaris Medical System])*

- **Heparin locks:** Short tubing filled with heparin, attached to a needle or catheter; they prevent clotting.

- **Infusion pumps:** Regulate medication flow into patients (see Figure 15–5).

- **Laminar airflow hoods:** Used to prepare sterile compounds by circulating air through HEPA filters to remove 99.97% of possible contaminants.

- **Large-volume parenterals:** Those greater than 100 mL.

- **Male/female adapters:** Used to mix two substances by attaching to syringes.

- **Minibags:** Those containing between 50 mL and 100 mL of solution.

- **Needles:** Used to inject substances; consisting of a hub and a shaft, they attach to syringes.

- **Piggybacks:** A small volume of solution added to a large-volume parenteral.

- **Sharps container:** A rigid plastic container used for sharps such as needles, glass slides, scalpel blades, or disposable syringes (see Figure 15–6).

- **Small-volume parenterals:** Those that are smaller than or equal to 100 mL.

- **Spikes:** Rigid pieces of plastic that insert into IV bags.

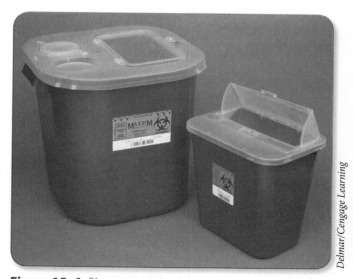

Delmar/Cengage Learning

Figure 15–6 Sharps containers.

- **Syringes:** The most common syringe sizes used in pharmacy for sterile compounding include 1 mL, 3 mL, 6 mL, 12 mL, 20 mL, 35 mL, and 60 mL.

- **Syringe caps:** Used to prevent contamination of syringes when they are moved between locations.

- **Tubing:** Used to conduct solutions between a container and a patient.

- **Vials:** Containers with rubber stoppers that contain medications.

- **¼ normal saline:** 0.225% sodium chloride.

- **5% dextrose, normal saline, and 0.45% sodium chloride:** For injection, USP.

- **70% isopropyl alcohol:** For cleaning surfaces.

- **Alcohol pads:** For cleaning ports, stoppers, skin surfaces, etc.

- **D10W:** 10% dextrose in water.

- **D5NS:** 5% dextrose in normal saline with 0.9% sodium chloride, for injection, USP.

- **D5W:** 5% dextrose in water.

- **LR:** Lactated Ringer's solution, for injection, USP.

- **NS:** Normal saline solution with 0.9% sodium chloride, for injection, USP.

- **SW:** Sterile water, for injection.

LAMINAR AIRFLOW HOODS

A laminar airflow hood is a piece of equipment designed for the handling of materials whenever a sterile working environment is required (see Figure 15–7). This device uses a system of circulating filtered air in parallel flow planes. Because room air may be highly contaminated, the system reduces the risk of bacterial contamination or exposure to chemical pollutants in surgical theaters, hospital

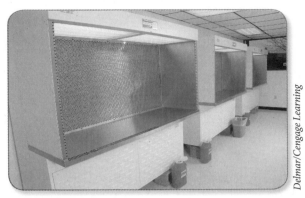

Figure 15–7 A laminar airflow hood.

pharmacies, laboratories, and food preparation areas. Sneezing, for example, produces up to 200,000 aerosol droplets, which can attach to dust particles and stay in the air for weeks! If operating properly, laminar airflow hoods are very effective for providing a clean area.

Types of Hoods

There are two types of laminar airflow hoods: vertical and horizontal (see Figures 15–8A and 15–8B). A horizontal airflow hood should be used for preparation of numerous types of parenteral medications and sterile product mixtures. Because of the direction of the airflow and the hood's specifications, a vertical airflow hood is used for all chemotherapeutic agents and can also be used to mix non-chemotherapeutic agents. However, chemotherapeutic agents should not be mixed in a horizontal airflow hood. Authorized inspectors must annually inspect the horizontal hoods used in hospital pharmacies to ensure the effectiveness of the filtering system.

Airflow in Hoods

Laminar airflow hoods basically have a box-like structure, with the top and sides made of Plexiglas, a transparent acrylic material. The work area is bathed by positive pressure (horizontal or vertical) flowing air called *laminar*, which has passed first through a prefilter that removes lint and dust and then through a high-efficiency particulate air

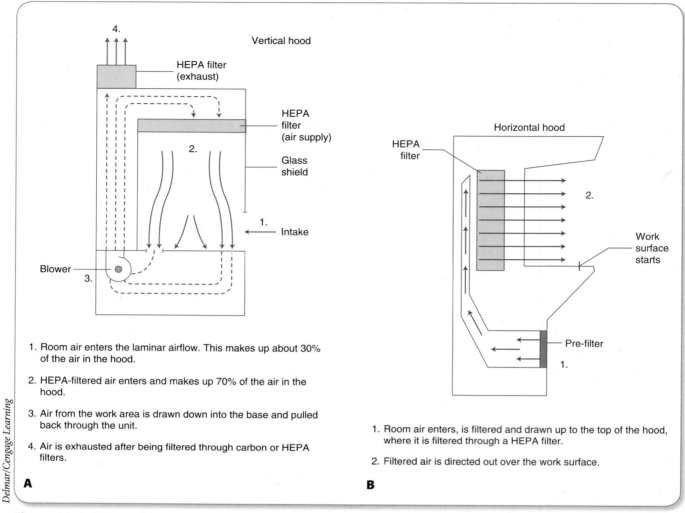

1. Room air enters the laminar airflow. This makes up about 30% of the air in the hood.

2. HEPA-filtered air enters and makes up 70% of the air in the hood.

3. Air from the work area is drawn down into the base and pulled back through the unit.

4. Air is exhausted after being filtered through carbon or HEPA filters.

A

1. Room air enters, is filtered and drawn up to the top of the hood, where it is filtered through a HEPA filter.

2. Filtered air is directed out over the work surface.

B

Figure 15–8 A. Vertical laminar airflow hood. B. Horizontal laminar airflow hood.

(HEPA) filter. This filter, the most important part of the system, removes microorganisms and small particles of matter (99.97% of all particles larger than 0.3 μm in size) from room air, compressing and redistributing the now ultraclean air into airflow streams that are parallel to each other.

The air moves at a rate of 90 to 120 linear feet per minute, with very little turbulence, at a uniform velocity. This process removes nearly all of the bacteria from the air. The HEPA filter is located at the rear of the work area, with a removable, perforated metal diffuser farther toward the front. HEPA filters cannot be cleaned or recycled and must be replaced every three to five years on average. Fluorescent lights illuminate the work area.

Location and Operation of Hoods

To minimize the potential for contamination, the controlled area should be a limited-access area sufficiently separated from other pharmacy operations and away from the major flow of materials and personnel into and out of the area. The hood's controlled air is a needed buffer from outside air. Air currents from briefly opened doors, from personnel walking past the laminar airflow workbench, or from the heating/ventilating/and air conditioning system can easily exceed the velocity of air from the laminar airflow workbench.

Laminar airflow hoods should be left on 24 hours a day and require regular maintenance. If turned off for any reason, the unit should be turned on for at least 30 minutes and then thoroughly cleaned before reusing. Also, all items to be used in procedures under the hood, including the operator's hands and arms, should be cleaned thoroughly before work begins. Excess dust must be avoided at all costs.

While performing procedures under the hoods, technicians should remove any jewelry from their hands and wrists, use gowns with knit cuffs, and wear rubber gloves. Personnel with a sensitivity to latex should use powder-free, low-latex protein gloves or latex-free (synthetic) gloves. Wearing gloves minimizes the shedding of skin flora into the work area. Also, because most people talk or may even cough or sneeze, technicians should wear masks. Conventional laboratory coats are not sufficient because their open cuffs allow entrapment of contaminated air between the wrists and forearms and inside the sleeves. As they work, technicians should keep their hands within the cleaned area of the hood as much as possible and not touch their hair, face, or clothing. Only materials essential for preparing the sterile product should be placed in the laminar airflow workbench or barrier isolator (see Figure 15–9).

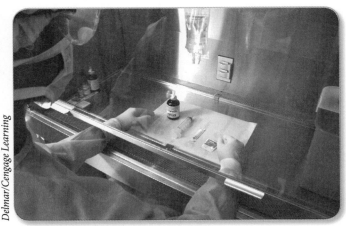

Figure 15–9 All materials used in the laminar airflow hood must be placed within the workbench clean area.

Delmar/Cengage Learning

Before placing materials in the workbench, technicians should disinfect the surface of ampules, vials, and container closures (e.g., vial stoppers) by swabbing or spraying them with alcohol. All aseptic procedures should be performed at least 6 inches inside the front edge of the laminar airflow workbench, in a clear path of unidirectional airflow between the HEPA filter and work materials (e.g., needles or closures). Technicians should avoid spraying or squirting solutions onto the HEPA filter, always aiming away from the filter when opening ampules or adjusting syringes. In a horizontal hood, technicians should place items away from the sides and HEPA filter. Nothing should touch the filter. Also, technicians should never place large objects near the back of the hood because they will contaminate everything downstream from them and disrupt the flow pattern of air.

Clean Up of Work Areas

Work areas should be cleaned after each use. Before and after a series of intravenous admixtures are prepared (the preparation of sterile products) or anytime something is spilled, the work surface of the laminar airflow hood should be thoroughly cleaned first with sterile water, and then disinfected with 70% isopropyl alcohol. This is a standardized method of cleaning according to USP 797. A long side-to-side motion should be used, starting at the ceiling of the hood. If it is a vertical flow hood, the cover over and around the filter should be cleaned at this time. The next step is to clean the back of the hood. If it is a horizontal flow hood, the cover over and around the filter should be cleaned at this time. Next, sides should be cleaned, working from the back of the hood to the front. Finally, the bottom of the hood should be cleaned, working from the back to the front (see Figures 15–10A through 15–10G here).

Also, the acrylic plastic sides should be cleaned periodically with appropriate solutions and by following the directions closely. Disinfectants should be alternated periodically to prevent development of resistant microorganisms. The HEPA filter should

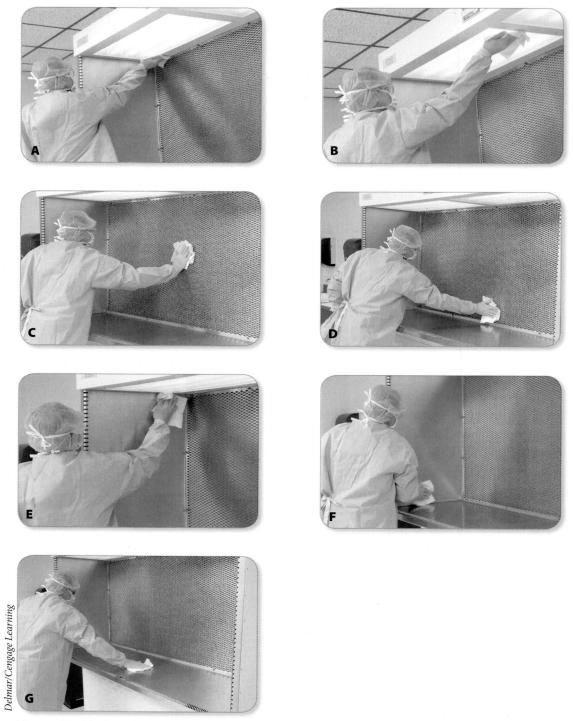

Delmar/Cengage Learning

Figure 15–10 A. and B. Clean the airflow hood with long strokes from left to right. C. and D. Working down from the top, clean the back of the airflow hood. E. and F. Clean each side of the airflow hood. G. Last, clean the countertop of the airflow hood.

be serviced and certified every six months. Active work surfaces in the controlled area (e.g., carts, compounding devices, and counter surfaces) should also be disinfected; and refrigerators, freezers, shelves, and other areas where pharmacy-prepared sterile products are stored should be kept clean. The floors of the controlled area should be nonporous and washable to enable regular disinfection.

COMPOUNDING A PARENTERAL PRODUCT

To avoid contamination, parenteral products must be prepared with strict controls. Contact with health-care personnel, the air supply, particle infiltration, and contaminants on equipment can all contaminate parenteral products. Giving a patient a contaminated product can cause serious adverse effects, including death. Parenteral medications account for more than 40% of all medications administered in institutional practice.

The following factors control the choice of a parenteral product's formulation and dosage form:

- **Route of administration:** The type of dosage form (intravenous, subcutaneous, intradermal, intramuscular, intraarticular, and intrathecal) will determine the route of administration, which places requirements on the formulation.

- **Pharmacokinetics:** Rates of absorption for any routes of administration besides intravenous or intra-arterial, rates of distribution, rates of metabolism, and rates of excretion will have an effect on the selected route of administration and type of formulation.

- **Solubility:** Solubility dictates the concentration of a drug in its dosage form. If the drug is insufficiently soluble in water at the required dosage, the formulation must contain a co-solvent or a solute that increases and maintains the drug in the solution.

- **Stability:** Drug concentration sometimes affects stability. If the drug has significant degradation problems in solution, then a freeze-dried or other sterile solid dosage form must be developed.

- **Compatibility:** A drug must be compatible with potential formulation additives. This requires preformulation screening studies to assure that additives will not cause additional problems with the preparation.

- **Packaging:** The desired type of packaging is often based on marketing preferences and competition. Formulation scientists should know the intended type of packaging early in the developmental process so that they may accomplish the correct formulation.

The extemporaneous compounding of sterile products is no longer confined only to the hospital environment. The term *sterile* means there are no living microorganisms present. Sterility can be achieved through heat, gas, or filtration methods. Community pharmacists engaged in home care practice now perform extemporaneous compounding of sterile products, and the pharmacy technician is an integral part of the production of parenteral products, both in hospitals and in the home care industry. Preparation of sterile products requires special skills and training, and without proper training, no one should attempt providing this service.

Sterile products must be prepared in a clean room, using aseptic technique. Dry powders of parenteral drugs for reconstitution are used for drug products that are unstable as solutions. It is important to know the correct diluents that can be used to yield a solution. Drug solutions for parenteral administration may also be further diluted before administration.

COMPOUNDING A TPN PRODUCT

Total parental nutrition (TPN) provides lipids, proteins, electrolytes, sugars, salts, vitamins, and essential elements designed to meet the patient's entire nutritional needs. It is indicated for patients with severe gastrointestinal (GI) distress, those with poor nutrient absorption, and for those who cannot eat. This system of nutrition may be used for patients who have AIDS, cancer, Crohn's disease, severe diarrhea, hyperemesis gravidarum, or surgical removal of the intestines. Premature neonates and comatose patients may also receive total parenteral nutrition. This method of nutrition is infused directly into a vein, usually over a 10- to 12-hour period.

Careful compounding procedures must be followed when working with total parenteral nutrition solutions. Levels of added ingredients must be carefully balanced to ensure that no harm will come to the patient. After pharmacy technicians have made the pertinent mixture calculations, the pharmacist must double-check them.

TPN solutions are compounded in laminar airflow hoods or in biological safety cabinets (BSCs). The base solution is composed of dextrose, amino acids, sterile water for injection, and sometimes lipids. Additives that are mixed into the base solution may include: electrolytes, minerals, vitamins, and other prescribed substances. Technicians may compound TPN solutions either by hand or by using automated mixing devices and should choose a bag into which the entire mixed solution will fit.

To ensure proper formulation, technicians must mix the base components in the following order: dextrose, amino acids, sterile water for injection (SWFI), and lipids. After the pharmacist performs a final check as to their accuracy, the additives are then injected separately into the TPN bag. The bag should be gently mixed in between the addition of each additive. Lipids should always be added last, because they can mask particulates or precipitation in the final solution. After injecting all additives, technicians can gently rotate or shake the bag to blend all the ingredients evenly.

A standard total parenteral solution is as follows: 42.5 g of amino acid and 250 g of dextrose (500 mL of an 8.5% amino acid solution and 500 mL of 50% dextrose) per liter. This formula provides 1000 calories per liter, with a non-protein-calorie to nitrogen ratio of 150:1. To prevent essential fatty acid deficiency, IV lipids are usually provided separately twice per week. Before administering the TPN solution, verify with the facility's procedures whether any in-line filters should be used.

Linked to computers to help control accuracy, automated filling devices may be used to compound total parenteral solutions. When pharmacists or pharmacy technicians receive an order for a total parenteral solution, they should enter the information from the prescription into the automated filling device's computer to calculate the amounts of each ingredient. The computer has automatic warning software that will alert the operator to any possible problems. Labels will be generated for the solution to be compounded, and these should be checked and rechecked. The compounding device should be programmed for the correct patient, and the TPN bag must be hung appropriately so that it can be filled.

The device weighs the filled bag to ascertain accuracy and pumps out each ingredient into the TPN bag in a specific sequence. The device can detect if the specific gravity is incorrect for any of the ingredients and will alert the operator if this occurs. Newer types of automated filling devices can handle more complex mixtures of TPN ingredients, which are composed of 50% dextrose, 20% fat, and 10% amino acids.

Preparing an IV Piggyback

Based on the type of equipment used, piggybacks may be prepared in several ways. In the traditional method, a vial of medication is added to an IV medication by removing the contents of the vial via a syringe and injecting it into the IV bag of medication. Many antibiotics are prepared as IV piggybacks. Generally, they are not activated and are mixed immediately before administration. These piggybacks are labeled "Activate when you want to administer." Therefore, they do not require refrigeration before being activated. However, once activated and if not used immediately, they should be refrigerated with a label stating "Do not freeze."

Today, vials of antibiotics are commonly attached to IV bags without actually mixing the contents before they are to be used. In this method, the medications are mixed at the time they are administered and not before. This technique usually allows for longer expiration dates than those in the traditional method.

Large-Volume Parenterals

Large-volume parenterals (LVP) are able to deliver large quantities of electrolytes, total parenteral nutrition solutions, chemotherapy, and other fluids. Popular large-volume parenterals include 0.9% sodium chloride, 5% dextrose in water (D_5W), lactated Ringer's, and 5% dextrose (Figure 15–11). Magnesium, lidocaine,

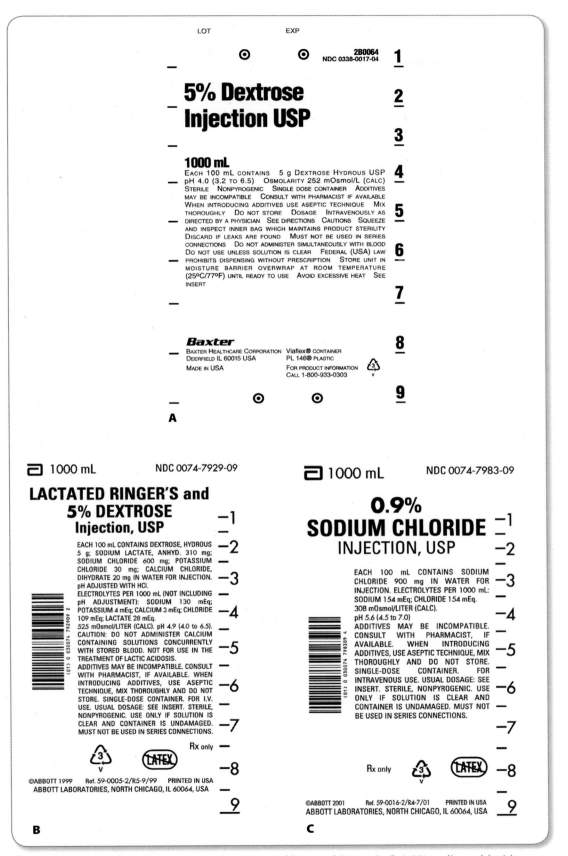

LOT   EXP

2B0064
NDC 0338-0017-04   **1**

5% Dextrose
Injection USP

2

3

1000 mL

EACH 100 mL CONTAINS   5 g DEXTROSE HYDROUS USP
pH 4.0 (3.2 TO 6.5)   OSMOLARITY 252 mOsmol/L (CALC)   **4**
STERILE   NONPYROGENIC   SINGLE DOSE CONTAINER   ADDITIVES
MAY BE INCOMPATIBLE   CONSULT WITH PHARMACIST IF AVAILABLE
WHEN INTRODUCING ADDITIVES USE ASEPTIC TECHNIQUE   MIX
THOROUGHLY   DO NOT STORE   DOSAGE   INTRAVENOUSLY AS   **5**
DIRECTED BY A PHYSICIAN   SEE DIRECTIONS   CAUTIONS   SQUEEZE
AND INSPECT INNER BAG WHICH MAINTAINS PRODUCT STERILITY
DISCARD IF LEAKS ARE FOUND   MUST NOT BE USED IN SERIES
CONNECTIONS   DO NOT ADMINISTER SIMULTANEOUSLY WITH BLOOD
DO NOT USE UNLESS SOLUTION IS CLEAR   FEDERAL (USA) LAW   **6**
PROHIBITS DISPENSING WITHOUT PRESCRIPTION   STORE UNIT IN
MOISTURE BARRIER OVERWRAP AT ROOM TEMPERATURE
(25ºC/77ºF) UNTIL READY TO USE   AVOID EXCESSIVE HEAT   SEE
INSERT

7

Baxter

BAXTER HEALTHCARE CORPORATION   Viaflex® CONTAINER   **8**
DEERFIELD IL 60015 USA   PL 146® PLASTIC
MADE IN USA   FOR PRODUCT INFORMATION
CALL 1-800-933-0303

9

A

━━━━━━━━━━━━━━━━━━━━━━━

1000 mL   NDC 0074-7929-09   1000 mL   NDC 0074-7983-09

LACTATED RINGER'S and
5% DEXTROSE   ## 0.9%
Injection, USP   ## SODIUM CHLORIDE
                                        ### INJECTION, USP

—1   —1

EACH 100 mL CONTAINS DEXTROSE, HYDROUS   —2   EACH 100 mL CONTAINS SODIUM   —2
5 g; SODIUM LACTATE, ANHYD. 310 mg;   CHLORIDE 900 mg IN WATER FOR
SODIUM CHLORIDE 600 mg; POTASSIUM   INJECTION. ELECTROLYTES PER 1000 mL:
CHLORIDE 30 mg; CALCIUM CHLORIDE,   —3   SODIUM 154 mEq; CHLORIDE 154 mEq.   —3
DIHYDRATE 20 mg IN WATER FOR INJECTION. 308 mOsmol/LITER (CALC).
pH ADJUSTED WITH HCl.   pH 5.6 (4.5 to 7.0)
ELECTROLYTES PER 1000 mL (NOT INCLUDING —4   ADDITIVES MAY BE INCOMPATIBLE.   —4
pH ADJUSTMENT): SODIUM 130 mEq;   CONSULT   WITH   PHARMACIST,   IF
POTASSIUM 4 mEq; CALCIUM 3 mEq; CHLORIDE AVAILABLE.   WHEN   INTRODUCING
109 mEq; LACTATE 28 mEq.   ADDITIVES, USE ASEPTIC TECHNIQUE, MIX
525 mOsmol/LITER (CALC). pH 4.9 (4.0 to 6.5).   THOROUGHLY AND DO NOT STORE.   —5
CAUTION: DO NOT ADMINISTER CALCIUM   SINGLE-DOSE   CONTAINER.   FOR
CONTAINING SOLUTIONS CONCURRENTLY   —5   INTRAVENOUS USE. USUAL DOSAGE: SEE
WITH STORED BLOOD. NOT FOR USE IN THE   INSERT. STERILE, NONPYROGENIC. USE   —6
TREATMENT OF LACTIC ACIDOSIS.   ONLY IF SOLUTION IS CLEAR AND
ADDITIVES MAY BE INCOMPATIBLE. CONSULT   CONTAINER IS UNDAMAGED. MUST NOT
WITH PHARMACIST, IF AVAILABLE. WHEN   BE USED IN SERIES CONNECTIONS.   —7
INTRODUCING   ADDITIVES,   USE   ASEPTIC   —6
TECHNIQUE, MIX THOROUGHLY AND DO NOT
STORE. SINGLE-DOSE CONTAINER. FOR I.V.
USE. USUAL DOSAGE: SEE INSERT. STERILE,
NONPYROGENIC. USE ONLY IF SOLUTION IS
CLEAR AND CONTAINER IS UNDAMAGED.   —7
MUST NOT BE USED IN SERIES CONNECTIONS.

Rx only   —   Rx only   —8

—8

©ABBOTT 1999   Ref. 59-0005-2/R5-9/99   PRINTED IN USA   —   ©ABBOTT 2001   Ref. 59-0016-2/R4-7/01   PRINTED IN USA   —
ABBOTT LABORATORIES, NORTH CHICAGO, IL 60064, USA   ABBOTT LABORATORIES, NORTH CHICAGO, IL 60064, USA

—9   —9

B   **C**

Figure 15–11 A. 5% dextrose. B. 5% dextrose and lactated Ringer's. C. 0.9% sodium chloride.
(Courtesy of Abbott Laboratories)

aminophylline, nitroglycerin, dopamine, and potassium are other ingredients that may be present in premixed solutions. Pharmacists must ensure the mixture's stability, compatibility, and safety and should verify *high doses of drugs or electrolytes* with the physician who orders a large-volume parenteral to be compounded.

Types of water that are commonly used when compounding large-volume parenterals include:

- **Bacteriostatic water for injection USP:** Sterile, with antimicrobial agents.

- **Sterile water for injection USP:** Sterile, but has no antimicrobial agents.

PREPARING IV ADMIXTURES

Consisting of several sterile products added into an IV fluid for administration, intravenous admixtures must be mixed using aseptic technique, which may be done inside a laminar airflow hood. Each sterile product should be added into the IV fluid with a fresh disposable syringe. Common ingredients used in various IV admixtures include sodium chloride 0.9%, water, dextrose 5% in water (D5W), dextrose 50%, and others.

UNITED STATES PHARMACOPEIA (USP) CHAPTER 797

Setting the standards for compounding, preparing, and labeling of sterile drug preparations, Chapter 797 of the United States Pharmacopeia has provisions that the FDA and state boards of pharmacy require and enforce. Some of these standards include beyond-use dating and the maintenance of quality sterile drug preparations once they leave the pharmacy.

A beyond-use date is calculated from the time that a sterile drug product is compounded until it is administered to a patient. There are three risk levels for contamination of sterile products under the USP 797 (see Table 15–1).

TABLE 15–1 Risk Levels for Contamination of Sterile Products

Risk	Time at Room Temperature	Refrigerate for
High	24 hours	3 days
Medium	30 hours	7 days
Low	48 hours	14 days

All compounded sterile products can be frozen for up to 45 days, but they cannot be shaken or exposed to excessive light or heat. If they need to keep them for use at home, patients and caregivers should be trained about the proper storage of sterile drug products.

NONINJECTABLE PRODUCTS

Certain noninjectable products must be sterile for use. These include ophthalmic products and irrigations.

Ophthalmics

Sterile preparations intended for direct administration into the conjunctiva of the eye, ophthalmics contain filtered elements that are safe to use. Ophthalmics are compounded in laminar airflow hoods in aseptic conditions, then autoclaved for sterilization. They are then cultured to assure that they contain no contaminants. The process for compounding ophthalmics properly takes from one to two weeks.

Irrigations

The most common sterile irrigations include: gentamicin irrigation solution and surgical antibiotic solution (SAS). These agents, which include sterile water, are used during surgery to irrigate open surgical sites. Although not truly aseptic in nature, they must be compounded in a sterile environment using sterile IV bottles or bags. The labels of these types of irrigations state that they are to be used *for irrigation only*, and they are never to be used intravenously.

COMPOUNDING RECORDS

Compounding records, also known as *mixing reports*, may be electronic or paper records and are used to document the activities undertaken during the compounding process. They should be stored along with patient charts. A compounding record includes: expiration dates of the substances used, lot numbers, stability information about the final mixture, and specific compounding instructions for the mixture.

POLICIES AND PROCEDURES FOR STERILE PRODUCT PREPARATION

Health-care personnel should read their facility's policies and procedures and verify by signature that they have done so prior to performing any sterile compounding. The policies and procedures manual should cover the following topics concerning sterile product preparation:

- **Job description:** Education level, certification, registration, experience, lifting various weights, pushing carts, handling rapid or repetitive manipulations with accuracy, work shifts, environment, garb, and compounding pharmaceutical products that are free of contaminants.

- **Job orientation:** Roles of employees, garb, facilities, equipment, area-specific techniques, and reference materials.

- **Training and education:** Aseptic technique, quality control, properties of drugs, good manufacturing practices, equipment operation, and product handling.

- **Competency evaluation:** Observation and/or testing methods, intervals between evaluations, aseptic technique, new equipment, and written math tests.

- **Acquisition:** Ingredient selection, bulk substance dating procedures, repackaging guidelines, ingredient testing, purchasing equipment, containers, and closures.

- **Storage:** Monitoring of temperatures, light, ventilation, and humidity; stock rotation and inspection; and locations of quarantined products.

- **Handling:** Proper removal of outer packaging, handling pouched supplies, decontaminating ampules and vials, disposal of used items, hazardous wastes and sharps, inspection of sterile ingredients and containers, handling expired drugs and supplies, and handling product recalls.

- **Facilities:** Cleaning procedures, traffic control, and safety.

- **Equipment:** Location, use, cleaning, allowable cart usage areas, laminar airflow hoods, and traffic.

- **Personal conduct and garb:** Eating, drinking, smoking, makeup and jewelry, hand washing and drying, infectious conditions, and garb policies and procedures.

- **Other important areas:** Product integrity, aseptic technique, work sheets, batch preparation records, sterilization methods, environmental monitoring, process validation, expiration dating, labeling, end-product evaluation, quality of compounded products, patient monitoring, housekeeping, quality assurance, and documentation records.

NONSTERILE COMPOUNDING

Extemporaneous compounding is the preparing, mixing, assembling, packaging, and labeling of a drug product based on a prescription order from a licensed practitioner for the individual patient. The pharmacist is responsible for preparing a quality pharmaceutical product, providing proper instructions about its storage, and advising the patient of any adverse effects. Compounding may have different meanings for different pharmacists, including the following:

- Preparation of oral liquids, topical preparations, and suppositories

- Conversion of one dose or dosage form into another

- Preparation of select dosage forms from bulk chemicals

- Preparation of intravenous admixtures, parenteral nutrition solutions, and pediatric dosage forms from adult dosage forms

- Preparation of radioactive isotopes

- Preparation of cassettes, syringes, and other devices with drugs for administration in the home setting

Equipment

The correct equipment is important when compounding. Therefore, pharmacy technicians should be familiar with those pieces of equipment that are necessary for compounding drugs. Many state boards of pharmacy have a required minimum list of equipment for compounding prescriptions. These pieces of equipment vary according to the amount of material needed and the type of compounded prescription. Several conventional pieces of equipment and instruments are available for pharmacists or pharmacy technicians to use for compounding. These include balances, forceps, spatulas, compounding slabs, mortars and pestles, graduates, and pipettes.

Class A Prescription Balances

Each pharmacy is required to have a **class A prescription balance** and/or an **electronic balance** (see Figure 15–12). Having a sensitivity requirement of 6 mg, a class A balance is a two-pan balance that

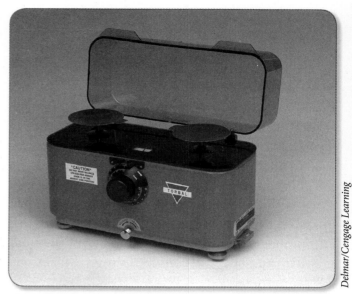

Figure 15–12 A class A prescription balance.

Delmar/Cengage Learning

may be used for weighing small amounts of drugs (not more than 120 g). Pharmacy balances must be certified every year.

Class B Balances

In the pharmacy, class B balances are used to weigh substances between 650 mg and 120 grams. They are considered "optional" pharmacy equipment because not all pharmacies will need to weigh these large amounts.

Counter Balances

Capable of weighing larger quantities, up to about 5 kg, a **counter balance**, a double-pan balance, is not indicated for prescription compounding. Rather, it is used for measuring bulk products.

Weights

Good-quality weights, preferably made from corrosion-resistant metals such as brass (see Figure 15–13), are essential and should be stored appropriately. Metric weights are in the front row; apothecary weights, in the back row. When transferring weights, technicians should be careful not to drop them and should always use forceps. Handling them with bare hands may cause a build up of oils on the weights, and these

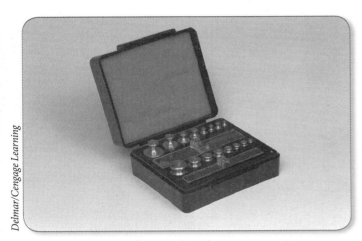

Figure 15–13 Weights used in pharmacy practice.

oils will alter their accuracy. In the pharmacy, while weighing various substances, pharmacists or technicians use sheets of moisture-resistant, nonabsorbent glassine "weighing" paper to keep balance pans clean. Weighing boats (sometimes called *weighing dishes*) are made of aluminum, plastic, or rubber.

Forceps

Resembling ice tongs and operating similarly to scissors or tweezers, *forceps* are instruments with two blades and a handle and are used for compressing, grasping, and handling many different items. Many different types of forceps designed for specific purposes are available.

Spatulas

Available in stainless steel, plastic, or hard rubber (see Figure 15–14), *spatulas* are used to transfer solid ingredients, such as ointments and creams, to weighing pans and to mix compounds on an ointment slab. Spatulas must be clean and have indented edges.

Compounding Slabs

Compounding slabs, also called *ointment slabs*, are plates made of ground glass with a hard, flat, and nonabsorbent surface for mixing compounds (see Figure 15–15).

Mortars and Pestles

A **mortar** is a cup-shaped vessel in which materials are ground or crushed by a **pestle** in the preparation of drugs. Mortars and pestles are available in three types: glass (see Figure 15–16A), Wedgwood, and porcelain (see Figure 15–16B), which is quite similar to Wedgwood in use and appearance. Because they are nonporous and nonstaining, glass mortars are preferred for mixing liquids and semisoft dosage forms. Being coarser and producing a finer trituration, Wedgwood and porcelain mortars and pestles are best used when triturating crystals, granules, and powders.

Heat Guns

Commonly used to shrink bands onto vials, *heat guns* resemble hair dryers and are used in a similar way. By slightly turning the end of the heat gun that emits heat, pharmacists or technicians can thoroughly apply heat to the vial's shrink band. Heat

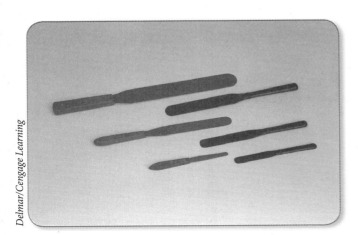

Figure 15–14 Spatulas.

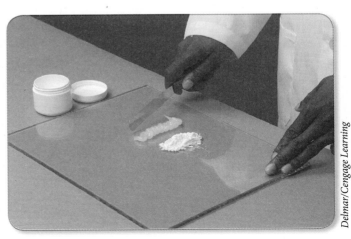

Figure 15–15 A compounding slab.

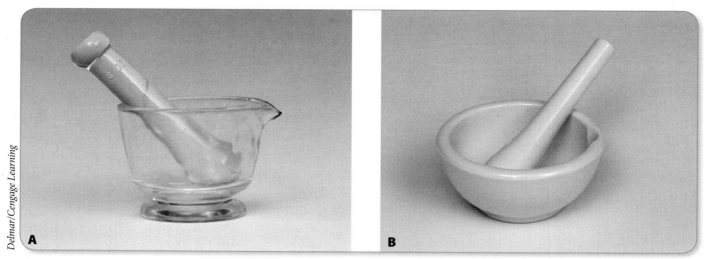

Figure 15–16 A. Glass mortar and pestle. B. Porcelain mortar and pestle.

guns may also be used for drying tablets during compounding.

Hot Plates

Resembling weight scales with flat ceramic or aluminum surfaces and front panels with controls, *hot plates* are used for quick heating of substances. Some hot plates even offer automated stirring technology. Varying in design, either intended for low-heat or high-heat use, hot plates are commonly used to melt cocoa butter or other substances for bases in compounding ointments or suppositories.

Heat Sealers

Commonly used to seal packages without damaging the chemicals, drugs, or other substances that these packages contain, *heat sealers* are available in various types. Some heat sealers may offer controls that affect temperature, sealing pressure, processing time, and automatic sample loading.

Crimpers

Resembling pliers (see Figure 15–17A), *crimpers* may be designed for manual use or for use with robotic machinery and are often found in pharmacies that handle extemporaneous compounding. Crimpers are commonly used to seal vials and other containers. Also, some crimpers are designed to be used as decappers (see the next paragraph).

Decappers

Decappers, also known as *decrimpers*, are used to remove seals placed onto vials and other containers (see Figure 15–17B). They may be used either manually or with robotic machinery.

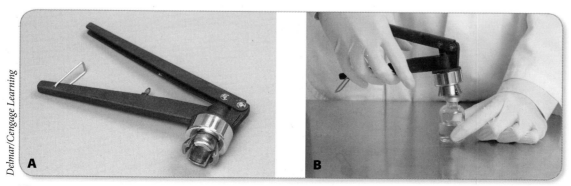

Figure 15–17 A. Crimper. B. Can also be used as a decapper.

Tablet Molds

Commonly made of metal, *tablet molds* have various sizes of plate cavities (ranging between 60 mg and 100 mg). Pharmacists or technicians use tablet molds by pressing a prepared, moistened powder mixture into the cavities (see Figure 15–18A). After filling the cavities (see Figure 15–18B), the pharmacist or technician applies pressure, forcing the formed tablets out of the cavities so that they can dry.

Suppository Molds

Suppository molds come in various types of aluminum, plastic, or rubber, and range from 1 g to 2.5 g in size. The aluminum type (see Figure 15–19A) is held together with screws or nuts and bolts. The plastic or rubber types (see Figure 15–19B), commonly used if the suppositories need to be refrigerated, allow the suppositories to be easily pushed out of each cavity once they have become firm.

Graduates and Pipettes

To measure liquids, pharmacists and technicians need equipment, which consists of conical graduates, cylindrical graduates, pipettes, or syringes. With their wide tops and wide bases that taper from top to bottom, conical graduates are easier to clean than cylindrical graduates, designed with a narrow diameter that is the same from top to base. More accurate than conical graduates, cylindrical graduates are generally calibrated in metric units (cubic centimeters), whereas conical graduates are mostly calibrated in both metric and apothecary units. Both types of graduates are used in different sizes, ranging from 5 mL to more than 1000 mL (1 liter). The smallest graduate available should always be used to measure a particular volume of liquid. The measure of a volume that is less than 20% of the graduate's capacity would not be accurate and therefore unacceptable. To measure volumes of liquids less than 1.5 mL, pharmacists or technicians use a

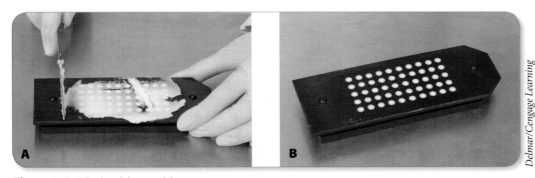

Delmar/Cengage Learning

Figure 15–18 A tablet mold.

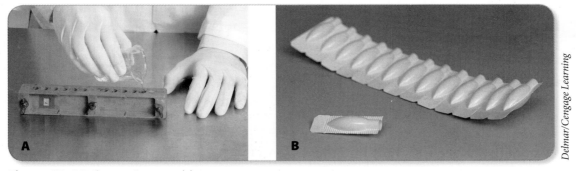

Delmar/Cengage Learning

Figure 15–19 Suppository molds.

pipette, a long, thin, calibrated, hollow tube made of glass. There are two types of pipettes: mouth or auto-pipettes.

Beakers

Usually cylindrical containers used to mix or melt liquids, *beakers* have flat bottoms and commonly range in size from 25 mL to 600 mL. They may be made of glass, plastic, or other materials specifically designed for laboratory use. Different from flasks, beakers have sides that are straight rather than sloped.

Beaker Tongs

Beaker tongs resemble ordinary ice tongs but may have either two or three "jaws." Used in the laboratory for lifting beakers onto and off of hot plates and other surfaces, beaker tongs are usually made of stainless steel and can handle beakers ranging from 50 mL to 2000 mL in size.

COMPOUNDING LIQUID DRUGS

Liquid dosage forms, the most common forms of compounded medications, include suspensions, solutions, elixirs, and emulsions. Active ingredients are dissolved in a liquid vehicle known as a solvent. Because they do not have to be weighed, liquid volumes are much easier to measure than solid volumes. The following sections discuss liquid dosage forms in detail.

Suspensions

A suspension is a liquid dosage form that contains solid drug particles floating in a liquid medium. Suspension are easy to compound; however, physical stability of the final product after compounding is problematic. The insoluble powders are triturated (reduced to a fine powder by friction). A small portion of liquid is used to levigate the powder (grind into a smooth surface with moisture); and the powders are triturated until a smooth paste is formed. The levigating agent is added slowly and mixed deliberately, and the vehicle containing the suspending agent is added in divided portions. A high-speed mixer greatly increases the dispersion, and the final mixture is transferred to a "light-resistant" bottle for dispensing to the patient. All suspensions should be dispensed with an auxiliary label reading "Shake well." Suspensions are not filtered, and the water-soluble ingredients, including flavoring agents, are mixed in the vehicle before mixing with the insoluble ingredients.

Solutions

Although similar to a suspension, a solution does not require shaking before use. Common types of solutions include sterile parenteral and ophthalmic solutions and nonsterile types include oral, topical, and otic solutions. When compounding solutions, the pharmacist or technician must know the solubility characteristics of each active ingredient so that it can be dissolved in the most soluble solvents. The compounding of solutions should not be rushed so that the proper mixing can occur. Measuring of solutions is accomplished by reading the liquid's lowest point or center, where the edges appear slightly higher than its center—this is known as the meniscus.

Elixirs

Sweetened liquids that contain alcohol and water, elixirs are made by dissolving alcohol-soluble ingredients in ethanol, dissolving water-soluble ingredients in water, and then combining the two solvents by adding the water solvent into the alcohol solvent. It is important to keep the alcohol concentration as strong as possible, hence, the water solvent is added into the alcohol solvent. When mixing elixirs, the pharmacist or technician should stir them constantly.

Emulsions

An emulsion is a type of suspension consisting of two different liquids and an *emulsifier*—an agent that holds them together. Oil-in-water emulsions are nongreasy and usually for oral use; whereas water-in-oil emulsions are greasy and usually for external use. Pharmacists or technicians can use two methods to create emulsions: the *dry gum* (Continental) method and the *wet gum* (English) method. Generally preferred, the dry gum method involves mixing gum acacia into the selected oil, mixing, adding all of the desired amount of water, and triturating until the color and sound of the mixture change. The wet gum method involves mixing water into gum acacia and then adding the selected oil, plus additional ingredients.

COMPOUNDING SEMISOLID DRUGS

Ointments, creams, pastes, and gels are semisolid dosage forms intended for topical application to the skin or mucous membranes. Ointments are characterized as being oily. Creams are generally oil-in-water or water-in-oil emulsions, and pastes are characterized by their high content of solids.

Ointments

Ointments are oil-based, whereas creams are water-based. Drugs in powder or crystal forms, such as hydrocortisone, salicylic acid, or precipitated sulfur, are often ordered to be mixed into ointment or cream bases. Mixing can be done either in a mortar or on an ointment slab. Liquids are incorporated by gradually adding them to an absorption-type base and mixing. Insoluble powders are reduced to fine powders and then added to the base, using geometric dilution. Water-soluble substances are dissolved with water and then incorporated into the base. The final product should be smooth and free of any abrasive particles.

Creams

Creams are usually used topically, and are combinations of oil with water. *Creams* are thicker than lotions, and may or may not contain a medication.

They may be dispensed from either a jar or a tube. Creams are compounded in the same manner as ointments.

Pastes

Intended for external use (except for toothpaste), *pastes* may or may not contain a medication and do not melt or soften at body temperature. Although similar to ointments, creams, and gels, pastes contain a higher amount of solids. Pastes are compounded in the same way as ointments.

Gels

Gels consist of suspensions made up of either small inorganic particles or large organic molecules interpenetrated by a liquid. Generally applied externally, gels may act solely on the surface of the skin to produce a local effect (e.g., an antifungal agent) or they can release the medication that penetrates into the skin (e.g., cortisol gel). These semisolid dosage forms may release medication for systemic absorption through the skin (e.g., nitroglycerin).

COMPOUNDING SUPPOSITORIES

Solid bodies of various weights, sizes, and shapes, *suppositories* are adapted for introduction into the rectal, vaginal, or urethral orifices of the human body. Suppositories are used to deliver drugs for local or systemic effects. The three common suppository bases are:

1. Cocoa butter, or theobroma oil, melts at body temperature. It is a fat-soluble mixture of triglycerides that is most often used for rectal suppositories.

2. Polyethylene glycol (Carbowax) derivatives are water-soluble bases suitable for vaginal and rectal suppositories.

3. Glycerinated gelatin is a water-miscible base often used in vaginal and rectal suppositories.

The first step to prepare suppositories is choosing the proper mold, which can be made of rubber, plastic, brass, stainless steel, or other suitable material. If appropriate, a "Refrigerate" label should appear on the container. Regardless of the base or medication used in the formulation, the patient should be instructed to store the suppositories in a cool, dry place.

COMPOUNDING SOLID DRUGS

Generally made using compression or trituration, solid drugs include capsules, tablets, and powders. Diluents used in compounding these types of drugs include various sugars and moistening agents.

Capsules

Capsules are solid forms in which the drug is enclosed within either a hard or soft soluble container or shell usually made from a suitable gelatin. Hard gelatin capsules may be manually filled for extemporaneous compounding. Capsule sizes for oral administration in humans range from number 5, which is the smallest, to number 000, the largest. Number 0 is usually the largest oral size suitable for patients. For preparation of hard and soft capsules, the pharmacist or technician must determine the correct size by trying different sizes, weighing, and choosing the appropriate size.

Before capsules are filled with the medication, the body and cap of the capsule are separated. Filling is accomplished by using the "punch" method. The powder formulation is compressed with a spatula on a pill tile, and the empty capsule body is repeatedly pressed into the powder until full. The capsule is then weighed to ensure an accurate dose. An empty tare capsule (the weight of an empty capsule used to compare to the full capsule) of the same size is placed on the pan containing the weights. For a large number of capsules, capsule-filling machines can be used for small-scale use to save time.

Tablets

Solid and small and usually cylindrically molded or compressed, **tablet triturates** are made of powders created by moistening the powder mixture with alcohol and water. They are used for compounding potent drugs in small doses. Tablet triturates are made in special molds consisting of a pegboard and a corresponding perforated plate. In addition to the mold, a diluent, usually a mixture of lactose, sucrose, and a moistening agent, is used. Moistening agents are usually a mixture of ethyl alcohol and water. The diluent is triturated with the active ingredients, and then a paste is made by using the alcohol and water mixture. This paste is spread into the mold, and the tablets are punched out and remain on the pegs until dry.

Powders

Powdered dosage forms are used when drug stability or solubility is a concern. These dosage forms may also be used when the powders are too bulky to make into capsules or when the patient has difficulty swallowing a capsule. Powder dosage forms may be unpleasant-tasting medications. Blending of powders may be accomplished by using trituration in a mortar, stirring with a spatula, and sifting. If needed, **geometric dilution** should be used. When heavy powders are mixed with lighter powders, the heavier powder should be placed on top and then blended (combined into one substance). When two or more powders are mixed, each powder should be pulverized (reduced in particle size by crushing or grinding) separately to about the same particle size before they are blended together.

EXPLORING THE WEB

Visit http://www.ascp.com; on its site, the American Society of Consultant Pharmacists (ASCP) offers links to practice resources and information on policy issues.

Visit http://www.ashp.org; the American Society of Health-System Pharmacists (ASHP) advances and supports the professional practice of pharmacists in hospitals and health systems and serves as their collective voice on issues related to medication use and public health.

Visit http://www.asepticsolutions.com; Aseptic Solutions, Inc., is a consulting firm offering specialized solutions to pharmaceutical manufacturers relative to sterility assurance, aseptic processing, and environmental control issues.

Visit http://www.medscape.com; on this site, do a search on "beyond-use date" to find some current articles on the issue.

Visit http://www.iacprx.org; the International Academy of Compounding Pharmacists (IACP) protects, promotes, and advances the art and science of the pharmacy compounding profession.

Visit http://www.fallonpharmacy.com; Fallon Wellness Pharmacy has been accredited by the Pharmacy Compounding Accreditation Board.

Visit http://www.paddocklabs.com; Paddock Laboratories, Inc., is a nationally recognized manufacturer, marketer, and distributor of generic pharmaceuticals.

Visit http://www.drugs.com; Drugs.com is a popular, up-to-date source of drug information online and provides free, peer-reviewed, and independent advice on more than 24,000 prescription drugs, over-the-counter medicines, and natural products.

Visit http://www.sterilizers.com; on Alpha Medical's site, you can learn more about the use of autoclaves.

REVIEW QUESTIONS

1. What is most commonly used for compounding IV antibiotics?

   A. intravenous piggybacks
   B. large-volume bags
   C. irrigations
   D. syringes

2. What is the base solution for compounding total parenteral nutrition?

   A. sterile water
   B. amino acid
   C. dextrose
   D. all of the above

3. According to the USP, for how long can a high-risk compounding product be refrigerated?

   A. 6 hours
   B. 24 hours
   C. 48 hours
   D. 72 hours

4. Which base component must be mixed last into a TPN bag?

   A. dextrose
   B. lipids
   C. sterile water
   D. amino acids

5. Why are ophthalmics compounded in laminar airflow hoods?

   A. for sterilization
   B. for destruction of spores
   C. for aseptic conditions
   D. for nonsterile products

6. Measuring of solutions is accomplished by reading the liquid's:

   A. highest point
   B. edges
   C. depth
   D. lowest point

7. A liquid dosage form in which active ingredients are dissolved in a liquid vehicle is known as a:

   A. solute
   B. solution
   C. suspension
   D. precipitate

8. What equipment can be used for weighing larger quantities?

   A. counter balance
   B. class A prescription balance
   C. slab
   D. graduate

9. Why do you avoid measurement of volumes that are less than 20% of the graduate's capacity?

   A. Contamination is more possible.
   B. Calibration is incorrect.
   C. Measurement requires more timing.
   D. Accuracy is unacceptable.

10. What is a semisolid, external dosage form with an oily base called?

   A. a suppository
   B. a cream
   C. a lotion
   D. an ointment

The Policies and Procedures Manual

GLOSSARY

Centers for Medicare and Medicaid Services (CMS) – the federal organization that administers Medicare and Medicaid; its official Web site offers information about programs, statistical highlights, and the full text of laws and regulations affecting the agency; formerly known as the Health Care Financing Administration (HCFA)

Department of Public Health (DPH) – an organization in which sciences, skills, and beliefs are combined and directed to the maintenance and improvement of the health of the general public

Joint Commission – a not-for-profit organization that sets standards to ensure effective quality services (e.g., optimal standards for the operation of hospitals)

Policies and procedures manual – a set of standard procedural statements or documents that aid an organization in operating effectively and efficiently and support the overall goals of the organization

State board of pharmacy (BOP) – the organization responsible for the registration of pharmacists, pharmacy interns, and pharmacy technicians

POLICIES AND PROCEDURES MANUAL

Hospitals today are very complex organizations. In addition, the hospital may be a member of an integrated health-care delivery system. This complexity dictates that the hospital and all its departments must have a set of standard operating statements to operate effectively and efficiently. The regulatory and quasi-legal organizations that oversee hospitals require a manual to fulfill this need. In support of the hospital and the health-care delivery system, the pharmacy department must develop guidelines for operations. This document is formally called the policies and procedures manual, which contains statements of the definite course or method of action selected to support the goals of the overall organization (policies) and statements of a series of steps to implement the policies of the department within the organization (procedures).

The policy and procedure statements in the manual should answer the following questions:

- What action must be undertaken?

- What is its purpose (why must it be done)?

- When must it be done?
- Where must it be done?
- Who should do it?
- How must it be done?

All pharmacy departments should create and implement its policies and procedures manual, and pharmacy personnel should use the manual as a guide for daily operations. However well organized and inclusive, a policies and procedures manual will never cover every situation that may arise and should never be used as a substitute for good judgment. For these situations, personnel must use their problem-solving skills and draw on their education and knowledge to formulate a course of action. There is no substitute for human judgment. All technicians must be familiar with the specific tasks that they may or may not perform and know which tasks the pharmacist is required to perform.

Need for Policies and Procedures

The primary reason for developing policies and procedures is that regulatory agencies require them. Governing the delivery of pharmaceutical services, the Food and Drug Administration (FDA) and state boards of pharmacy not only require development of certain policies and procedures, but also many times prescribe the content of the document. The Joint Commission and the American Society of Health-System Pharmacists (ASHP), quasi-legal organizations, have defined a standard of practice for pharmacy departments that includes certain policies and procedures with a defined content. Table 16–1 lists the policies and procedures that various organizations require.

Regulatory Agencies Overseeing the Hospital Pharmacy

The agencies that oversee all aspects of hospital operations, including the pharmacy department, are as follows:

- **Joint Commission:** Formerly known as the Joint Commission on Accreditation

TABLE 16–1   Specific Policies and Procedures Required by Various Organizations

Organization	Policies and Procedures Required
Food and Drug Administration (FDA)	Investigation of drug policies and procedures in hospital pharmacies Policies and procedures for drug recall
Drug Enforcement Agency (DEA)	Policies and procedures showing proper handling of controlled substances
Occupational Safety and Health Administration (OSHA)	Policies and procedures that ensure the health and safety of people in the workplace
Joint Commission	Policies and procedures that guide the pharmacy department in providing safe, effective, and cost-effective drug therapy
American Society of Health-System Pharmacists (ASHP)	Policies and procedures showing implementation of its guidelines and standards of practice

of Healthcare Organizations, the Joint Commission surveys and accredits health-care services. All health-care organizations must undergo this accreditation process every three years. Identifying specific guidelines for every department within the hospital, the Joint Commission evaluates and accredits more than 17,000 health-care organizations and programs in the United States.

- **State Board of Pharmacy (BOP):** Following guidelines that its state government establishes, each state's board of pharmacy registers pharmacists, pharmacy interns, and pharmacy technicians. An up-to-date list of each state board of pharmacy is available at the National Association of Boards of Pharmacy website, listed near the end of this chapter.

- **Centers for Medicare and Medicaid Services (CMS):** The CMS inspects and approves hospitals to provide care for Medicaid patients. Approval by this organization is required to receive reimbursement for any patients covered by Medicaid and Medicare. The mission of CMS is to ensure effective and up-to-date health-care coverage, as well as to promote quality care for beneficiaries.

- **Department of Public Health (DPH):** Each state or local DPH oversees hospitals, including the pharmacy department. In addition to inspecting hospitals to ensure compliance with laws concerning hospital practice, the DPH works with the CDC and other health organizations to combat outbreaks of disease and, in general, to protect the health of the general public.

Benefits of a Policies and Procedures Manual

The primary benefit of having a policies and procedures manual is to document compliance with the rules of accrediting, certifying, and regulatory bodies. The second most beneficial effect of having a policies and procedures manual is to create a more effective departmental management program. Other benefits include:

- Establishing standards of practice for delivering pharmaceutical services
- Coordinating use of resources
- Improving intradepartmental relationships
- Providing consistency in orientation and training of personnel
- Providing a reference guide to all personnel in the performance of daily activities
- Creating a positive work environment, including increased job satisfaction and productivity

A department with a well-developed policies and procedures manual will operate more efficiently and effectively. In addition, the policies and procedures manual provides information about every aspect of the technician's job, listing in step-by-step form how technicians are to complete various procedures properly.

Every year the United States Pharmacopeia (USP) updates their policies and procedures regarding sterile compounding. These updates are available via downloadable software and can be assimilated into any pharmacy's policies and procedures manual. Pharmacy technicians should be aware of any change or update to USP's policies and procedures.

DEVELOPING THE POLICIES AND PROCEDURES MANUAL

Working cooperatively with and with the approval of the hospital director, chief executive officer or president, and the pharmacy and therapeutics committee, the pharmacy director initiates and develops the policies and procedures for the pharmacy department. The policies and procedures manual should be continually revised to reflect changes in procedures and organization, and all pharmacy personnel should be familiar with the manual's contents. The minimum standards for pharmacies in the hospital include the following:

- Preparing a comprehensive operations manual
- Clearly defining lines of authority and areas of responsibility
- Having written job descriptions that are developed and revised as needed
- Updating the manual with revisions that include continuing changes
- Familiarizing all personnel with the contents of the manual
- Obtaining input from other disciplines

Policies and procedures should relate to the selection, distribution, and safe and effective use of drugs in the facility. The director of pharmaceutical services, the medical staff, the nursing service, and the administration should conjointly establish policies and procedures, which will be either administrative or professional. Administrative policies and procedures are related to the control of resources (human resources, financial resources, supplies and equipment, job descriptions, and the physical plant) and relationships with other departments and administration. Professional policies and procedures pertain either directly or indirectly to patient care services. Representing the major portion of the manual, this section should include all dispensing and clinical functions. A list of the topics contained in a policies and procedures manual is found in Table 16–2.

Writing Policies and Procedures

Seeking input from all affected parties and the staff of other departments, the pharmacy director must create and write policies and procedures that either the hospital administration or the pharmacy and therapeutics committee should approve. In presenting the information, the pharmacy director should write clearly, directly, and simply. The content, format, and design of policies and procedures manuals vary by organization.

Most policies and procedures manuals include general information and an index of the information each policy and procedure covers. Some method of tracking the origination date and the dates of reviews and revisions of each policy or procedure should be established. Because the practices of medicine and pharmacy are ever-changing, the policies and procedures manual should always be in a state of development. Hence, it would be beneficial to have a dedicated staff member who is analytical and skilled in the process of creating and managing a policies and procedures manual. The policies and procedures manual should inform and guide but not suppress professional judgment, personal initiative, or creativity.

To make the policies and procedures manual available to any department employee, a copy of the policies and procedures manual needs to be located in each area of the pharmacy department. The document should start with a policy title followed by a policy statement. The next section of the document should contain the step-by-step procedure for placing the policy into operation. A section should be devoted to references to source material used in the creation of the policies and procedures manual. After the policies and procedures have been defined, signatures indicating proper approvals should be obtained.

REVIEW AND REVISION OF THE POLICIES AND PROCEDURES MANUAL

The information in the policies and procedures manual must not only be current and reliable, but also flexible and adaptable to change accordingly; hence, the manual must be readily revisable. The entire contents should be reviewed or revised at least annually. Reasons for this are to ensure currency and conformity with new laws, rules, and regulations of government agencies and to ensure compliance with the standards of the Joint Commission.

The policies and procedures should clearly identify the method for handling revisions to the manual. The method established should address who can initiate change, how change is accomplished, who reviews and comments on change, and how to process revision of outdated material.

EXPLORING THE WEB

Visit http://cms.hhs.gov; the Centers for Medicare and Medicaid Services ensure effective, up-to-date health-care coverage and promotes quality care for beneficiaries.

Visit http://www.companymanuals.com to review a sample policies and procedures manual.

Visit http://www.nabp.net to find a listing of the state boards of pharmacy.

Visit http://www.cdc.gov; each state has its own department of public health. Search for the department in your state by using the CDC's Web site.

Visit http://www.jointcommission.org to learn more about the Joint Commission and its standards.

TABLE 16–2 Hospital Pharmacy—Policies and Procedures Manual

Section 1: Introduction	Section 2: Organizational Structure	Section 3: Administration	Section 4: Clinical Pharmacy	Section 5: Dispensing	Section 6: Drug Distribution Systems	Section 7: Safe Use of Medications	Section 8: Pharmacy Communications	Section 9
Purpose	Hospital	Develops budget	Patient care	Inpatients	Floor stock			Index
Hospital	Pharmacy	Purchasing and inventory control	Research	Outpatients	Unit doses			
Mission/vision statement		Medical service representative and pharmacy relations	Teaching	Ancillary supplies	Automation			
Pharmacy		Drug charges	Pharmacy and therapeutics committee	Controlled substances	Mixed systems			
Mission/vision statement		Pharmacy policies and procedures manual	Formulary	After hours				
Scope of practice		Accreditation—Joint Commission	Drug research studies	Intravenous admixtures				
		Physical plant and facilities	Drug utilization and evaluation	Pharmacist and radioisotopes				
		Professional practices and relations	Pharmacy library—drug information center	Prepackaging				
		Preparation of annual report		Manufacturing—bulk and sterile				
		Human resources						
		Job descriptions						
		Performance evaluations						
		Quality improvement						

REVIEW QUESTIONS

1. A statement of a series of steps to implement the pharmacy department's policies is called:

    A. organization
    B. regulation
    C. benefits of a policy
    D. procedures

2. Which is not a benefit of having a policies and procedures manual?

    A. creating a negative work environment
    B. documenting compliance with the rules of accrediting, certifying, and regulatory bodies
    C. coordinating use of resources
    D. providing consistency in the orientation and training of personnel

3. Which agencies oversee all aspects of hospital operations, including the pharmacy department?

    A. Centers for Medicare and Medicaid Services (CMS)
    B. National Association of Boards of Pharmacy (NABP)
    C. Joint Commission
    D. A and C

4. The information in the policies and procedures manual must be:

    A. written by pharmacy technicians
    B. written by physicians
    C. current, reliable, flexible, and adaptable to change
    D. written by patients

5. Who has the responsibility for providing a policies and procedures manual?

    A. pharmacy technician
    B. director of pharmacy
    C. director of the hospital
    D. director of human resources

6. Who should approve all pharmacy policies and procedures in the hospital?

    A. pharmacy and therapeutics committee
    B. state government
    C. hospital administration
    D. A and C

7. How often should the entire contents of a policies and procedures manual be reviewed or revised?

    A. daily
    B. weekly
    C. monthly
    D. annually

8. Which organization accredits health-care services?

    A. Centers for Medicare and Medicaid Services (CMS)
    B. Joint Commission
    C. Department of Public Health (DPH)
    D. State Board of Pharmacy (BOP)

9. Which agency or organization registers pharmacists and pharmacy technicians?

    A. State Board of Pharmacy (BOP)
    B. Department of Public Health (DPH)
    C. Joint Commission
    D. Centers for Medicare and Medicaid Services (CMS)

10. Which regulatory agency requires specific policies and procedures for drug recalls?

    A. Drug Enforcement Agency (DEA)
    B. State Board of Pharmacy (BOP)
    C. Centers for Disease Control and Prevention (CDC)
    D. Food and Drug Administration (FDA)

Management of Pharmacy Operations

OUTLINE

GLOSSARY

Batch repackaging – the reassembling of a specific dosage and dosage form of medication at a given time

Cost control – the implementation of managerial efforts to achieve cost objectives

Inventory – the stock of medications a pharmacy keeps immediately on hand

Invoice – a form describing a purchase and the amount due

Purchase order – the document created when an order is placed

Time purchase – the time that the purchase order was made but not paid at the time of purchase

Unit-of-use packaging – the packaging from bulk containers into patient-specific containers

Want book – a list of drugs and devices that routinely need to be reordered

MANAGING THE PHARMACY

The concept of managerial effectiveness is extremely important for anyone involved in the management process. If it is to survive, an organization must effectively provide a product or service that fits customers' needs; this is critical. Management of pharmacy operations encompasses all of the experience, skills, judgment, abilities, knowledge, contacts, risk taking, and wisdom of the manager and other individuals associated with an organization. A complete understanding of strategic sources of competitive advantages must include an analysis of the organization's internal strengths, opportunities, and weaknesses. The most important concerns of the pharmaceutical organization are productivity, quality, service, and price.

COST ANALYSIS

The pharmacist or manager is responsible and accountable for the finances of the pharmacy. In general, the process of cost analysis involves the gathering of information and data, the establishment of standards based on this information, and the adjustment of operations to conform to the standards developed. Cost analysis involves all information of the disbursements of an activity, agency department, or program.

Cost control is the implementation of managerial efforts to achieve cost objectives. This process of monitoring and regulating an agency's or institution's expenditure of funds includes budget reports and cost-accounting procedures, which are performed to achieve cost control. Several factors should be considered when performing a cost analysis study. These include cost finding, cost factors, and cost-benefit analysis. Generally, cost control studies are performed for one of two purposes:

1. To estimate the total cost of an operational or proposed system, or

2. To compare two or more methods or systems to determine which is more advantageous (profitable).

PURCHASING PROCEDURES

The pharmacy must order and buy the products for use or sale, which is usually carried out in one of two ways: independent purchasing or group purchasing. *Independent purchasing* means that the pharmacist or technician works alone and deals directly with representatives of pharmaceutical companies or wholesalers to negotiate price, quantity, and delivery.

In *group purchasing*, a number of hospitals or pharmacies join together to obtain or negotiate discounts for high-volume purchases. A purchase order, the document created when an order is placed, should contain complete information for each item ordered such as the name, brand, dosage form, size of the box or the package, strength, and quantity of product.

Ordering

Regular drugs, devices, and supplies may be ordered electronically by fax or telephone or online by computer. The order is normally submitted as a purchase order. The decision to order a drug or item depends on how well it sells in the pharmacy. Many pharmacies have a list of drugs and devices that routinely need to be reordered. Previously called the want book, the list is now commonly referred to as an "electronic inventory control system." Information to be specified when ordering includes:

- Item name and manufacturer (for a drug product, the generic or brand name must be specified)

- Strength and dosage form of the drug (or size, if ordering a device)

- Quantity of drug dosage forms per package (e.g., bottle of or boxes of 100, package of two or more)

- Type of packaging

- Number of bottles, packages, or devices being ordered

Invoice

An invoice is a paper describing a purchase and the amount due. When the pharmacy makes a time purchase, that is, when the item is not paid for at the time of purchase, the vendor usually includes a packing slip with delivery of the merchandise. A packing slip describes the item enclosed. The vendor may also enclose an invoice. Invoices should be placed in a special folder until paid. The pharmacy may be making more than one purchase from the same vendor during the month. Some vendors request that payment be made from the invoice; others may later send a statement, or a request for payment.

RECEIVING

Receiving is one of the most important parts of the pharmacy operation. When products that have been ordered arrive at the pharmacy, a system for checking purchases and receiving should be in place. Generally, the individual who ordered the products should not do the checking and receiving also. All items must be carefully checked against the purchase order. When pharmaceuticals or medical supplies are received, the following procedure should be followed:

- Verify and compare the delivery against the purchase order for name of product, quantity of boxes, and package size. Examine delivery for any gross damage of boxes.

- For drug products, check the name, brand, dosage form, size of package, strength, quantity, and expiration date.

- NOTE: Only the pharmacist, not a pharmacy technician or other pharmacy employee, can receive Schedule II drugs.

After receiving and checking the products, pharmacists or pharmacy technicians place them in an appropriate storage location. Products requiring refrigeration or freezing should be processed first. Suppliers may provide special bags or similar containers designed to contain refrigerated or frozen medications, as well as chemotherapeutics.

Returning Products

For damaged, or incorrect shipments, or for expired medications, the manufacturer should be notified immediately and a return merchandise authorization should be requested for the return of the rejected shipment.

RECORD KEEPING

A modern record-keeping system has three key components:

1. Symbols on the outside of the jacket or folder to indicate the active or inactive status of records,

2. Safeguards to prevent misfiling, and

3. A filing technique that allows quick, accurate retrieval and proper refilling.

Files may be kept as hard copies (on paper), scanned into the computer system, or kept on computer disks. Most medical facilities and pharmacies use a combination of computer and hard-copy filing. The most popular system today is color coding on open shelves, and some records are kept in card or tray files. Regardless of the type or style of filing system equipment, purchasing the best-quality product is always recommended. Some considerations in record keeping are size, type, and volume of records.

It is also important to ensure confidentiality requirements and at the same time maximize retrieval speed. At the time of payment, pharmacy technicians should compare the statement with the invoice(s) to verify accuracy and fasten the statement and invoices together. After writing the date and check number on the statement, technicians place it in the paid file.

Disbursements are recorded and distributed to specific expense accounts such as the following:

- Dues and meetings
- Equipment
- Insurance
- Medical supplies
- Pharmacy expenses
- Printing, postage, and stationery
- Rent and maintenance
- Salaries
- Taxes and licenses
- Travel
- Utilities
- Miscellaneous

All records for wholesale distributors need to be kept separate and distinct from the records for the rest of the pharmacy operations. These records should not be filed by prescription number. The inventory and records of purchase from wholesale transactions must be made available at the time of DEA inspections, for which they should be centrally maintained. Wholesale records (purchase and sale) must be maintained for a minimum of two years from the date of disposition of the prescription drugs. Also, if notified that an investigation is underway, the pharmacy may have to keep required records for prescription drugs more than two years after the date of disposition.

INVENTORY CONTROL

Inventory is a list of articles in stock, along with the description and quantity of each. In other words, inventory is the entire stock of products on hand at a given time in the pharmacy. Closely associated with the function of purchasing, inventory control is important to pharmacists because it is the means by which they assure that all medications and products are accounted for and used legitimately, that adequate stocks are available when needed, and that the costs of excessive inventory are reduced (Figure 17–1). Several factors and issues with regard to inventory are important:

1. How much inventory should be maintained?

2. When should inventory levels be adjusted?

3. Where should inventory be stored?

In an ideal system, pharmaceutical products would arrive shortly before they are needed (*just-in-time [JIT] system*).

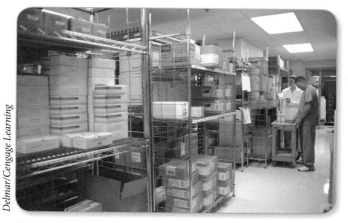

Figure 17–1 The pharmacy technician is responsible for maintaining inventory in the pharmacy.

Delmar/Cengage Learning

Computerized Inventory System

Today, most pharmacies use computers to manage their inventory and may even use electronic "auto-order" or reordering programs that automatically handle orders and reorders when supplies reach specified amounts. Considered old-fashioned, the traditional purchasing and inventory control system does not involve computers; and maintaining all information accurately is more expensive and difficult, in addition to being more time-consuming. For these reasons, some pharmacists have implemented more sophisticated purchasing and inventory control systems. Computers and computerized inventory systems increase accuracy, generate more data, and require less time than do traditional systems. However, when a computer system fails or orders quantities in error, humans must still check actual quantities available and needed and communicate with suppliers to correct the situation.

The basis of the computerized purchasing and control system is the medication database. The medication master file contains all of the information needed for ordering, maintaining inventory, pricing, and distributing pharmaceuticals. Most computerized systems provide all of the information needed to write a purchase requisition, and a few systems actually produce the final purchase order. The real advantage of computerized inventory control systems is the *time savings* for the pharmacy and the business office.

Perpetual Inventory

Perpetual inventory systems are being used today to show when it is time to reorder materials. Not only do these systems allow pharmacists to review drug use monthly, but they also allow better monitoring of all information, including monitoring of the budget. Board regulations require that pharmacists keep a perpetual inventory of each Schedule II controlled substance that has been received, dispensed, or disposed of, in accordance with the Comprehensive Drug Abuse Prevention and Control Act, discussed in Chapter 2. A perpetual inventory is commonly reconciled twice a year, or approximately every six months.

The perpetual inventory is a written record of the amount of Schedule II controlled substances that are physically contained with the pharmacy or pharmacy department. Technicians must keep in mind that the computer system is only effective when all input information is accurate.

Drug Formulary

Drug formularies are lists or catalogs of drugs that are approved for use either within a hospital or for reimbursement by a third-party payer. Formularies were developed to eliminate therapeutic duplication and to provide patients with the best drug at the lowest cost. In the past, hospitals used formularies to control drug inventories and to provide prescribers a list of drugs of choice for various conditions. The absence of a drug from the formulary was not usually a great barrier to a prescriber's obtaining it for a patient. The prescriber could make a special request to a member of the pharmacy and therapeutics committee of the hospital and would usually obtain the drug for the patient.

However, when managed-care organizations and pharmacy-benefit management companies began to use formularies, circumventing them became much more difficult. The use of formularies to restrict drug availability has led to a number of important ethical questions. For example, does the use of generic drugs for therapeutic substitution violate the patient's and/or the prescriber's autonomy? Is the use of such substitution a violation of informed consent? Does the use of formularies violate the ethical principles of beneficence (doing good) and nonmaleficence (avoiding harm)?

Point of Sale

The most suitable, flexible, and open-ended system on the market, the point-of-sale (POS) master can increase overall profitability and can be installed in all of the computers at the main pharmacy. In addition to controlling stock in the pharmacy accurately, the system can handle a significant volume of customers and transactions and all the orders, credits, interstore transfers, and returns. A major benefit of the POS master is that it can cover every area that a user could conceivably be interested in and is driven by practical requests of the users themselves. Probably the best system and the best support team of the business, the POS master can enhance every area of the pharmacy and is really easy to use.

REPACKAGING

As pharmaceutical manufacturers began to prepare, package, and distribute commonly prescribed medications, the pharmacist's role changed from formulator and packager to repackager of commercially prepared medication. Therefore, pharmacists and technicians repackage bulk containers of medication into patient-specific containers of medication.

The course of therapy generally predicates the amount of medication that is repackaged into the patient container. This type of packaging from bulk containers into patient-specific containers is called unit-of-use packaging, sometimes referred to as *repackaging*, and is a suitable concept for inpatient or outpatient dispensing. This type of dispensing process allows pharmacists to prepare medications for administration before their anticipated use. As the standard by which all other distribution systems are measured, the unit-dose system of dispensing medication in organized health-care settings has been the driving force behind repackaging programs as we know them today.

Always containing the dose of the drug for a given patient, a single-dose package may contain two tablets or two capsules in one package or container, if the dose calls for two tablets or two capsules. In contrast, single-unit packages will contain only one tablet or one capsule. A major advantage of unit-dose drug distribution systems is that they decrease the total cost of medication-related activities. Repackaging medications in advance of when they are needed allows pharmacists to take advantage of periods of reduced staff activity to lessen the demands of peak activity. Batch repackaging is defined as the repackaging of a specific dosage and dosage form of medication at a given time.

Specific Guidelines for Repackaging

Drug packages must have four basic functions:

1. Protect their contents from deleterious environmental effects.

2. Protect their contents from deterioration resulting from handling.

3. Identify their contents completely and precisely.

4. Permit their contents to be used quickly, easily, and safely.

Manufacturers of repackaging materials and repackaging equipment describe their products based on the type of package that is achievable. There are four classes—A, B, C, and D—with class A being the best and class D the worst. The package types most often found in hospital pharmacy departments include those used for oral solids, oral liquids, injections, respiratory medications, and topical medications. Compounded and repackaged products typically have short expiration dates, ranging from days to months. Because expired compounded or repackaged pharmaceuticals cannot be returned, they must be disposed of properly.

EXPLORING THE WEB

Visit http://www.pharmacypurchasing.com for the National Pharmacy Purchasing Association and PPO's website.

Visit http://www.ncpanet.org/members/pdf/ownership-managinginventory.pdf for tips on managing pharmacy inventory.

Visit http://www.phpni.com/memberinfo/pharmacy/drugformulary.aspx for information on pharmacy drug formularies.

Visit http://rxshowcase.com/repackaging_unit_dose_pharmaceutical.html for detailed information and sources for pharmacy repackaging.

REVIEW QUESTIONS

1. What is the implementation of managerial efforts to achieve cost objectives called?

    A. purchasing procedures
    B. cost control
    C. ordering
    D. record keeping

2. What action should pharmacy technicians immediately take if they discover that deliveries of drugs or supplies are damaged, shipped incorrectly, or contain expired medications?

    A. Inform a co-worker.
    B. Take the packing slip to the purchasing department.
    C. Notify the manufacturer.
    D. Enter the information in the logbook.

3. What is the list of articles in stock called?

    A. in-stock items
    B. inventory
    C. items on record
    D. want book

4. What is a major advantage of unit-dose drug distribution systems?

    A. decrease in the total cost of medication-related activities
    B. decrease in the total dosage for patients
    C. increase in the effectiveness of medications
    D. increase in the absorption of medications

5. A list of drugs approved for use either within a hospital or for reimbursement by a third-party payer is called a:

    A. drug inventory
    B. drug formulary
    C. drug prescription
    D. drug file

6. What type of purchasing occurs when the pharmacist or technician works alone and deals directly with pharmaceutical companies' representatives to negotiate prices, quantities, and deliveries?

    A. control purchasing
    B. group purchasing
    C. independent purchasing
    D. inventory purchasing

7. What is the list of drugs and devices that routinely need to be reordered called?

    A. red book
    B. white book
    C. want book
    D. green book

8. What activity is one of the most important parts of the pharmacy operation?

    A. ordering office supplies
    B. receiving invoices
    C. receiving products
    D. returning products

9. The repackaging of a specific dosage and dosage form of medication at a given time is called:

    A. batch repackaging
    B. unit-of-use repackaging
    C. manufacturer repackaging
    D. none of the above

10. What is the basis of the computerized purchasing and control system?

    A. the repackaging database
    B. the expired medications
    C. the medication database
    D. the manufacturers' database

CHAPTER 18

Financial Management and Health Insurance

OUTLINE

GLOSSARY

Accounting – a system of recording, classifying, and summarizing financial transactions for preparing a pharmacy budget

Amortize – to spread the cost of services out over a period of several years

Assignment of benefits – an authorization to an insurance company to make payment directly to the pharmacy or physician

CHAMPVA – Civilian Health and Medical Program of the Veterans Administration; a program to cover medical expenses of the dependent spouse and children of veterans with total, permanent service-connected disabilities

Coordination of benefits – the prevention of duplicate payment for the same service

Copayment – most policies have a coinsurance, or cost-sharing requirement, that is the responsibility of the insured

Deductible – a specific amount of money that a policyholder must pay each year before the policy benefits begin (e.g., $50, $100, $300, or $500)

Dependents – the insured's spouse and children under the terms of the policy

Dispensing fee – a pricing mechanism calculated by adding the operating expenses and profit margin and dividing by the total work units, either unit doses or inpatient prescriptions

Eligibility – the specific terms of coverage under a policy

Health insurance – a contract between a policyholder and an insurance carrier or government program to reimburse the policyholder for all or a portion of the cost of medical care that health-care professionals render

Independent practice association (IPA) – a type of health maintenance organization (HMO) in which the HMO contracts directly with physicians, who continue in their existing practices

Markup fee system – a pricing mechanism in which the price charged to the patient is calculated by adding a percentage markup, in addition to a dispensing fee, to the drug's acquisition cost

Medicaid – a federal/state medical assistance program to provide health insurance for specific populations; it is a type of Medigap insurance policy

Medicare – a federal health insurance program created as part of the Social Security Act

Overpayment – payment by the insurer or by the patient of more than the amount due

Percentage markup system – a system of establishing price that assumes that total operating expenses are directly related to the acquisition cost

Point-of-service (POS) – payment of services outside of an insurance plan at the time the service is rendered

Policy limitation – policies that exclude certain types of coverage

Policy terms and financial obligations – policy that becomes effective only after the company offers the policy and the person accepts it and pays the initial premium

Preauthorization – the requirement of notification and permission to receive additional types of services before one obtains those services

Preferred provider organization (PPO) – a managed care organization that contracts with a group of providers, who are called *preferred providers*, to offer services to the managed care organization's members

Premium – the cost of the coverage that the insurance policy contains; this may vary greatly, depending on the individual's age and health and the type of insurance protection

Subscriber – the individual or organization protected in case of loss under the terms of an insurance policy

Third-party payer – the fee for services provided is paid by an insurance company and not by the patient

Time limit – the amount of time from the date of service to the date (deadline) the claim can be filed with the insurance company

TRICARE – a federally funded comprehensive health benefits program for dependents of personnel serving in the uniformed services

Waiting period – the period of time that an individual must wait to become eligible for insurance coverage (e.g., 30 days) before coverage commences or for a specific benefit

FINANCIAL ASPECTS OF PHARMACY PRACTICE

The practice of pharmacy is a business, as well as a profession, and pharmacy technicians often have the responsibility of conducting the detailed business aspects of a pharmacy. Although service to the patient is the primary concern of the medical profession, a pharmacist must charge and collect a fee for such services to continue providing medical care. As a business, a pharmacy must charge competitive and fair prices for services and must receive payment for those services in cash or in a timely fashion. Patients or customers with medical insurance should be fully informed about the practice's fees and payment policies; they are ultimately responsible for the bill if the insurance company refuses to pay or does not cover the full amount.

Financial Issues

A pharmacy's business records are the key to good management practice. Pharmacy technicians who can keep accurate financial records and who will conduct the nonclinical side of the practice in a business-like fashion are genuinely needed and appreciated. Complete, correct, and current financial records are essential for:

- Prompt billing and collection procedures
- Professional financial planning
- Accurate reporting of income to federal and state agencies

Purchasing

The pharmacy department's complexity dictates the level of involvement that it has with the purchasing department. Pharmacies that provide intravenous infusion programs, central supply services, or other services, such as supplying orthopedic assistance, will have continued involvement with purchasing in the buying of equipment and supplies. Pharmacies with limited services may have little involvement, particularly if purchasing medications is the pharmacy's responsibility. Regardless of the frequency of involvement, the purchasing department can provide valuable assistance to the pharmacy.

The purchasing department in a hospital or retail pharmacy deals with sales representatives, negotiates contracts, purchases and stores supplies, and acts as a liaison between departments within the hospital or retail pharmacy and the manufacturers. The department provides expertise concerning quality of supplies. Although the selection of drugs must always remain with the pharmacist, the purchasing department may prepare the actual purchase orders.

Accounting

A system of recording, classifying, and summarizing financial transactions for preparing a pharmacy budget, accounting is an important function that must be carried out on an annual basis. Good accounting principles provide for an efficient department. The accounting department or section can be instrumental in supplying the pharmacy with data that depicts expenses, revenues, dollar volume of inventory, cost per patient day of pharmacy operations, and cost/revenue relationships to previous periods of operation. This information will save pharmacists a great deal of time when they need to justify new programs or when they need financial comparisons.

Pricing

To understand the wide variations in prescription prices, it is important to understand various pricing mechanisms in the pharmacy setting. The three basic pricing mechanisms are:

1. Percentage markup system
2. Dispensing fee system
3. Markup fee system

Percentage Markup System

The oldest and probably least-equitable pricing mechanism is the percentage markup system. *Markup,* defined as "the difference between the cost price and the selling price," is computed as a percentage of either the selling price or the cost price. The following example shows the steps involved in calculating the percentage of markup.

Example:

If a prescription drug costs $35.00 and retails for $50.00, what is the percentage of markup ?

Step 1:

Subtract the drug's cost from its retail price to find the markup amount.

$$\$50.00 - \$35.00 = \$15.00$$

Step 2:

Divide the markup amount by the drug's cost.

$$\$15.00/\$35.00 = 0.428 \text{ (rounded)}$$

Step 3:

Change this answer into a percentage by multiplying by 100 and rounding to the nearest whole number which shows that the percentage of markup is 43%.

$$0.428 \times 100 = 42.8\%, \text{ or } 43\% \text{ rounded}$$

The entire formula looks like this:

$$15/35 \times 100 = 43\%$$

In tying the medication's price to the drug's cost, one assumes that total operating expenses are directly related to the acquisition cost. This is not a valid assumption. Although the inventory cost of an expensive medication may be slightly greater than that of a less expensive drug, other operating expenses such as salaries, expendable supplies, and so forth, remain relatively stable. This system also relates the pharmacy charge directly to the product and does not consider the services involved. Another disadvantage of this system is that it does not separate different categories of operating expenses such as dispensing cost, administrative cost, clinical cost, and others.

Dispensing Fee System

The second and probably most commonly used pricing mechanism is the dispensing fee. This fee is calculated by determining the operating expenses, including salaries, overhead, supplies, and equipment cost, which is amortized over a period of time.

A desired profit margin is added to this figure. A unit charge is then calculated by adding the operating expenses and profit margin and dividing by the total work units, either unit doses or inpatient prescriptions. The end result is a dispensing fee that is added to the medication's acquisition cost to determine the total price charged to the patient. The advantage of this system is its lack of a direct relationship among the price charged, the patient, and the medication's acquisition cost. Hence, the system does not encourage the dispensing of a more expensive medication.

Markup Fee System

A third pricing mechanism that hospital pharmacies have used to price medications is a combination of the first two, namely, the markup fee system. In this system, the price charged to the patient is calculated by adding a percentage markup, in addition to a dispensing fee, to the drug's acquisition cost. The sum of these costs yields the total charge to the patient for the medication. For example, if the acquisition cost of a medication is $1.00, the percentage markup is 20%, and the dispensing fee is $0.75, the total charge for the medication would be $1.95.

$$\$1.00 + (\$1.00 \times 20\%) + \$0.75 = \$1.95$$

As a result, this system may appear to provide the best of both worlds.

HEALTH INSURANCE

Health insurance is a contract between a policyholder and an insurance carrier or government program to reimburse the policyholder for all or a portion of the cost of medical care that health-care professionals render. This care includes medically necessary care and preventative treatment. The purpose of health insurance is to help offset some of the high costs that patients accrue from an injury or illness. Patients may receive coverage under different types of private, state, or federal programs; and each patient may have a different type of health insurance policy with various benefits. Therefore, pharmacy technicians should be familiar with different types of patient insurance coverage.

A person can acquire health insurance three ways:

1. Enrolling in a prepaid health plan
2. Obtaining insurance through a group plan
3. Paying the premium on an individual basis

Insurance Policy

An *insurance policy*, a legally enforceable agreement, is also called an *insurance contract*, regardless of whether it is a group, individual, or prepaid contract. Although there is no standard health insurance contract, state laws regulate the way policies are written and the minimum requirements of coverage.

Health Insurance Terminology

Pharmacy technicians should be familiar with the following terms that are commonly used in health insurance:

- Assignment of benefits: An assignment of benefits is an authorization to an insurance company to make payment directly to the pharmacy or physician.
- Copayment: Most policies have a coinsurance, or cost-sharing requirement, which is the insured's responsibility.
- Coordination of benefits: A coordination of benefits prevents duplicate payment for the same service. For example, if a child has coverage through both parents' insurance policies, a primary carrier is designated to pay benefits according to the terms of its policy, and the secondary plan may cover whatever charges are still left. If the primary carrier pays $145 of a $180 charge, the most the secondary carrier will pay is $35.
- Deductible: A policyholder must pay a specific amount of money each year before the policy benefits begin (e.g., $50, $100, $300, or $500). The higher the deductible, the lower the cost of the policy; the lower the deductible, the higher the cost of the policy.

- **Dependents**: A policy might also include the spouse and children of the insured. These are called the *dependents* of the insured.

- **Eligibility**: By contacting the insurance company, one can verify that the patient indeed has coverage, or eligibility. Contact may be done over the telephone, via a voice-automated system, by using computer software, over the Internet, or by checking an eligibility list for a managed care plan.

- **Overpayment**: The insurer or the patient may pay more than the amount due, or make an *overpayment*.

- **Policy limitation**: Some patients or individuals may have exclusion health insurance policies. Some exclusions are acquired immunodeficiency syndrome (AIDS), attempted suicide, cancer, losses as a result of injury on the job, and pregnancy.

- **Policy terms and financial obligations**: The policy becomes effective only after the company offers the policy and the person accepts it and pays the initial premium.

- **Preauthorization**: Many private insurance companies and prepaid health plans have certain requirements that patients, providers, or institutions must meet before they will approve diagnostic testing, hospital admissions, inpatient or outpatient surgical procedures, specific procedures, and specific treatment or medications.

- **Premium**: The *premium* is the cost of the coverage that the insurance policy contains and may vary greatly, depending on the individual's age and health and the type of insurance protection.

- **Subscriber**: The individual or organization protected in case of loss under the terms of an insurance policy, the subscriber is known as an *insured* or a *member*, *policyholder*, or *recipient*.

- **Time limit**: The *time limit* is the amount of time from the date of service to the date (deadline) a claim can be filed with the insurance company. Each insurance program has specific time limits that must be adhered to, or the insured party will not be able to collect from the insurance company.

- **Waiting period**: A *waiting period* or *elimination period* is the period of time that an individual must wait to become eligible for insurance coverage (e.g., 30 days) before coverage commences or for a specific benefit (e.g., an employee must wait nine months before seeking maternity benefits).

Types of Health Insurance

Many forms of health insurance coverage are available in the United States. Health insurance may include private insurance, government plans, managed care contracts, and workers' compensation—all referred to as third-party payers, or groups or agencies that provide payment for services instead of the patient. The three major third-party payers are:

1. Third-party full payment groups (private insurance companies)

2. Third-party contractual payment groups (Blue Cross®, Medicare, and Medicaid)

3. Cash payment groups

Private Health Insurance

Having a variety of managed care plans, numerous private insurance companies across the United States offer health insurance to individuals and groups. Examples of private insurance include:

- Blue Cross Blue Shield

- Worker's compensation

- Managed care programs, including the Kaiser Foundation and various health maintenance organizations (HMOs and PPOs)

A nationwide federation of local nonprofit service organizations, the Blue Cross Blue Shield Association (BCBSA) offers prepaid health-care services to subscribers. Under prepaid health coverage plans, carriers pay for specified medical expenses if subscribers pay premiums in advance. The Blue Cross of BCBSA covers hospital services, outpatient and home care services, and other institutional care; whereas the Blue Shield plans cover physician and dental services, vision, and other outpatient benefits. Now, however, both offer full health-care coverage for their subscribers. In most states, they have become a single corporation; although in some states, they remain separate.

Blue Cross Blue Shield offers a variety of plans, including individual and family, group, preventative care, and managed care plans. Some local BCBSA organizations help the government administer Medicare, Medicaid, and TRICARE programs. There are 86 local BCBS plans in the United States, each with its own claim form. Plans make direct payments to member physicians, but they may make payments to the subscriber (patient) if the physician is a nonmember. Many small groups and individuals who may not be able to get coverage elsewhere can join a Blue Cross Blue Shield plan, which may offer coverage regardless of medical condition during special periods of time. Plans must get permission from the state to raise their rates.

Government Plans

Government plans sponsor insurance coverage for eligible individuals. The federal government provides coverage under Medicare, Medicaid, TRICARE or CHAMPUS, and CHAMPVA.

Medicare is the largest single medical benefits program in the United States. Congress authorized this federal program, and the Centers for Medicare and Medicaid Services (CMS) administers it. Medicare provides health insurance to citizens aged 65 and older and to younger patients who are blind or widowed or who have serious long-term disabilities such as kidney failure. The Medicare program has four distinct parts (A, B, C, and D), as described below:

- **Medicare Part A:** Under the Medicare program, Part A covers hospital, nursing facility, home health, hospice, and inpatient care. Those who are eligible for Social Security benefits are automatically enrolled in Medicare Part A.

- **Medicare Part B:** Under the Medicare program, Part B covers outpatient services, services by physicians, durable medical equipment, and other services and supplies. Medicare Part B coverage is optional and voluntary. By paying monthly premiums, everyone eligible for Part A can choose to enroll in Part B. Deductibles must be met in Parts A and B before payment benefits begin. Some federal employees and former federal employees who are not eligible for Social Security benefits and Part A may still enroll in Part B. Many Medicare enrollees also carry private supplemental insurance that pays the deductible and the 20% copayment. If a patient has both Medicare and Medicaid, charges must be filed with Medicare first; Medicaid is the secondary payer.

- **Medicare Part C:** Known as the *Medicare + Choice* plan, Part C of Medicare was created to offer a number of health-care options, in addition to those available under Medicare Part A and Part B. This plan receives a fixed amount of money from Medicare to spend on its members. Some variations of Medicare Part C require members to pay a premium, similar to the Medicare Part B premium. Patients who choose Part C do not need coverage under Part A or Part B. Medicare Part C offers the following plans:

  o Health maintenance organization (HMO) plan

  o Medicare medical savings account (MSA—pilot program)

  o Point-of-service (POS) plan

  o Private fee-for-service (PFFS) plan

  o Provider-sponsored organization (PSO) plan

  o Religious fraternal benefit society (RFBS)

- **Medicare Part D:** Designed to cover the costs of medications and to give patients better access to required drugs to obtain medications in retail pharmacies, Part D is offered to all Medicare recipients. To join Medicare Part D, patients must first join a plan run by an insurance company or another private company that Medicare approves. Various types of plans under Part D exist, offering different costs and covered drugs. Monthly premiums usually apply.

When patients are first eligible for Medicare, they have a choice of joining into Part D. However, if patients later change their minds, a penalty applies. Additional financial assistance is available for individuals with limited finances to help pay for their Part D coverage. Like many outpatient drug plans, Part D uses the "cost plus fee" technique. This means that a drug's cost is combined with a dispensing fee of approximately $4.50 to determine the drug product's final price. Because it relates to coverage of prescription drugs, Part D is an important component of the Medicare program that pharmacy technicians must especially understand.

Medicaid is a health benefit program designed for low-income people (those receiving welfare payments or other forms of public assistance), the blind, those who have disabilities, and members of families with dependent children deprived of the support of at least one parent and financially eligible on the basis of income and resources. Each state decides what services are covered and what the reimbursement will be for each service. Two types of copayment requirements may apply to the Medicaid patient. Some states require a small fixed copayment that the patient pays the provider at the time of service (e.g., $1.00 or $2.00). This policy was instituted to help pay some of the administrative costs of physicians participating in the Medicaid program. Certain groups of patients may be exempt from this copayment requirement (e.g., persons under 18 years of age or women receiving perinatal care).

The TRICARE program is a comprehensive health benefits program offering three (tri) types of plans for dependents of men and women in the uniformed services (military). Under the basic TRICARE program, individuals have the following three options:

- TRICARE standard, fee-for-service (cost-sharing plan)
- TRICARE extra, preferred provider organization (PPO) plan
- TRICARE prime, health maintenance organization (HMO) plan with a point-of-service option

TRICARE replaced the Civilian Health and Medical Program of the Uniformed Services (CHAMPUS), which was a health-care benefit for families of uniformed personnel and retirees from the uniformed services.

The Civilian Health and Medical Program of the Veterans Administration (CHAMPVA) covers the expenses of the families of veterans with total, permanent service-connected disabilities. It also covers the expenses of surviving spouses and dependent children of veterans who died in the line of duty. The nearest Veterans Affairs medical center determines eligibility and issues identification cards. The insured persons are then free to choose their own private physicians. Benefits and cost-sharing features are the same as those for TRICARE beneficiaries who are military retirees or their dependents and dependents of deceased members of the military.

Workers' Compensation

All state legislatures have passed workers' compensation laws to protect wage earners against the loss of wages and the cost of medical care resulting from occupational accidents or disease. Compensation benefits include medical care benefits, weekly income replacement benefits for temporary disability, permanent disability settlements, and survivor benefits when applicable. The providers, such as physicians, hospitals, therapists, or pharmacies, accept the workers' compensation payment as payment in full and do not bill the patient. Time limitations are set for the prompt reporting of workers' compensation cases.

The employee is obligated to promptly notify the employer of an injury; the employer, in turn, must notify the insurance company and must refer the employee to a source of medical care. Individuals entitled to workers' compensation insurance coverage are private business employees, state employees, and federal employees such as postal workers, coal miners, and maritime workers. Workers' compensation insurance coverage provides benefits to employees and their dependents if employees suffer work-related injury, illness, or death.

Managed Care Programs

During the past six decades, many reforms of the health-care system have been made. Medical practices have made transitions from rural to urban, from generalist to specialist, from solo to group practice, and from fee-for-service to capitated reimbursement. The expansion of health-care plans to a number of different types of delivery systems that try to manage the cost of health care has resulted in managed care. Managed care organizations manage, negotiate, and contract for health care with the goal of keeping costs down. Managed care organizations sign up health-care providers who agree to charge a fixed fee for services. The managed care organization or the government agency responsible for managed care sets these fixed fees.

Health maintenance organizations (HMOs) were the first type of managed care organizations developed to control the expenditure of health-care dollars and to manage patient care. The HMO contracts with employers to provide health service for their employees. The member of an HMO selects a primary care physician (PCP) from the medical group. The HMO is responsible for all but limited administrative needs of a PCP, including processing of capitation (a system of payment that managed care plans use, paying physicians and hospitals a fixed, per capita amount for each patient enrolled over a stated period of time, regardless of the type and number of services provided) and fee-for-service checks.

An independent practice association (IPA) is a closed-panel HMO. Instead of maintaining its own staff and clinic buildings, the IPA contracts with independently practicing physicians. The IPA may pay each physician a set amount per patient in advance (capitation), or the fees charged for services to group members may be billed directly to the IPA, rather than to the patient. Fees for services to nonmember patients are handled the same as any other fee for service. A physician may contract with several IPAs.

In a preferred provider organization (PPO), a type of managed care plan, enrollees receive the highest level of benefits when they obtain services from a physician, hospital, or other health provider designated by their program as a preferred provider. Enrollees receive reduced benefits when they obtain care from a provider who is not designated as a preferred provider (or an out-of-network provider) by their program. PPO patients may see specialists without prior authorization from their primary care physicians. HMOs offering point-of-service options are more like PPOs. Point-of-service (POS) is an option added to some HMO plans that allows patients to choose a physician outside the HMO network and to pay increased deductible and coinsurance fees.

The Kaiser Foundation Health Plan is a type of prepaid group practice (HMO). The Kaiser Foundation was a pioneer of nonprofit prepaid group practice beginning in California in 1933. The plan owns the medical facilities and directly employs the physicians and other providers.

VIOLATING HIPAA'S PRIVACY RULE

The Health Insurance Portability and Accountability Act (HIPAA) sets standards for the privacy of individually identifiable health information. Collectively, these standards are known as the *HIPAA Privacy Rule*. Protecting medical records and other personal health information, HIPPA requires covered entities to:

- Create privacy practices that are appropriate for the services offered

- Educate employees about these privacy practices

- Have a privacy official who oversees these privacy practices

- Carefully control patients' records to avoid breaches of privacy

- Notify patients about how their information can be disclosed or used

Anyone whose privacy has been compromised in any way can file a complaint with the Department of Health and Human Services (DHHS). Complaints can be filed regardless of how the patient's privacy was compromised. Complaints cover misuse or disclosure of personal health information by actual health-care providers, clearinghouses, or health plans. Penalties include fines up to $250,000 and/or up to 10 years in prison *per offense*.

FRAUD

The intentional deception or misrepresentation of health information that results in unauthorized benefits to an individual or organization, *fraud* is a felony, potentially resulting in large fines or long terms of imprisonment. Each state has its own laws governing fraud. When Medicare or TRICARE is involved, the fraud may involve federal laws, making it a federal offense. Two types of intentional actions must be proven in a fraud case:

1. There must be intent to practice the fraudulent act

2. There must be intent to commit a major offense

Fraud does not require that an individual receive monetary compensation. Fraud can be proven as the outcome of any of the following examples:

- Altering fee amounts on claim forms

- Applying for duplicate payments

- Billing for services that were not provided

- Intentionally leaving information off of a claim form

- Using another patient's insurance card

EXPLORING THE WEB

Visit http://www.bcbs.com; the Blue Cross Blue Shield Association (BCBSA) is a national federation of 39 independent, community-based and locally operated Blue Cross and Blue Shield companies.

Visit http://cms.hhs.gov; the Centers for Medicare and Medicaid Services (CMS) has the mission to ensure effective, up-to-date health-care coverage and to promote quality care for beneficiaries.

Visit http://www.kaiserinsurance.com; this is the Kaiser Insurance's home page geared to members of its plan.

Visit http://www.medicare.gov; members can follow links on Medicare's home page to enroll in the program, to enroll in a prescription drug plan, to file a grievance, and to learn the basics about Medicare, among other topics.

Visit http://www.tricare.mil; TRICARE offers its members comprehensive, affordable health coverage with several health plan options, a robust pharmacy benefit, dental options, and other special programs.

REVIEW QUESTIONS

1. If a person is covered under both Medicare and Medicaid, to which program should the claim be sent first?

   A. Medicaid
   B. Medicare
   C. A and B
   D. Kaiser Foundation Health Plan

2. Which group will TRICARE not cover?

   A. employees of the National Oceanic and Atmospheric Administration
   B. families of uniformed personnel
   C. families of veterans with service-related disabilities
   D. members of the Coast Guard

3. An authorization to the insurance company to make payments directly to the physician is called:

   A. coordination of benefits
   B. service benefit plan
   C. tracker
   D. assignment of benefits

4. Medicare Part D is designed to cover the costs of:

   A. physician copayment
   B. hospital administration
   C. patient medications
   D. laboratory procedures

5. What is Medicaid?

   A. a governmental insurance plan with which all physicians must comply
   B. a secondary carrier when the patient has Medicare
   C. always the primary carrier
   D. a type of Medigap insurance policy

6. What does Medicare Part B cover?

   A. nursing facility care
   B. hospice care
   C. hospital care
   D. outpatient services

7. Which association or program is a federation of nonprofit organizations offering private insurance plans?

   A. CHAMPVA
   B. Medicare
   C. Blue Cross and Blue Shield Association
   D. TRICARE

8. TRICARE was formerly known as:

   A. CHAMPUS
   B. CHAMPVA
   C. BCBSA
   D. Medicaid

9. The term *point-of-service* refers to:

   A. the preauthorization some HMOs require
   B. the geographic place where a medical service is performed
   C. an option added to some HMO plans that allows patients to choose physicians outside the HMO network
   D. a type of Medicare

10. Which pricing mechanism is the most commonly used?

    A. markup fee
    B. percentage markup
    C. dispensing fee
    D. none of the above

CHAPTER 19

Computer Technology and Automation

OUTLINE

GLOSSARY

Automation – machinery controlled by computers that completes many tasks involved in prescription compounding and dispensing

Biometrics – a system of computerized identification that involves the use of hardware devices that read users' fingerprints

Cassette system – the most common type of prescription filling robot; it can hold hundreds or thousands of dosage units

Data – the raw facts the computer can manipulate

Hardware – the parts of the computer that you can touch

Modems – devices used to transfer information from one computer to another

Personal digital assistants (PDAs) – handheld electronic devices that interface with computer systems to handle data such as patient charts, medical histories, and drug information

Protected health information (PHI) – all of a patient's private information that is protected from unauthorized use

Software – a set of electronic instructions that tell the computer what to do

Telepharmacy – the use of electronic communications to bring pharmacy services to patients who are not located close to a pharmacy.

COMPUTER USE IN THE PHARMACY

Computers have revolutionized the world of pharmacy. It is impossible to imagine any future scenario that does not involve the use of new technologies such as automation. This is true regardless of the type of pharmacy practice. Computers are the main components of pharmacy practice. Computer applications, which include programs for drug distribution, administration, clinical practice, and ambulatory care, have been developed in each retail pharmacy and for each segment of the hospital pharmacy. Development of programs related to administrative applications has been given the most attention because these programs have the most impact on the pharmacy's financial health. Development of programs to improve drug distribution has also been a primary focus because this has been considered the primary problem area in pharmacy practice.

COMPUTER COMPONENTS

Computers are data processors that receive input, process that input, and produce output. A computer system consists of hardware and software components.

Hardware

Software systems control the hardware components of a computer. Consisting of interconnected electronic devices that control the computer's operations, hardware includes the computer's processor, memory, storage, and input/output devices.

Software

Defined as a set of instructions that tell the computer's hardware how to operate, computer software can be divided into *operating systems* and *applications*. Operating systems such as *Microsoft Windows* control all hardware operations, whereas applications support activities such as those found in the practice of pharmacy.

Computer Input Devices

Computer input devices include the keyboard, a pointing device (such as a mouse or trackball), and a scanner (see Figure 19–1). Other less common devices used for input include microphones. Becoming more popular in pharmacies and other medical settings, touch screens are also input devices that allow users to input data by selecting choices on the actual computer monitor itself. The keyboard is the most common device to input information into the computer.

Computer Output Devices

The most common output device is a monitor (or display), and speakers and printers are other common output devices used in the pharmacy setting. Modems are both input and output devices that allow communications between computers in different locations. However, modems (which use telephone lines to work) are becoming outdated as new technology is developed allowing direct connections between computer terminals.

COMPUTERIZED SYSTEMS IN THE PHARMACY

Computerization helps pharmacists by providing a systematic method of order entry, development of patient profiles, production of labels, detection of patient's allergies and sensitivities, verification of dosage, and determination of drug-drug and drug-food interactions. The computer also offers pharmacists or technicians the ability to confirm the accuracy of drug dosages, generic and trade names of drugs, contraindications, adverse effects, and other information that is essential to the patient's well-being. Aside from the computer's clinical uses, it is also used to transfer charges to the patient's account, control inventory, and track unused drugs returned to the pharmacy.

Pharmacy technicians are involved in all aspects of the pharmacy setting's computerization. Hospitals and community pharmacies have been using information

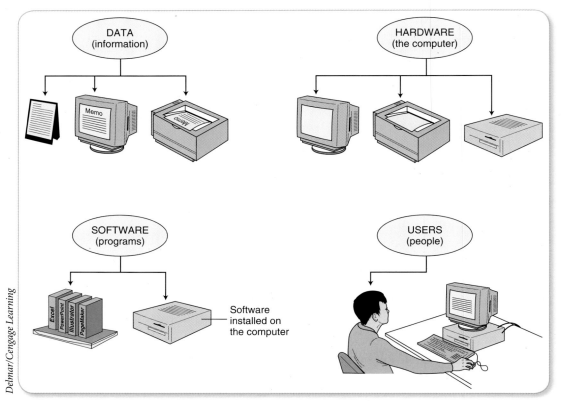

Delmar/Cengage Learning

Figure 19–1 Components of a computer.

systems to improve productivity and the quality of pharmaceutical care for many years. Today, computerized systems create new opportunities for pharmacists and technicians in the health-care delivery process. The network system in hospital pharmacy, computers have created a need for pharmacy operations to link more closely with other departments within the hospital to communicate better and faster.

In large retail pharmacies, networked computers have created much better communication and access to shared data or to the Internet. The processes of dispensing, record keeping, pricing, creating new prescriptions, and refilling prescriptions have become faster and easier. Computer applications are also helpful in drug use control. The processes of ordering, stocking, mixing medications, and preparing sterile intravenous medications all benefit from the use of computer applications.

Benefits of Computer Use in the Pharmacy

Computer technology helps to make many aspects of work in the pharmacy—such as claims processing, billing for prescriptions, researching drug interactions, and cross-referencing, among others—more efficient in many ways. In the future, computers may link the person preparing the prescription directly with the physician's office, increasing formulary compliance, simplifying pharmaceutical administration, and reducing dispensing or other errors related to illegible handwritten prescriptions.

Use of computers will, most importantly, increase patient satisfaction. Also, the physician will be able to give and receive feedback about the patient's plan, the formulary used, prior authorization requirements, and treatment guidelines. By linking insurance companies with this system, the physician can also check on drugs that the insurance company prefers with just the click of a button. This new system would benefit physicians, pharmacists, and patients by reducing complications before the patient arrives, saving time from missed phone calls for prescription changes, and the like.

Drug Information

Pharmacy technicians, as well as pharmacists, can use various computerized sources to access drug information. The Internet is a great resource to access drug information through websites such as the U.S. National Library of Medicine/National Institutes of Health (which offers the "MedLine" website at www. nlm.nih.gov) and the Mayo Clinic (www.MayoClinic. com). Information about drugs that can be accessed at these and other websites includes generic and trade names, drug dosages, the most commonly prescribed drugs, controlled substances lists, drug-food inter-actions, drug-drug interactions, sound-alike and look-alike drugs, and actual pictures of tablets and capsules. Book sources such as physician desk refer-ences (PDRs) and "Drug Facts and Comparisons" are also now available in computerized forms.

TELEPHARMACY

Telepharmacy involves bringing pharmaceutical care and information to patients who are not located close to a suitable pharmacy setting. Dispensing of medica-tions can be done using electronic communications equipment. In this manner, pharmacists who do not work in the actual location where the pharmaceutical products are dispensed can oversee the dispensing activities. Remotely located pharmacists can control and verify the products that are dispensed without physically being at the dispensing location. They can also counsel patients and monitor drug regimens and patient outcomes with accuracy.

AUTOMATION AND ROBOTICS

Automation uses computers to control storing, pack-aging, compounding, dispensing, and distributing medications and other drug products. Automation can save time, reduce labor costs, and greatly increase accuracy—especially for repetitive, time-intensive tasks. Automated machinery and robots can also reduce stress in the workplace, increase documentation of operations, and enhance security. Most automated machinery in the pharmacy is involved in the counting, packaging, and labeling of drug products. Although most robots can easily repackage and shrink-wrap a wide variety of products, some robots can load bulk medication containers into themselves so that desired amounts of medications can be dispensed.

Counting Drugs

Pharmacy technicians should always count drugs a minimum of two times to ensure accuracy. In addition, pharmacists should count Schedule II drugs following the pharmacy technician's counts. Most pharmacies require this manual counting and recounting for Schedule II drugs. When using count-ing machines, the accuracy of counting is higher than it is in manual counting. One type of counting machine counts the number of tablets or capsules, for example. Pharmacists or technicians pour the drugs into a receptacle; and as each tablet or capsule falls past the "eye" of the machine, it counts them, showing the total count on a digital display. Other machines use the weight of one capsule or tablet as a basis to determine how many total units are being dispensed. This method offers the highest accuracy available.

As well as Schedule II drugs, penicillin and drugs containing sulfur should not be counted automatically to prevent cross-contaminating the machinery and, hence, other drugs that are counted in the machinery after them.

Bar-coding Equipment

Bar-coding equipment increases accuracy and patient safety. A bar code scanner scans the bar codes on medication bottles to determine that the drugs they contain match the prescription order. Each bar code identifies the drug, its dosage form and strength, and can alert the user to any errors.

Prescription Filling Robots

The most common type of prescription filling robot is the cassette system, which can hold hundreds or thousands of dosage units. Pharmacy technicians select the correct cassette that contains the desired medication and attach it to the counting machinery. After technicians select the number of dosage units, the machine automatically drops the correct amount into the prescription vial. Other types of cassette systems have a counting device inside each drug cassette.

Many institutional pharmacies use robots that handle the complete counting of medications without pharmacy technicians or other personnel required to intervene. These robots can quickly and accurately select the desired medication cassette and perform all necessary movements to dispense the desired amount. Though large in size and cost, these robots can accurately fill up to 130 prescriptions per hour. Examples of prescription filling robots include Baker Cassettes/Baker Cells® by McKesson and the SP 200® by ScriptPro (see Figure 19–2). Pyxis Medstation is an automated dispensing device kept on the nursing unit. Baker Cells are used in outpatient pharmacies, and OmniLink Rx is a physician order entry system.

Medication Order Process

In hospitals, physicians write patient medication orders, which nurses send to the hospital pharmacy. Usually, pharmacy technicians enter each order into the computer system for the pharmacist's review and then send the completed medication order back to the nursing unit. Automated delivery systems help speed up the medication order process by decreasing the delivery time. Software interfaced with the automated machinery helps increase accuracy and decrease the time needed to process each order. Security is also increased by automation.

Inventory Control

Providing inventory usage reports that track medications and hospital supplies, automated systems have the ability to inform pharmacy directors and other personnel of the exact inventory available in the hospital at any time and can easily compile and save the usage

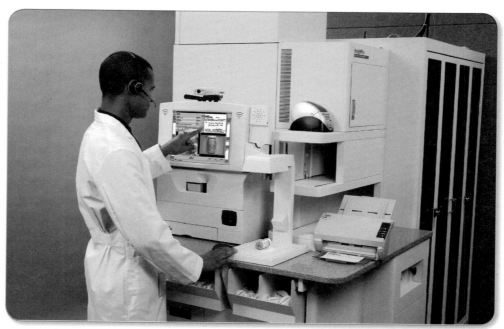

Figure 19–2 Computerized pharmacy system. *(Courtesy of ScriptPro)*

history of each product. All users are required to have a username and a password, making it easy to check who is responsible for each action involving inventory. With automated systems, inventory may also be automatically ordered from suppliers by using preset "order points" that trigger the system to place orders.

Automated Compounding

The majority of hospitals and other institutional facilities in the United States now use automated compounding devices for the compounding of parenteral nutrition products and intravenous admixtures. Automated compounding involves the use of either gravity-based flow systems that mix desired ingredients or volume-based systems that use pumps to control flow of ingredients. The primary area of concern with these automated devices is ensuring that ingredients being mixed remain uncontaminated by anyone who works with the machinery or by any component of the machinery itself.

Personal Digital Assistants

Handheld, battery-powered, electronic devices that interface with computer systems to handle massive amounts of very detailed data, **personal digital assistants (PDAs)** are seen in most physician offices in the form of electronic patient charts, complete with each patient's medical history. Each time the physician updates the PDA, the device saves and stores the changes until it is reconnected with the computer server. At this point, the PDA uploads the new information into the patient chart on the server. Prescriptions can then be sent out to the patient's pharmacy or be printed. PDAs also contain detailed drug information books for easy drug referencing, and pharmacists may use PDAs as a resource for accurate pharmaceutical information.

SECURITY OF COMPUTERS

Automated computer systems offer high security levels for hospitals and other institutional facilities. By issuing passwords and using **biometrics** (hardware devices that read fingerprints), each user can be identified and tracked. User identification badges or cards are also used to increase security protection. Some systems dispense controlled medications only in unit doses or in "units-of-use," allowing only the exact amounts needed to be dispensed.

Passwords

A password can protect each item inside an automated dispensing cabinet. Each user's activity is then easily tracked by checking which passwords were used to obtain which medications and other drug products. Only licensed staff members are issued passwords, limiting the access to drug products.

CONFIDENTIALITY AND PATIENT PRIVACY

Confidentiality and privacy are concepts associated with patients' rights. Often there is a misconception about the meaning of these terms, and sometimes they are misused or interchanged. Privacy is usually understood to mean the right of individuals to limit access by others to some aspect of their **protected health information (PHI)**. For health data, the focus is on informational privacy. *Confidentiality*, on the other hand, is based on special doctor-patient or pharmacist-patient relationships and refers to the expectation that the information collected will be used for the purpose for which it was gathered.

With confidentiality, the patient expects that information shared with a health-care provider will be used for its intended purpose (diagnosis and treatment) and that this information will not be disclosed to others unless the patient is first made aware and consents to its disclosure. In understanding the importance of the privacy and confidentiality of patients, pharmacy technicians also must deal with the security of health information when working with computers. The three principal goals for the security of patients' health information are:

1. Protecting the informational privacy of patient-related data

2. Ensuring the integrity of information

3. Ensuring the availability of information to the appropriate individuals in a timely manner

Access to the computer system is limited by password or other security measures. Following security and confidentiality rules, technicians are not allowed to provide information about treatment or patients to anyone unless the pharmacist in charge gives them specific guidance.

EXPLORING THE WEB

Visit http://www.comptechdoc.org; this site contains computer documentation and information in various technical areas, including markup and Web languages, operating systems, hardware, programming, and networking, for beginners to experts.

Visit http://www.ama-assn.org; the American Medical Association's site offers much information about confidentiality and patient privacy, among other topics.

Visit http://www.mckesson.com; McKesson provides services and products to health-care providers and payers, from pharmaceuticals and supplies to sophisticated medical workflow solutions.

Visit http://www.uspharmd.com; this site offers more information on pharmacy computer systems.

Visit http://www.roboticmagazine.com; search for "prescription filling robots" to learn more about this aspect of automation in the pharmacy.

Visit http://telepharmacy.blogspot.com; this site is a blog for medical professionals interested in the evolving field of remote pharmacy practice, or telepharmacy.

REVIEW QUESTIONS

1. *Software* refers to:
   A. the part of the computer you can touch
   B. the raw facts the computer can manipulate
   C. people who are working with computer
   D. the set of electronic instructions that tell the hardware what to do

2. Which is not a principal goal for security of patients' health information?
   A. ensuring the availability of information to the appropriate individuals in a timely manner
   B. ensuring the unavailability of information to the appropriate individuals
   C. ensuring the integrity of information
   D. protecting the informational privacy of patient-related data

3. Which item limits access to the computer system?
   A. modem   C. password
   B. hardware   D. software

4. Which device transfers information from one computer to another through telephone lines?
   A. modem   C. laptop
   B. scanner   D. motherboard

5. A pharmacist who does not work in the actual location where pharmaceutical products are dispensed can oversee dispensing activities by using:
   A. retail pharmacy
   B. advanced pharmacy
   C. mail-order pharmacy
   D. telepharmacy

6. Which device or practice controls storing, packaging, compounding, dispensing, and distributing medications using computers?
   A. personal digital assistant
   B. automation
   C. bar code scanner
   D. password

7. The most common type of prescription filling robot is the:
   A. counting machine
   B. bar code scanner
   C. order point system
   D. cassette system

8. What is *Microsoft Windows*?
   A. output device
   B. computer hardware
   C. operating system
   D. central processor

9. Which device cannot help confirm the accuracy of generic and trade names of drugs, dosages, and contraindications?
   A. computer
   B. drug reference
   C. bar-coding equipment
   D. PDR

10. How many prescriptions per hour can robots accurately fill?
    A. up to 95   C. up to150
    B. up to 130   D. up to 220

Inventory Control and Management

OUTLINE

GLOSSARY

Inventory control – controlling the amount of product on hand to maximize the return on investment

Inventory turnover rate – a mathematical calculation of the number of times the average inventory is replaced over a period of time (usually annually)

Perpetual inventory systems – inventory control systems that allow monthly drug use reviews

Point-of-sale (POS) master – an inventory control system that allows inventory to be tracked as it is used

INVENTORY CONTROL

Inventory control is of vital importance to pharmacies of all types. Inventory is typically a pharmacy's largest asset. Because so much is invested in inventory, proper inventory control has a strong and direct effect on a pharmacy's return on investment.

Inventory control is also important because a pharmacy must have the correct inventory to properly serve its patients. It must have those products that patients need

and in the quantities they need. Although this aspect of inventory control is much harder to quantify and control, it is equally important. If a community pharmacy does not have the products that its patients need, at the time they need them, loss of sales will occur. If this happens often, the pharmacy will lose clients.

The two goals of effective inventory control are minimizing total inventory investment and carrying the right mix of products to satisfy patient demand. *Inventory* is a list of articles in stock with the description and quantity of each. It is discussed in detail in Chapter 17. Examples of popular inventory control systems in the pharmacy include:

- **AutoPharm (by Talyst):** This system controls inventory, patient safety, and workflow by managing pharmacy inventory from arrival to delivery.

- **Beacon (by TCGRX Products):** Beacon is a pharmacy shelving and retrieval system that organizes medications by activity, zones, and processes.

- **MedBoard (by Baxa Corporation):** This system uses bar code technology to prioritize orders, manage workflow, and track all medication delivery activities.

Inventory Turnover

To determine the effectiveness of their inventory control system, many pharmacy departments use the inventory turnover rate. This is a mathematical calculation of the number of times the average inventory is replaced over a period of time, usually annually. The target figure is 10 to 12 times per year. This generally means that the entire inventory value is turned over once a month:

$$\text{Inventory turnover rate} = \text{Purchases over a period of time} \div \text{Average inventory for the period}$$

Example:

A pharmacy has purchased 550 products over a period of three months. If its average inventory was 235 products in a three-month period, the pharmacy's inventory turnover rate for this period may be calculated as follows:

$$\text{Purchases (550 over 3 months)} \div \text{Average inventory (235 over 3 months)} = 2.34$$

This is the pharmacy's inventory turnover rate.

The formula for calculating average inventory is as follows:

$$\frac{\text{Beginning inventory for period} + \text{Ending inventory for period}}{2}$$

Example:

For the period of January through June, a pharmacy had a beginning inventory of 312 products and an ending inventory of 336 products.

Step 1:

Using the above formula, find the total number of products during the period.

$$\text{Beginning inventory (312 products)} + \text{Ending inventory (336 products)} = 648 \text{ products}$$

Step 2:

Then, to find the average inventory for this 6-month period, divide by 2, as follows:

$$648 \div 2 = 324$$

So, the pharmacy's average inventory over the 6-month period is 324 products.

INVENTORY MANAGEMENT

The pharmacy department must select a method of inventory management. Many various types of inventory management systems exist. The following common management systems will be discussed in this chapter:

1. Order book system

2. Economic order quantity (EOQ)/economic order value (EOV) system

3. Computerized inventory system

4. Minimum/maximum (min/max) level system

5. Perpetual inventory system

6. Point-of-sale (POS) system

Common inventory management errors may be made by: miscounting the final (ending) inventory, creating labels that are not easily read, having poorly marked or unmarked locations for storage, having improper storage as a result of poor lighting, inputting data with errors, not documenting when a drug product is used, trying to read illegible handwriting, malfunctioning of computers, and having insufficient space.

Order Book System

One of the simplest and most widely used methods of inventory control is a *want book*, which is simply a list of items that the pharmacist or technician needs to order. Before the operations of most pharmacies and wholesalers were computerized, a want book typically consisted of a notebook kept in a convenient place. As the items were sold or dispensed, pharmacists or technicians recorded product names or item numbers and quantities to be ordered. Then, directly from the information recorded in the want book, the pharmacist or technician in charge of ordering made orders to the wholesaler or manufacturer. Now, the want book is more likely to be a handheld electronic device (resembling a large cellular phone) into which pharmacists or technicians enter item numbers and quantities. These devices are also commonly referred to as *personal digital assistants (PDAs)* or *palmtop computers.*

An example of a *pharmacy order entry form* that may be part of a want book is shown in Figure 20–1. The pharmacist or technician records the needed items in this device just as in the notebook, and the order can now be placed electronically.

Economic Order Quantity (EOQ)/ Economic Order Value (EOV) System

Minimizing total inventory costs, the economic order quantity (EOQ)/economic order value (EOV) system is based on the following conditions:

- Constant ordering costs, rates of demand, and purchase prices
- Fixed lead times
- Complete orders delivered at one time

In this system, total inventory cost equals the cost of the order, plus the transportation cost from the supplier to the pharmacy. Total ordering costs equal the number of orders multiplied by the cost per order. The total transporting costs equal the average level of inventory multiplied by the price per unit, multiplied by the carrying cost (a percentage). The "lead time" is assumed to be zero, as orders to replenish stock are made when the inventory level reduces to zero or another predetermined "critical" level. The basic idea of this system is to order as many units (with a predetermined minimum level per order) of a desired product at one time so that the stock remains as full as possible. This not only helps ascertain that ordering costs remain the same, but it also helps suppliers determine exactly when pharmacies will be ordering their regularly stocked products.

Computerized Inventory System

Considered old-fashioned, the traditional purchasing and inventory control system does not involve computers, and maintaining all information is more expensive and difficult, in addition to being more time-consuming. For these reasons, most pharmacists have implemented more sophisticated purchasing and inventory control systems.

Computer systems use sales and inventory information to calculate and record points, to identify low turnover items that should be dropped from inventory, and to generate orders to be sent to wholesalers or manufacturers. The basis of the computerized purchasing and control system is the medication database. For further information, see Chapter 17.

Minimum/Maximum (Min/Max) Level System

The minimum/maximum (min/max) level system involves ordering products when a specified minimum level is reached, not to exceed a maximum amount of storable products—meaning, the total amount that the pharmacy can actually have on hand (as a result of size and space requirements). An example of a *reorder point (ROP) system*, the min/max system uses an anticipated demand for a product over a specific time period, allowing for a small extra amount in case the anticipated demand is unexpectedly higher. When inventory drops to the minimum set level, an automatic reorder of the product is made. An *EOQ* is ordered to replenish the item in stock. Less popular than the perpetual inventory system, the min/max system is flawed somewhat in that it assumes that demand is basically the same most of the time.

Melbourne Medical Center Pharmacy
4321 Practice Street, Melbourne, Florida 32901
(321) 555-9876

PHARMACY ORDER ENTRY								
CODE							QTY.	DESCRIPTION
Wholesaler #1								
Wholesaler #2								
Special Order								

Delmar/Cengage Learning

Figure 20–1 Pharmacy order entry form.

PERPETUAL INVENTORY SYSTEM

Perpetual inventory systems used today show when it is time to reorder materials. These systems are discussed in detail in Chapter 17.

POINT OF SALE

The most suitable, flexible, and open-ended system on the market, the point-of-sale (POS) master can increase overall profitability and can be installed in all of the computers at the main pharmacy. Point-of-sale systems are discussed in detail in Chapter 17.

EFFECT OF INVENTORY ERRORS ON FINANCIAL STATEMENTS

When an inventory error occurs, the pharmacy's income statement and balance sheet are affected, as well as the cost of products that are sold and the pharmacy's gross profit. Inventory errors often occur because of shipping terms and consigned inventory. *Consigned inventory* means products that manufacturers ship to the pharmacy but still own because the pharmacy did not purchase them outright to sell. For example, if a manufacturer asked a pharmacy to sell a plastic device that reminds patients when to take their daily medications, and the pharmacy did not think the item would be a strong seller, the manufacturer may ask the pharmacy to stock the item without paying for it up front. Then, when the item sold, the pharmacy would owe the manufacturer a predetermined amount per item sold. Hence, during the time the item is stocked, the manufacturer actually still owns it, not the pharmacy.

When an inventory count is understated, the calculation of the pharmacy's assets is also understated. Obviously, the reverse situation is also true. Miscalculating finances can lead to the perception that the pharmacy is being managed incorrectly or even illegally. If authorities such as the Internal Revenue Service (IRS) perceive any financial miscalculations to be fraudulent, this can be detrimental to the pharmacy practice. Also, the state board of pharmacy could start an investigation if financial statements seem incorrect or possibly suspect. Therefore, it is important to understand that strict accuracy in inventory management, inventory counts, and related financial statements must be maintained.

ORDERING

The process of pharmacy ordering is usually done via computer, either manually or automatically. When predetermined stock levels and reorder points are reached, the computer automatically reorders drug products, and pharmacy staff members should verify these automatic orders. The next step is to send the order form electronically to the supplier(s) via the computer or, in fewer situations, by fax.

When using computers for ordering, the supplier's computer system interacts directly with the pharmacy's computer system to communicate quickly. The order is analyzed item by item, the inventory of the supplier is verified, and the pharmacy is sent a confirmation of whether the order will be complete or partial. Confirmations should be printed so that the pharmacy has a hard copy of the supplier's information about the order. Sometimes, items are omitted from an order, most commonly because the items are temporarily out of stock, are on back order, or have been discontinued by the supplier. Once it ships the order, the supplier will communicate to the pharmacy about the type of shipping, cost, number of packages, and future dates of shipments of back-ordered items.

RECEIVING

When the pharmacy receives the items, they should be checked and verified individually; and the printed copy of the items actually received should be kept on hand. If there are any errors, the pharmacy should contact the supplier immediately. If too many items are received compared with the order, the supplier will have an established policy for returning items and receiving credit if any overbilling occurred. When opening a received package, pharmacy staff members must be extremely accurate in verifying the items received. They should look for incorrect, damaged, outdated, or missing items.

Bar codes can easily determine each received item and its associated information—and they can verify correctness. Items should be reconciled with invoices and purchase orders, and the amount of each item and correct drug strengths must be verified. Any price changes must be identified and determined if they are correct. If controlled substances have been ordered, they will be shipped separately from other drug products; and the pharmacist on duty should receive them. Any material safety data sheets must be stored in the pharmacy's approved location for these items.

STOCKING

Most drug products are received in bulk "stock bottles," whereas some are packaged in "unit-dose" packaging and should be stored in a separate area from bulk products. Items must be stocked according to their specific storage requirements. This means that room temperature, humidity, ventilation, and light must all be taken into consideration for each drug product. Some drugs require refrigeration or freezing for storage. Both refrigerators and freezers must be calibrated and checked for temperature accuracy on a regular basis, according to the pharmacy's policy. The proper temperatures at which certain drugs are to be stored are defined as follows:

- **Drugs to be stored "cold":** Temperature must not exceed 46°F (8°C).

- **Drugs to be stored "cool":** Temperatures must be between 46°F (8°C) and 59°F (15°C).

- **Drugs to be stored "at room temperature":** Temperatures must be between 59°F (15°C) and 86°F (30°C).

- **NOTE:** "Warm" temperatures are defined as being between 86°F (30°C) and 104°F (40°C), whereas "excessive heat" is defined as any temperature above 104°F (40°C).

Pharmacy technicians must always follow manufacturer guidelines or their employer's policies and procedures manual regarding the proper temperatures for storing individual drugs.

Many retail pharmacies stock their drug products by manufacturer name. Other pharmacies alphabetically organize drugs by generic name or, less commonly, trade name. Each drug product should be stocked in a way so that the oldest items are taken from stock first, and expiration dates must always be verified so that expired drugs are not dispensed. So that each drug product's location is numbered and stored in the computer, a locator system should be in place. Space should be ample so that products can be stored with enough room to avoid breakage or confusion with other drugs too close to them. Hospital pharmacies often stock medications in dispensing units known as *supply stations* or *med-stations*. All withdrawals from stock must be thoroughly and completely documented in the computer system.

EXPIRED STOCK

Expired, deteriorated, contaminated, or other non-reusable drug products should be removed immediately from usable pharmacy stock, placed into containers labeled with "Expired Drugs—DO NOT USE" (or a similar, clearly understood warning), and promptly discarded. Disposal requirements for most drugs that have an expiration date are listed in the package inserts or on a material safety data sheet (MSDS). Expired drugs and their disposal methods should be documented, regardless of whether the drugs are put into biohazard bags for collection by

Self-Evaluation: Test 1

1. The suffix –*kinesia* means:

   A. mind
   B. muscle
   C. movement
   D. pain

2. The metric system employs a uniform scale based on powers of:

   A. 1
   B. 10
   C. 50
   D. 100

3. Which Medicare program covers hospital charges?

   A. Part A
   B. Part B
   C. Part C
   D. Part D

4. Who developed the Model State Pharmacy Practice Act (MSPPA), which can provide a greater degree of uniformity between states in regards to the practice of pharmacy?

   A. boards of pharmacy
   B. Food and Drug Administration (FDA)
   C. National Association of Boards of Pharmacy (NABP)
   D. Department of Health and Human Services

5. Which formula for calculating pediatric dosages is most accurate and is based on the child's weight?

   A. West's Rule
   B. Clark's Rule
   C. Young's Rule
   D. Fried's Rule

6. Which statement is true about a HEPA filter?

   A. It removes 85% of possible contaminants.
   B. It removes 90% of possible contaminants.
   C. It removes 95% of possible contaminants.
   D. It removes 99% of possible contaminants.

7. A potassium chloride supplement contains 10 mEq per tablet. There are 75 mg of potassium chloride per mEq. How many milligrams are in three 10-mEq tablets?

   A. 1150 mg
   B. 2000 mg
   C. 2250 mg
   D. 750 mg

8. Which drug is a Schedule V drug that requires a prescription?

   A. Lomotil
   B. cough syrup with codeine (10 mg/5 mL)
   C. Morphine
   D. Imodium

9. Which word is misspelled?

   A. vacsine
   B. sphincter
   C. parietal
   D. osseous

10. How is vancomycin usually given?

    A. intravenously
    B. subcutaneously
    C. intramuscularly
    D. intradermally

11. Approximately how many days prior to its expiration should an application for reregistration for a DEA license be mailed?

    A. 14 days
    B. 30 days
    C. 60 days
    D. 120 days

12. What size of insulin syringe is most commonly used?

    A. 40-unit size
    B. 60-unit size
    C. 80-unit size
    D. 100-unit size

13. If a total cost of delivering a prescription changes unexpectedly, which factor would most likely be to blame?

   A. turnover rate of employees
   B. change in utility costs from the electric company
   C. increase in health insurance premiums for employees
   D. change in costs of prescription labels

14. The suffix –scope means an instrument for:

   A. measuring
   B. viewing
   C. recording
   D. illuminating

15. A 10-month-old child weighing 26.5 lbs is prescribed a medication for which the normal adult dose is 50 mg. Using Fried's Rule, how much should the child's dose be?

   A. 3.3 mg
   B. 8.8 mg
   C. 3.25 mg
   D. 5.6 mg

16. Pharmacists must be registered with the DEA if they:

   A. work in a pharmacy that dispenses controlled drugs
   B. own a pharmacy that is incorporated
   C. own a pharmacy as a sole proprietor
   D. worked previously for a drug manufacturer

17. For what is a vertical laminar airflow hood used?

   A. chemotherapeutic agents
   B. sterile product mixtures
   C. unit-dose parenteral medications
   D. nonsterile products

18. Chronic dilation and distention of the bronchial walls is called:

   A. hemoptysis
   B. atelectasis
   C. bronchiectasis
   D. pneumoconiosis

19. A pharmacy technician was asked to convert 30 grains of medication into the metric system. Which amount represents an accurate conversion?

   A. 2 grams
   B. 2 drams
   C. 3 ounces
   D. 3 grams

20. According to the USP, how long can a low-risk compounding product be refrigerated?

   A. 1 day
   B. 3 days
   C. 7 days
   D. 14 days

21. When checking in an order from a supplier, it is NOT necessary to:

   A. check for the expiration date
   B. write down the lot number
   C. put away refrigerated items first
   D. compare the items received with items listed on the purchase order

22. How long must the blower run in a laminar airflow hood prior to use?

   A. 10 minutes
   B. 20 minutes
   C. 30 minutes
   D. 60 minutes

23. A patient is prescribed 15 units of 70/30 insulin to be given subcutaneously every morning. How many units of NPH insulin is the patient receiving per dose?

   A. 3.2 units
   B. 9.5 units
   C. 10.5 units
   D. 20.5 units

24. The abbreviation stat means:

   A. immediately
   B. stay on alert
   C. statistics
   D. daily

25. The Pure Food and Drug Act of 1906 was believed inadequate for the following reasons, EXCEPT:

   A. This act did not extend to cosmetics.
   B. This act did not permit the authority to ban unsafe drugs.
   C. A manufacturer could not make false statements about a drug.
   D. Labels were not required to identify the contents of a drug.

26. Atropine 0.2 mg SC was ordered stat. The drug is available at a dosage of 0.4 mg/mL. For the correct required dosage, how many mL of atropine should be administered?

   A. 0.25
   B. 0.5
   C. 0.75
   D. 1.25

27. The organs of the respiratory system include all of the following, EXCEPT the:

    A. larynx
    B. pharynx
    C. trachea
    D. thoracic duct

28. Which organization has helped direct the implementation of bar coding in the pharmacy?

    A. DEA
    B. FDA
    C. ISMP
    D. CDC

29. The most common sterile irrigations include:

    A. gentamicin irrigation solution
    B. neomycin irrigation solution
    C. hydrochloride irrigation solution
    D. chloride potassium solution

30. Enfuvirtide is classified as which of the following HIV antiviral agents?

    A. nucleoside reverse transcriptase inhibitor (NRTI)
    B. non-nucleoside reverse transcriptase inhibitor (NNRTI)
    C. protease inhibitor (PI)
    D. fusion inhibitor (FI)

31. What is a medication applied in patch form called?

    A. buccal
    B. topical ointment
    C. transdermal
    D. tine test

32. How many 500 mg doses can be prepared from a 10 g vial of cefuroxine?

    A. 10 doses
    B. 15 doses
    C. 20 doses
    D. 35 doses

33. Which suffix means "lack of strength"?

    A. –tomy
    B. –asthenia
    C. –trophy
    D. –phasia

34. Patient counseling, as required by the Omnibus Budget Reconciliation Act of 1990, should include:

    A. the name and description of the drug
    B. all possible side effects of the drug
    C. the name of the manufacturer
    D. the pharmacokinetics of the drug

35. Glucophage is the trade name for:

    A. glipizide
    B. glimepiride
    C. miglitol
    D. metformin

36. Which term means "cell eating"?

    A. pinocytosis
    B. phagocytosis
    C. exocytosis
    D. endocytosis

37. Which drug recall level indicates that the drug may cause serious harm or death?

    A. Class I
    B. Class II
    C. Class III
    D. Class IV

38. What is the study of natural drugs called?

    A. pharmacology
    B. toxicology
    C. posology
    D. pharmacognosy

39. How many types of asepsis are used in the hospital?

    A. 2
    B. 3
    C. 4
    D. 5

40. For how long must wholesale records (purchasing and sale) be maintained?

    A. 1 year
    B. 2 years
    C. 4 years
    D. indefinitely

41. Bacteria that are permanent and beneficial residents in the human body are called:

    A. pathogens
    B. hosts
    C. normal flora
    D. parasites

42. The medication vial contains 1,000,000 units of penicillin G. The label directions state: "Add 2.3 mL of sterile water to the vial, 1.2 mL = 500,000 units." How many milliliters equal 200,000 units?

    A. 0.24 mL
    B. 0.48 mL
    C. 0.64 mL
    D. 0.88 mL

43. An expandable organ that stores urine is the:

    A. urinary bladder
    B. kidney
    C. urethra
    D. nephron

44. Schedule IV controlled substances include drugs with:

    A. a high abuse potential and no accepted medical use
    B. a high abuse potential with a legitimate medical use
    C. a low abuse potential such as certain hypnotics and minor tranquilizers
    D. the lowest abuse potential such as some narcotic drugs generally for their antitussive properties

45. What is the most effective method for destruction of all types of microorganisms?

    A. a laminar airflow hood
    B. an autoclave
    C. an oven
    D. an alcohol pad

46. Diltiazem, an antianginal drug, is classified as which of the following?

    A. beta-adrenergic blocker
    B. calcium channel blocker
    C. angiotensin II receptor blocker
    D. nitrate

47. The prefix *ab-* means:

    A. without
    B. toward
    C. against
    D. away from

48. Who creates the standards for child-resistant packaging as required by the Poison Prevention Packaging Act (PPPA)?

    A. Food and Drug Administration (FDA)
    B. Drug Enforcement Agency (DEA)
    C. United States Pharmacopoeia (USP)
    D. Consumer Product Safety Commission (CPSC)

49. Using Clark's Rule, if a child weighs 15 kg and the adult dose is 75 mg, how many milligrams should be given?

    A. 6.2 mg
    B. 9.8 mg
    C. 16.5 mg
    D. 22.5 mg

50. What is true concerning unit-of-use packaging?

    A. It increases the cost of medication-related activities.
    B. It is suitable only for inpatient pharmacies.
    C. It will allow pharmacists to prepare medications before they are needed.
    D. It may increase staffing demands during peak activity.

51. Water intoxication may result in which of the following conditions?

    A. stroke
    B. fatigue
    C. insomnia
    D. swelling of the brain cells

52. Which drug is a natural penicillin?

    A. dicloxacillin sodium
    B. ampicillin
    C. penicillin V potassium
    D. amoxicillin clavulanate potassium

53. Drugs with high abuse potential and no accepted medical use are classified in Schedule:

    A. I
    B. II
    C. III
    D. IV

54. A 1-gram vial of ceftriaxone states that if 10 mL of sterile water is added for reconstitution, the final concentration will be 980 mg per mL. How many milliliters of water would be required for a 245 mg dosage?

    A. 0.15 mL
    B. 0.25 mL
    C. 0.35 mL
    D. 0.45 mL

55. Which cell is the largest white blood cell?

    A. lymphocyte
    B. monocyte
    C. erythrocyte
    D. thrombocyte

56. How far inside a laminar airflow workbench should all aseptic procedures be performed?

    A. 3 inches from the front edge
    B. 6 inches from the front edge
    C. 9 inches from the front edge
    D. 12 inches from the front edge

57. Augmentin is the trade name of:

    A. nafcillin
    B. penicillin V potassium
    C. penicillin G benzathine
    D. amoxicillin/clavulanate potassium

58. Which health plan does the federal government fund?

    A. Blue Cross and Blue Shield
    B. Aetna
    C. TRICARE
    D. Starmark

59. The combined effect of two drugs that is less than the effect of either drug taken alone is called:

    A. synergism
    B. dependence
    C. antagonism
    D. idiosyncrasy

60. The "Administrative Simplification" provision of the Health Insurance Portability and Accountability Act (HIPAA) consists of:

    A. Electronic Health Transaction Standards
    B. standards for setting insurance premiums
    C. Privacy and Confidentiality Standards
    D. both A and C

61. Excessive amounts of fluoride in drinking water may cause discoloration of the:

    A. skin
    B. teeth
    C. nails
    D. tongue

62. Under which of the following circumstances is it permissible to release information from a patient's records?

    A. when the patient signs a release
    B. when a physician calls to request it
    C. when the insurance company signs a release
    D. when the patient is in an accident

63. A physician ordered 120 mg of a drug that comes only in 30 mg tablets. How many tablets constitute a dose?

    A. 3
    B. 4
    C. 6
    D. 12

64. The abbreviation q.o.d., as used in prescriptions, means:

    A. every hour
    B. every two hours
    C. every other day
    D. four times a day

65. A piece of paper describing a purchase and the amount due is known as a(n):

    A. inventory
    B. disbursement
    C. vendor
    D. invoice

66. A patient has an order for heparin 1000 units per hour by continuous infusion for a deep venous thrombosis. The pharmacy keeps a stock solution of 25,000 units of heparin in 250 mL of NS. How many mL would be required for 24 hours of therapy?

    A. 75 mL
    B. 140 mL
    C. 175 mL
    D. 240 mL

67. Which endocrine gland releases calcitonin?

    A. pancreas
    B. thyroid gland
    C. hypothalamus
    D. anterior pituitary gland

68. What is one of the greatest barriers to communication?

    A. the inability to communicate well
    B. complaining
    C. assertiveness
    D. stress

69. Which amendment or act required manufacturers to register and list their products?

    A. Medical Device Amendment
    B. Kefauver-Harris Amendment
    C. Durham-Humphrey Amendment
    D. Omnibus Budget Reconciliation Act

70. Manipulating estrogen and progesterone levels can prevent:

    A. breast cancer
    B. pregnancy
    C. prostate cancer
    D. abortion

71. Pharmacists or technicians are required by law to file which form for all eligible Medicare patients?

    A. HCPCS
    B. ICD-9
    C. RBRVS
    D. CMS-1500

72. A 3% sodium chloride solution is often administered intravenously to patients with severe hyponatremia. How many grams of sodium chloride are in a 250 mL bag of 3% sodium chloride?

    A. 4.5 grams
    B. 5.5 grams
    C. 6.5 grams
    D. 7.5 grams

73. What should pharmacy technicians do when new supplies are received?

    A. Throw out the old ones.
    B. Place them in the front of the supply area.
    C. Place them in the back of the supply area.
    D. Inventory all supplies.

74. The FDA now requires physicians and pharmacists to register and use a specific Web site in order to receive which of the following medications?

    A. ibuprofen (Motrin)
    B. isoniazid (Isoniazid)
    C. isotretinoin (Accutane)
    D. isoflurane (Forane)

75. Which drug is a sedative?

    A. phenothiazine
    B. lithium
    C. barbiturate
    D. levodopa

76. How many milliliters are found in a 1.5 L bag of an intravenous solution?

    A. 15 mL
    B. 150 mL
    C. 1500 mL
    D. 15,000 mL

77. A solution of water, sugar, and a drug is called a(n):

    A. emulsion
    B. elixir
    C. liniment
    D. syrup

78. By federal law, all medications should have a unique identifying number that must appear on the label. What is this number called?

    A. UPC (Universal Product Code)
    B. NDC (National Drug Code)
    C. UDC (Universal Drug Code)
    D. BN (Batch Number)

79. Which of the following words is misspelled?

    A. nueron
    B. malaise
    C. humerus
    D. glaucoma

80. Which of the following is NOT a proton pump inhibitor?

    A. rabeprazole
    B. omeprazole
    C. sulfisoxazole
    D. lansoprazole

81. The normal dosage for amoxicillin is 45 mg/kg/24 hours administered in divided doses. What would the dosage be for a 44-pound child if the dose is ordered b.i.d?

    A. 250 mg
    B. 350 mg
    C. 450 mg
    D. 650 mg

82. Cromolyn is used to treat:

    A. pneumonia
    B. tuberculosis
    C. allergies
    D. asthma

83. Which law is an extension of the Patriot Act?

    A. Medicare Modernization Act
    B. Combat Methamphetamine Epidemic Act
    C. Dietary Supplement Health and Education Act
    D. Anabolic Steroid Control Act

84. Expired compounded pharmaceuticals must be:

    A. returned
    B. disposed of
    C. repackaged
    D. sold immediately

85. The presence of raised or abnormal levels of lipoproteins and lipids in the blood is called:

    A. hypertension
    B. hyperlipidemia
    C. hyperkalemia
    D. hypernatremia

86. The generic name of Prozac is:

    A. fluoxetine
    B. imipramine
    C. nadolol
    D. lidocaine

87. Butenafine is prescribed to treat:

    A. depression
    B. constipation
    C. osteoporosis
    D. athlete's foot

88. An example of an intentional tort is:

    A. negligence
    B. malpractice
    C. libel
    D. battery

89. An infusion of the antibiotic vancomycin is currently running at 70 gtts/min. What is the rate in mL/hr if the tubing being used is rated 20 gtts/mL?

    A. 110 mL/hr
    B. 210 mL/hr
    C. 250 mL/hr
    D. 310 mL/hr

90. An example of a Class III antiarrhythmic drug that interferes with potassium outflow is:

    A. lidocaine
    B. amiodarone
    C. acebutolol
    D. verapamil

91. Balance weights should only be handled with:

    A. latex gloves
    B. a spatula
    C. forceps
    D. none of the above

92. Compounding slabs are also known as:

    A. glass slabs
    B. hard slabs
    C. ointment slabs
    D. cream slabs

93. The prefix *retro-* means:

    A. behind
    B. around
    C. below
    D. before

94. Furosemide is prescribed for:

    A. congestive heart failure
    B. nephrotic syndrome
    C. hypercalcemia
    D. all of the above

95. When an angry patient confronts you, you should always:

    A. learn how to cause anger
    B. focus on the patient's mental capacity
    C. stay very close to the patient while talking
    D. remain calm

96. A doctor orders 2 liters of hydration fluids to be infused intravenously over 4 hours. How many milliliters per hour should be infused?

    A. 250 mL/hr
    B. 350 mL/hr
    C. 500 mL/hr
    D. 575 mL/hr

97. Which body system does the condition vitiligo affect?

    A. respiratory
    B. reproductive
    C. endocrine
    D. integumentary

98. The generic name of Tofranil is:

    A. citalopram
    B. imipramine
    C. sertraline
    D. paroxetine

99. A Class II drug recall is one in which:

    A. the use or exposure to the produce will cause severe adverse reactions or death
    B. the use or exposure to the product may cause temporary or medically reversible adverse health hazards
    C. the use or exposure to the product is not likely to cause adverse health hazards
    D. none of the above

100. Which of the following is the trade name of amlodipine?

    A. Norvasc
    B. Plendil
    C. Nisocor
    D. Edecrin

Self-Evaluation: Test 2

1. What is the generic name for Prilosec?

   A. simvastatin
   B. atorvastatin
   C. ranitidine
   D. omeprazole

2. The unauthorized disclosure of client information is called:

   A. invasion of privacy
   B. unethical protocol
   C. breach of contract
   D. battery

3. Ranitidine is classified as an:

   A. H_2 blocker
   B. alpha blocker
   C. antihistamine
   D. ACE inhibitor

4. For what conditions is Bupropion used?

   A. depression
   B. epilepsy
   C. smoking cessation
   D. A and C

5. A pregnant woman was prescribed 60 mg of Fergon daily. Her cumulative monthly dose (30 days) would be approximately how many grams?

   A. 0.8 g
   B. 1.8 g
   C. 2.8 g
   D. 4.8 g

6. The suffix –*penia* means:

   A. increase
   B. enlargement
   C. formation
   D. abnormal reduction

7. The hypothalamus releases:

   A. prolactin
   B. testosterone
   C. vasopressin
   D. insulin

8. What is the generic name of Nasonex?

   A. fenofibrate
   B. metformin
   C. mometasone
   D. temazepam

9. How many mL equal 2 gallons?

   A. 954
   B. 1908
   C. 2816
   D. 7680

10. Which medication is contraindicated in patients with electrolyte imbalances, anuria, and hepatic coma?

    A. metolazone (Mykrox)
    B. folic acid (Folacin)
    C. digoxin (Digitek)
    D. cephalexin (Keflex)

11. Estradiol is classified as a(n):

    A. beta blocker
    B. antibiotic
    C. hormone
    D. antihistamine

12. What is the generic name of Xanax?

    A. diltiazem
    B. alprazolam
    C. amlodipine
    D. enalapril

13. How long must the blower run in a laminar airflow hood prior to use?

A. 10 minutes
B. 20 minutes
C. 30 minutes
D. 45 minutes

14. The United States classifies "clean" or "critical" room environments as "Class 100" or:

A. "Grade A"
B. "Grade B"
C. "Grade C"
D. "Grade D"

15. A pediatrician ordered Benadryl 25 mg orally every 8 hours for a 2-year-old child who weighs 16 kg. Pediatric dosage range is 5 mg/kg/day. If this drug is available as 12.5 mg/5 mL, how many milliliters should be given?

A. 2.5 mL
B. 5 mL
C. 7.5 mL
D. 10 mL

16. Of which department is the FDA a branch?

A. U.S. Department of Agriculture
B. U.S. Department of Health
C. U.S. Department of Labor
D. U.S. Department of Health and Human Services

17. Metamucil is classified as a(n):

A. laxative
B. antacid
C. antiflatulent
D. antiulcer medication

18. Which of the following is vitamin B_9?

A. cyanocobalamin
B. thiamine
C. folic acid
D. ascorbic acid

19. "Good" cholesterol is:

A. LDL
B. HDL
C. VLDL
D. NVCT

20. Which type of anemia may cause neurologic damage by impairing myelin formation?

A. iron deficiency
B. folic acid deficiency
C. aplastic
D. pernicious

21. Which law was the first to regulate the importation, manufacture, sale, and use of narcotic drugs?

A. Harrison Narcotic Act
B. Pure Food, Drug, and Cosmetic Act
C. Pure Food and Drug Act
D. Controlled Substance Act

22. A special container made of gelatin that is sized for a single dose is called a:

A. tablet
B. troche
C. suppository
D. capsule

23. The following medication is prescribed for a patient: erythromycin, 500 mg b.i.d × 7 days. The pharmacy technician only has the 250 mg dose in stock. How many 250 mg capsules will the technician dispense to the patient?

A. 7
B. 14
C. 21
D. 28

24. Which of the following abbreviations should appear on a written prescription?

A. Tx
B. Rx
C. Hx
D. Fx

25. For which scheduled drugs must dispensing records be kept on file for two years?

A. I
B. II
C. III
D. IV

26. Emergency pharmaceutical supplies should include which basic drugs?

A. vaseline
B. antibiotics
C. epinephrine
D. antitussives

27. How many grams are equal to 326 mg?

A. 3.26
B. 32.6
C. 0.36
D. 0.326

28. Most of the furniture inside a clean room should be cleaned with which of the following?

    A. 10% bleach
    B. 20% isopropyl alcohol
    C. 70% isopropyl alcohol
    D. 100% isopropyl alcohol

29. Sales – Costs = Gross Profit. What is the gross profit for a pharmacy whose sales total $199,991 and whose costs total $19,191?

    A. $108,072
    B. $188,000
    C. $180,080
    D. $180,800

30. Which type of injection is used to administer antibiotics in a patient with streptococcal pharyngitis?

    A. subcutaneous
    B. intradermal
    C. intramuscular
    D. intravenous

31. Which type of drug decreases appetite?

    A. antiemetics
    B. analgesics
    C. anorectics
    D. naleptics

32. Flushing of the ear canal to remove impacted cerumen is called:

    A. ear instillation
    B. ear irrigation
    C. tympanectomy
    D. Rinne test

33. How many Tbsp are equal to 12 tsp?

    A. 2
    B. 3
    C. 4
    D. 5

34. The smallest capsule is which of the following sizes?

    A. 0
    B. 1
    C. 3
    D. 5

35. What is the generic name of Zanaflex?

    A. simvastatin
    B. atorvastatin
    C. azithromycin
    D. tizanidine

36. Which act established the five controlled substance "schedules"?

    A. Harrison Narcotics Tax Act
    B. Drug Regulation Reform Act
    C. Drug Listing Act
    D. Comprehensive Drug Abuse Prevention and Control Act

37. Which type of environment should a laminar airflow hood provide?

    A. Class 100 area
    B. Class 1000 area
    C. Class 10,000 area
    D. Class 100,000 area

38. What is the trade name of fluoxetine?

    A. Paxil
    B. Elavil
    C. Nexium
    D. Prozac

39. A medication order label must contain all of the following information, EXCEPT the:

    A. generic and trade name of the medication
    B. expiration date of the medication
    C. name of the pharmacist who dispensed the medication
    D. refill number

40. The nurse increases a lidocaine infusion of 2 g in 250 mL D_5W to 30 mL/hr to control the patient's dysrhythmia. He should document that the patient is now receiving how many milligrams per minute?

    A. 2
    B. 3
    C. 4
    D. 5

41. Which syringe should be used to administer 1 mL of ampicillin pediatric drops?

    A. tuberculin syringe
    B. insulin syringe
    C. oral syringe
    D. low-dose syringe

42. The last two numbers represented in an NDC number signify the:

    A. drug product
    B. drug manufacturer
    C. drug package type
    D. drug selection

43. How frequently must HEPA filters be certified?

    A. 2 months
    B. 4 months
    C. 6 months
    D. 2 years

44. Which law was passed to establish clear criteria for classifications of legend and OTC drugs?

    A. Kefauver-Harris Amendment
    B. Durham-Humphrey Amendment
    C. Harrison Narcotics Tax Act
    D. Pure Food and Drug Act

45. Which dispensing device may be kept on the nursing unit?

    A. Pyxis Medstation
    B. Safety Pak
    C. Omni Link Rx
    D. Baker cells

46. The temperature of 86 degrees Fahrenheit is equal to how many degrees Celsius?

    A. 15
    B. 20
    C. 25
    D. 30

47. Which temperatures may be considered a "warm" environment?

    A. Above 45° Celsius
    B. Above 35° Celsius
    C. Above 25° Celsius
    D. Between 8° and 15° Celsius

48. Which agency oversees controlled substances and recommends prosecution for individuals who illegally distribute them?

    A. FDA
    B. CDC
    C. DEA
    D. HIPAA

49. Paxil is used for:

    A. diabetes
    B. depression
    C. asthma
    D. inflammation

50. A type of cholesterol that may put patients at risk of heart disease is called:

    A. cholesterolemia
    B. high-density lipoprotein
    C. low-density lipoprotein
    D. atherosclerosis

51. Peptic ulcers may be caused by:

    A. *Escherichia coli*
    B. *Streptococcus*
    C. *Helicobacter*
    D. *Staphylococcus*

52. Which white blood cells kill parasites and help control allergic reactions?

    A. neutrophils
    B. monocytes
    C. eosinophils
    D. lymphocytes

53. How many 4-tsp doses may be prepared from 1 L of a solution?

    A. 50
    B. 100
    C. 250
    D. 500

54. Clarithromycin is used for the treatment of:

    A. respiratory allergies
    B. pneumonia
    C. anxiety
    D. hypotension

55. The process of digestion begins in the:

    A. small intestine
    B. stomach
    C. large intestine
    D. mouth

56. Which vitamin is an antioxidant?

    A. D
    B. B_3
    C. E
    D. A

57. Atenolol is used for:

    A. diabetes
    B. anxiety
    C. hypertension
    D. osteoporosis

58. What part of a prescription contains the names and quantities of the ingredients?

    A. inscription
    B. superscription
    C. subscription
    D. signature

59. Using Clark's Rule, the usual adult dose for Celebrex is 100 mg twice daily for a total dose of 200 mg/day. How much should a child weighing 52 lb receive per dose?

   A. 49.34 mg
   B. 59.34 mg
   C. 69.34 mg
   D. 82.26 mg

60. Cocaine is a:

   A. Schedule I drug
   B. Schedule II drug
   C. Schedule III drug
   D. Schedule IV drug

61. A needle has all of the following parts, EXCEPT a:

   A. hub
   B. shaft
   C. flange
   D. lumen

62. What is the percentage of a 1:40 (W/V) solution?

   A. 1.5%
   B. 2.5%
   C. 4%
   D. 40%

63. Which type of agents do physicians use to prevent cell growth in a malignant form?

   A. beta-adrenergic blockers
   B. anticoagulants
   C. antineoplastics
   D. antimicrobials

64. Thrombolysis is:

   A. the surgical reconstruction of blood vessels
   B. the destruction of a clot
   C. the blockage of blood vessels
   D. the surgical removal of a clot

65. What is the best clinical example of a "genetic engineering" substance?

   A. insulin
   B. penicillin
   C. aspirin
   D. vitamin A

66. The abbreviation "Sig" means:

   A. the doctor's signature line
   B. the doctor's license number
   C. write on label
   D. number of refills

67. A pediatrician prescribes 250 mg q.i.d. for 10 days. How many milliliters of ampicillin oral suspension containing 250 mg/5 mL should be dispensed?

   A. 100 mL
   B. 125 mL
   C. 150 mL
   D. 200 mL

68. Which of the following is/are considered to be the drug(s) of choice for chronic asthma?

   A. theophylline
   B. albuterol
   C. antihistamine
   D. glucocorticoids

69. Acetaminophen with codeine is classified in which drug schedule?

   A. II
   B. III
   C. IV
   D. V

70. Which word is misspelled?

   A. pleurisy
   B. puritos
   C. pneumonia
   D. cirrhosis

71. Medication errors should be reported to which agency by using the program called MedWatch?

   A. CMS
   B. FDA
   C. DEA
   D. State Board of Pharmacy

72. A pharmacy technician wants to prepare 1 L of 5% W/V solution. He has an 80% solution in hand. How much diluent will be needed?

   A. 50 mL
   B. 180 mL
   C. 537 mL
   D. 937.5 mL

73. What is the generic name of Cialis?

   A. metaxalone
   B. famotidine
   C. valsartan
   D. tadalafil

74. Impairment of speech caused by a brain lesion is referred to as:

    A. dysphasia
    B. aphasia
    C. amnesia
    D. akinesia

75. What kind of organism is responsible for athlete's foot?

    A. fungi
    B. virus
    C. bacteria
    D. protozoa

76. How many grams of sodium chloride are in 100 mL of normal saline solution?

    A. 9 g
    B. 0.9 g
    C. 0.09 g
    D. 0.009 g

77. The simplest dosage forms compounded extemporaneously are:

    A. solutions
    B. suspensions
    C. emulsions
    D. elixirs

78. Epinephrine is also called:

    A. prolactin
    B. vasopressin
    C. estrogen
    D. adrenaline

79. The "four Ds of negligence" include each of the following, EXCEPT:

    A. direct cause
    B. depth of cause
    C. derelict
    D. damages

80. Which number would be a correct DEA number for Dr. Smith?

    A. CS 3076216
    B. AS 135879
    C. MS 1578926
    D. FS 224545

81. The gonadotropins are released from the:

    A. ovaries
    B. hypothalamus
    C. anterior pituitary
    D. testicular interstitial cells

82. Used for diaper rash, 40% zinc oxide is an example of a:

    A. paste
    B. gel
    C. ointment
    D. cream

83. A child was prescribed 5 mL of cough syrup, four times a day, as needed. The child's mother wanted to know how many teaspoon(s) should be given per dose. The correct answer is:

    A. 1
    B. 1 ½
    C. 2
    D. 2 ½

84. Which law required that pharmaceutical manufacturers file a New Drug Application with the FDA?

    A. Durham-Humphrey Amendment
    B. Kefauver-Harris Amendment
    C. Poison Prevention Packaging Act
    D. Food, Drug, and Cosmetic Act

85. Which is the most appropriate method for administration of Nitrostat tablets?

    A. SC
    B. SL
    C. PO
    D. PRT

86. How must significant losses of controlled substances be reported?

    A. in writing to the DEA within 7 days
    B. in writing to the DEA within 72 hours
    C. immediately by phone to the nearest DEA office
    D. immediately by phone to the local Health Department

87. The process of destruction of all microorganisms is called:

    A. disinfection
    B. filtration
    C. sanitization
    D. sterilization

88. A label shows that a medication is dispensed in a 6-oz container and is a 2% solution. How much medication is in the container?

    A. 3.6 g
    B. 6.6 g
    C. 12.6 g
    D. 22.6 g

89. What is the single most active agent against breast cancer?

    A. dactinomycin
    B. mitomycin
    C. doxorubicin
    D. bleomycin

90. What is the generic name for Tylenol?

    A. ibuprofen
    B. naproxen
    C. aspirin
    D. acetaminophen

91. Wrong doses can easily be avoided by using:

    A. unit-dose systems
    B. expired drugs
    C. Internet pharmacies
    D. generic drugs

92. According to the USP, for how long can a high-risk compounding product be refrigerated?

    A. 6 hours
    B. 24 hours
    C. 48 hours
    D. 72 hours

93. Which organization is responsible for employee safety?

    A. OBRA
    B. OSHA
    C. HIPAA
    D. TJC

94. How many tablets, each containing 500 mg of an antibiotic, are needed to provide 50 mg/kg/day for 10 days for an adult weighing 194 lb?

    A. 18
    B. 68
    C. 88
    D. 128

95. Which of the following is NOT an adrenergic drug?

    A. dobutamine
    B. epinephrine
    C. dopamine
    D. atropine

96. What is the trade name of benzonatate?

    A. Telfast
    B. Tessalon
    C. Tenoretic
    D. Tussionex

97. Cancer in which site is the leading cause of cancer death in males?

    A. prostate
    B. pancreas
    C. lung
    D. colon

98. Which was the first enforceable nationally published standard for sterile compounding of drugs?

    A. USP 797
    B. TJC
    C. HIPAA
    D. CDC

99. How many grams are in 90 gr?

    A. 0.85 g
    B. 5.85 g
    C. 12.85 g
    D. 125.85 g

100. Which of the following drugs are contraindicated in patients with hypertension, asthma, hyperthyroidism, and peptic ulcer?

    A. cholinergic agonists
    B. anticholinergics
    C. adrenergic blockers
    D. adrenergic agonists

Self-Evaluation: Test 3

1. Which agency regulates the transporting of hazardous materials?

    A. Food and Drug Administration (FDA)
    B. Department of Transportation (DOT)
    C. Environmental Protection Agency (EPA)
    D. Drug Enforcement Agency (DEA)

2. A pharmacy balance must be certified every:

    A. 3 months
    B. 6 months
    C. 12 months
    D. 24 months

3. Which piece of equipment may be used to measure volumes less than 1.5 mL?

    A. syringe
    B. pipette
    C. beaker
    D. cylindrical graduate

4. Which is the most effective method of communication?

    A. telephone
    B. E-mail
    C. writing a letter
    D. face-to-face

5. Which area is the most appropriate for storage of finished radiopharmaceutical products?

    A. compounding area
    B. disposal area
    C. packaging area
    D. outside the pharmacy

6. Which of the following is represented by an NDC number?

    A. drug manufacturer, drug strength, and drug name
    B. drug manufacturer, drug product, and package size
    C. drug product and package size
    D. drug product and controlled substance schedule

7. What is the allowable number of refills for a Schedule II drug?

    A. 0
    B. 2
    C. 3
    D. 5

8. Which may be a base for an ointment?

    A. oleaginous base
    B. oil-in-water emulsion
    C. water-in-oil emulsion
    D. all of the above

9. Simple liquid containers that may be cylindrical in shape are known as:

    A. beakers
    B. droppers
    C. graduates
    D. funnels

10. Which agency establishes radiation safety standards?

    A. National Board of Pharmacy
    B. Occupational Safety and Health Administration
    C. State Board of Pharmacy
    D. Centers for Disease Control

11. Spring-based Class A balances have a weighing capacity that ranges from:

    A. 3 mg to 45 g
    B. 6 mg to 90 g
    C. 6 mg to 120 g
    D. 60 g to 5 kg

12. If 1 gram of dextrose provides 3.4 kilocalories, how many kilocalories will 300 mL of a 50% dextrose solution provide?

    A. 35 kcal
    B. 75 kcal
    C. 510 kcal
    D. 475 kcal

13. What is the brand name for ranitidine?

    A. Tagamet
    B. Axid
    C. Pepcid
    D. Zantac

14. Which is the most common form of compounded medications?

    A. liquid drugs
    B. creams
    C. tablets
    D. capsules

15. Examples of substances commonly available in capsule form include all of the following, EXCEPT

    A. vitamin E
    B. BENADRYL
    C. phenergan
    D. cod liver oil

16. What is the brand name for esomeprazole?

    A. Nexium
    B. AcipHex
    C. Protonix
    D. Prevacid

17. 25 degrees Celsius is equal to:

    A. 32° F
    B. 47° F
    C. 65° F
    D. 77° F

18. Which vitamin deficiency may cause beriberi?

    A. B_{12}
    B. A
    C. D
    D. B_1

19. Dry baths allow both cooling and heating, with commonly available temperatures as low as:

    A. –30° C
    B. –20° C
    C. –10° C
    D. 0° C

20. A pharmacy's inventory turnover rate indicates which of the following?

    A. how many times in a week that the inventory has been used or replaced
    B. how many times in a month that the inventory has been used or replaced
    C. how many times in a year that the inventory has been used or replaced
    D. none of the above

21. A physician ordered 56 mEq of calcium carbonate to be added to an IV solution. The technician has a 25 mL vial of calcium carbonate 4.4 mEq/mL. How many milliliters of this concentration does the technician need to add to the IV solution?

    A. 12.7
    B. 10.4
    C. 7.5
    D. 5.6

22. The total number of dosage units of controlled substances that a pharmacy distributes to another registrant during a 12-month period should NOT exceed:

    A. 1% of its total amount
    B. 5% of its total amount
    C. 10% of its total amount
    D. 15% of its total amount

23. What is the trade name for zidovudine?

    A. Zerit
    B. Ziagen
    C. Retrovir
    D. Reyataz

24. How often should laminar airflow hoods be thoroughly cleaned?

    A. 1 hour
    B. 3 hours
    C. 5 hours
    D. 8 hours

25. Which is an example of the fight-or-flight syndrome?

    A. fear
    B. emotion
    C. empathy
    D. projection

26. Which vitamin is necessary for formation of prothrombin in the liver and is essential to blood clotting?

    A. vitamin E
    B. vitamin C
    C. vitamin K
    D. vitamin A

27. When following CSA requirements, how often does each DEA registrant need to create a complete controlled substances stock record?

    A. every year
    B. every two years
    C. every three years
    D. every five years

28. Which dosage form is prepared by using the "punch method"?

    A. tablet
    B. capsule
    C. plaster
    D. troche

29. Which drug schedule allows prescriptions to be faxed to a pharmacy?

    A. II
    B. III
    C. IV
    D. all of the above

30. Which law contained important amendments affecting Medicare and Medicaid?

    A. Omnibus Budget Reconciliation Act
    B. Prescription Drug Marketing Act
    C. Orphan Drug Act
    D. Patriot Act

31. The abbreviation "NPI" means:

    A. National Pharmacopeia Index
    B. National Provider Identifier
    C. National Pharmacy Institute
    D. National Pharmaceutical Institute

32. Which medication should NOT be chewed?

    A. fexofenadine (Allegra)
    B. ascorbic acid (Vita-C)
    C. azelastine (Astelin)
    D. benzonatate (Tessalon)

33. Which drug is derived from a plant drug source?

    A. insulin
    B. pepsin
    C. meperidine
    D. morphine

34. What is the abbreviation that means "nothing by mouth"?

    A. NOC
    B. NBM
    C. NPO
    D. PRN

35. The drug of choice for Parkinson's disease is:

    A. levodopa
    B. aspirin
    C. amantadine
    D. pyridoxine

36. A pharmacy technician was asked to mark up a drug by 25%. How much would an item with this markup cost if its original cost was $3.50?

    A. $3.18
    B. $4.38
    C. $5.85
    D. $6.68

37. What is the meaning of the word root *lachry*?

    A. tear
    B. finger
    C. artery
    D. gland

38. What is the newest drug in the group of hydantoins?

    A. phenytoin (Dilantin)
    B. valproic acid (Depakene)
    C. fosphenytoin (Cerebyx)
    D. felbamate (Felbatol)

39. HEPA filters need to be certified every 6 months unless they become:

    A. wet
    B. dry
    C. dusted
    D. all of the above

40. The *Physician's Desk Reference* is published every:

    A. six months
    B. year
    C. two years
    D. three years

41. Which form is used when ordering Schedule II narcotics?

    A. Form 224
    B. Form 41
    C. Form 106
    D. Form 222

42. Which components are found in total nutrient admixtures?

   A. dextrose, amino acids, and vitamins
   B. dextrose, amino acids, and minerals
   C. dextrose, amino acids, and lipids
   D. dextrose, amino acids, and proteins

43. Which part of the brain controls emotions, sleep, water balance, body temperature, and appetite?

   A. medulla oblongata
   B. hypothalamus
   C. midbrain
   D. cerebellum

44. What is the flow rate for 1 L of 5% dextrose and 0.9% sodium chloride over 24 hours?

   A. 25 mL/hr
   B. 41 mL/hr
   C. 54 mL/hr
   D. 71 mL/hr

45. What is the correct route of administration for heparin?

   A. oral
   B. intramuscular
   C. intra-arterial
   D. intravenous

46. To avoid soiling balance pans, what should be placed underneath substances to be weighed?

   A. legal paper
   B. wrapping paper
   C. glassine paper
   D. aluminum foil

47. Which is a side effect of an antihistamine?

   A. runny nose
   B. hypertension
   C. drowsiness
   D. tachycardia

48. To grind a powder into a smoother mixture, using moisture, requires a process called:

   A. pasteurization
   B. agitation
   C. suspension
   D. levigation

49. In what schedule are anabolic steroids classified?

   A. II
   B. III
   C. IV
   D. V

50. The law limits sales of pure ephedrine or pseudoephedrine (which are precursors of methamphetamine) to how many grams per month per person?

   A. 2 g
   B. 5 g
   C. 9 g
   D. 45 g

51. The invoice or packing slip for Schedule III, IV, or V drugs must be kept in a separate, secure location in the pharmacy for a minimum of:

   A. 6 months
   B. 12 months
   C. 24 months
   D. 6 years

52. The two-pan type of Class A prescription balance requires external weights for measurements exceeding:

   A. 1 mg
   B. 10 mg
   C. 1 g
   D. 10 g

53. In which body organ(s) is the corpus callosum located?

   A. lungs
   B. kidneys
   C. liver
   D. brain

54. Which hormone is related to carbohydrates?

   A. vasopressin
   B. glucagon
   C. prolactin
   D. oxytocin

55. What is the trade name for fluoxetine?

   A. Zoloft
   B. Paxil
   C. Prozac
   D. Celexa

56. The percent equivalent of a 1:20 ratio is:

   A. 0.25%
   B. 0.05%
   C. 0.5%
   D. 5%

57. Which law prohibits the sale or trade of drug samples?

    A. Prescription Drug Marketing Act
    B. Omnibus Budget Reconciliation Act
    C. FDA Safe Medical Devices Act
    D. Orphan Drug Act

58. Which health professionals make notations in Medication Administration Records (MARs) in a hospital?

    A. physicians
    B. pharmacists
    C. nurses
    D. phlebotomists

59. What is the correct DEA number for Dr. Alan Smith?

    A. BA2456681
    B. CS2141632
    C. KS1677825
    D. DS4725941

60. Which solution is the most concentrated?

    A. 45%
    B. 25%
    C. 20%
    D. 0.25%

61. Approximately 5% of people allergic to cephalosporins are also allergic to:

    A. tetracyclines
    B. aminoglycosides
    C. penicillins
    D. macrolides

62. The sensitivity of a Class A balance is:

    A. 2 mg
    B. 6 mg
    C. 12 mg
    D. 25 mg

63. Considered a medical emergency, an extremely high temperature is called:

    A. hyperkalemia
    B. hyperpyrexia
    C. hypertension
    D. hyperhydrosis

64. What is the most common anemia?

    A. folic acid deficiency
    B. aplastic anemia
    C. iron deficiency anemia
    D. pernicious anemia

65. How many refills are allowed for a Schedule IV drug?

    A. 0
    B. 2
    C. 3
    D. 5

66. Which DEA form must be used when returning Schedule II substances?

    A. Form 222
    B. Form 224
    C. Form 106
    D. Form 41

67. The official authority that sets standards for all prescriptions and OTC medications is the:

    A. BOP
    B. USP
    C. DOH
    D. NABP

68. A painless but highly contagious local lesion of syphilis is called a:

    A. chancroid
    B. papule
    C. pastule
    D. chancre

69. What is the generic name of Biaxin?

    A. clindamycin
    B. clarithromycin
    C. tobramycin
    D. azithromycin

70. How many days will the medication last for amoxicillin 500 mg if a physician orders 36 capsules to take orally every 8 hours?

    A. 8 days
    B. 10 days
    C. 12 days
    D. 15 days

71. What temperature is equivalent to 102.6 degrees F?

    A. 36° C
    B. 38° C
    C. 39.2° C
    D. 41.4° C

72. What is the generic name for Glucotrol?

    A. glipizide
    B. glyburide
    C. pioglitazone
    D. metformin

73. How far inside a laminar airflow hood should a pharmacy technician prepare a sterile product?

   A. 3 in.
   B. 6 in.
   C. 8 in.
   D. 12 in.

74. How many milliliters of water must be added to 250 mL of a 0.9% (W/V) stock solution of sodium chloride if the pharmacy technician is required to prepare a ½ NS solution?

   A. 150 mL
   B. 250 mL
   C. 350 mL
   D. 450 mL

75. All of the following drugs are NSAIDS, EXCEPT:

   A. ibuprofen
   B. meloxicam
   C. indomethacin
   D. colchicine

76. What does the suffix –stomy mean?

   A. surgical opening
   B. incision
   C. turning
   D. enlargement

77. What is the disadvantage of an oral dosage form?

   A. ease of administration
   B. first-pass metabolism
   C. convenience of use
   D. cheap to administer

78. Which DEA form is used to complete the destruction of noncontrolled substances?

   A. 224
   B. 222
   C. 106
   D. none of the above

79. Which drug recall signifies that the death of a person occurred?

   A. Class I
   B. Class II
   C. Class III
   D. Class V

80. MSDS is required for what types of drugs?

   A. intravenous admixtures
   B. investigational drugs
   C. hazardous chemicals and drugs
   D. none of the above

81. Which dosage form can be either water-in-oil or oil-in-water?

   A. suspensions
   B. solutions
   C. elixirs
   D. emulsions

82. A nosocomial infection may occur:

   A. in a hospital
   B. in a school
   C. at home
   D. because of cold temperature

83. How many gr are equal to 4 g?

   A. 15.3
   B. 30.7
   C. 50.2
   D. 60.4

84. For mixing liquids, a mortar and pestle should be made out of:

   A. Wedgwood
   B. glass
   C. porcelain
   D. any of the above

85. The Joint Commission may certify all of the following pharmacy settings, EXCEPT:

   A. retail pharmacies
   B. hospitals
   C. long-term care services
   D. nursing homes

86. What do the first five numbers represent in an NDC number?

   A. drug product
   B. drug packaging
   C. drug manufacturer
   D. drug expiration date

87. What is the largest endocrine gland?

   A. thyroid
   B. liver
   C. adrenal cortex
   D. parathyroid

88. What is the generic name of Zyrtec?

   A. fexofenadine
   B. cetirizine
   C. brompheniramine
   D. pseudoephedrine

89. A drug has a concentration of 40 mg/mL. How many grams of the drug are found in ½ L of solution?

    A. 5 g
    B. 10 g
    C. 15 g
    D. 20 g

90. Which law mandates that a prescription label must be placed onto a medication container?

    A. Poison Prevention Packaging Act
    B. Comprehensive Drug Abuse Prevention and Control Act
    C. Food, Drug, and Cosmetic Act
    D. Drug Regulation Reform Act

91. Which drugs are contraindicated with potassium-sparing diuretics?

    A. nitrates
    B. ACE inhibitors
    C. beta-adrenergic blockers
    D. calcium channel blockers

92. Which cells release histamine?

    A. lymphocytes
    B. eosinophils
    C. basophils
    D. monocytes

93. Which antibiotics are contraindicated in children younger than 8 years of age?

    A. cephalosporins
    B. aminoglycosides
    C. sulfonamides
    D. tetracyclines

94. What is the trade name of meperidine?

    A. Demerol
    B. Dolophine
    C. Talwin
    D. Hycodan

95. Which is NOT the best example of a solution?

    A. syrup
    B. emulsion
    C. liniment
    D. elixir

96. What number does a manufacturer provide to identify a particular batch of medicine?

    A. lot number
    B. NDC number
    C. both A and B
    D. neither A or B

97. Which aminoglycoside is the most nephrotoxic?

    A. tobramycin
    B. neomycin
    C. kanamycin
    D. gentamicin

98. If a 4-year-old weighing 37 lb took a bottle of 50 aspirin tablets, with each tablet containing 81 mg, how much aspirin did the child ingest on a milligram per kilogram basis?

    A. 104
    B. 165
    C. 241
    D. 274

99. Abnormally large growth of body tissue as a result of an excess of growth hormone during childhood is called:

    A. dwarfism
    B. acromegaly
    C. gigantism
    D. myxedema

100. Which is a major complication of heparin administration?

    A. hypertension
    B. angina pectoris
    C. bronchospasms
    D. bleeding

Self-Evaluation: Test 4

1. Which reference book gives information about drug prices?

   A. *National Formulary*
   B. *Drug Topic Orange Book*
   C. *United States Pharmacopeia*
   D. *Drug Topics Red Book*

2. What is the trade name of propoxyphene?

   A. Demerol
   B. Darvon
   C. Dilaudid
   D. Talwin

3. Type 2 diabetes is also called:

   A. NIDDM
   B. IDDM
   C. GDM
   D. Juvenile DM

4. Which is an example of a protozoal infection?

   A. genital herpes
   B. toxic shock syndrome
   C. trichomoniasis
   D. syphilis

5. The general root *xero* means:

   A. white
   B. dry
   C. yellow
   D. tumor

6. Where are sebaceous glands found?

   A. pancreas
   B. prostate
   C. spleen
   D. skin

7. A technician receives a prescription to compound 6 fl oz of a 15% solution, and there is a 25% solution on hand. How much diluent must the technician add to fill this order?

   A. 72 mL
   B. 108 mL
   C. 112.5 mL
   D. 180 mL

8. The prefix *milli-* means:

   A. one-hundredth
   B. one-thousandth
   C. one-tenth
   D. many

9. What is the generic name of Adalat?

   A. naratriptan
   B. dicyclomine
   C. nifedipine
   D. dolasetron

10. The formula that explains the composition of a drug is known as its:

    A. brand name
    B. chemical name
    C. generic name
    D. biological name

11. Which is a solid dosage form?

    A. elixir
    B. plaster
    C. emulsion
    D. spirit

12. The term *hypokalemia* means:

    A. high potassium
    B. high sodium
    C. low sodium
    D. low potassium

13. Keflex 500 mg p.o. q.i.d. has been ordered. On hand is Keflex 250 mg per 5 mL. How many milliliters should be administered per dose?

    A. 2 mL
    B. 5 mL
    C. 10 mL
    D. 20 mL

14. The first branches of the ascending aorta are called the:

    A. coronary arteries
    B. carotid arteries
    C. subclavian arteries
    D. brachiocephalic arteries

15. What is the generic name of Catapres?

    A. clonidine
    B. citalopram
    C. loratadine
    D. hydralazine

16. When the brain experiences shrinkage and exhibits senile plaques, the condition is called:

    A. Parkinson's disease
    B. Addison's disease
    C. Alzheimer's disease
    D. Cushing's syndrome

17. A pediatrician ordered 35 mg/kg of a drug q6h for an infant weighing 16.4 lb. How many milligrams of the drug are needed for each dose?

    A. 120
    B. 180
    C. 230
    D. 260

18. Who must review Investigational New Drug Applications?

    A. DEA
    B. EPA
    C. FDA
    D. BOP

19. Which medications may cause constipation, dry mouth, and difficulty in urinating?

    A. beta blockers
    B. anticholinergics
    C. alpha blockers
    D. none of the above

20. What is the trade name of metronidazole?

    A. Floxin
    B. Folvite
    C. Fungizone
    D. Flagyl

21. A cancer of the epithelial cells is called a:

    A. carcinoma
    B. sarcoma
    C. metastasis
    D. endometriosis

22. What are the most common causes of pelvic inflammatory disease?

    A. chlamydia and gonorrhea
    B. *staphylococcus* and chlamydia
    C. *streptococcus* and chlamydia
    D. all of the above

23. How many milliliters are there in 75 cc?

    A. 15 mL
    B. 25 mL
    C. 50 mL
    D. 75 mL

24. What is the generic name of Lasix?

    A. triamcinolone
    B. furosemide
    C. naproxen
    D. hydrochlorothiazide

25. Which drug is classified in Schedule IV?

    A. diphenoxylate
    B. anabolic steroid
    C. methadone
    D. benzodiazepine

26. How many ounces are equivalent to 240 mL?

    A. 4 oz
    B. 6 oz
    C. 8 oz
    D. 12 oz

27. Which form is used to report the theft of controlled substances?

    A. 224
    B. 222
    C. 106
    D. 41

28. A chronic condition characterized by raised red patches covered with white scales is referred to as:

    A. seborrheic dermatitis
    B. eczema
    C. psoriasis
    D. atopic dermatitis

29. How many refills are allowed for Schedule II prescriptions?

    A. 0
    B. 1
    C. 2
    D. 5

30. What is the trade name of procainamide?

    A. Pronestyl
    B. Prozac
    C. Prilosec
    D. Minipress

31. Which may cause goiter?

    A. hyperglycemia
    B. hyperthyroidism
    C. hypogonadism
    D. hypoglycemia

32. Trisomy 21 is also called:

    A. polydactyly
    B. galactosemia
    C. Down syndrome
    D. Turner's syndrome

33. A patient is taking Pepcid 20 mg, and the instructions read "i PO tid." What is the total daily dose?

    A. 20 mg
    B. 40 mg
    C. 60 mg
    D. 80 mg

34. What is the trade name of famotidine?

    A. Maxalt
    B. Tagamet
    C. Axid
    D. Pepcid

35. The Poison Prevention Act allows a pharmacist to dispense which medications in a non-child-resistant container?

    A. nitroglycerin
    B. amlodipine
    C. diltiazem
    D. atenolol

36. The abbreviation for the word *diagnosis* is:

    A. D&C
    B. DG
    C. Dx
    D. Diag

37. Which agent is contraindicated in young males?

    A. sertraline (Zoloft)
    B. trazodone (Desyrel)
    C. diazepam (Valium)
    D. trifluoperazine (Stelazine)

38. The flow rate of 1500 mL of Ringer's lactate to be infused over 10 hours is:

    A. 25 mL/hr
    B. 50 mL/hr
    C. 75 mL/hr
    D. 150 mL/hr

39. What is the trade name of glyburide?

    A. Diamox
    B. DiaBeta
    C. Glucotrol
    D. Hytrin

40. What is the most potent topical corticosteroid?

    A. ointment
    B. patch
    C. lotion
    D. gel

41. Which prescription medication does NOT require a patient package insert to be given?

    A. progesterones
    B. metered-dose inhalers
    C. ACE inhibitors
    D. Accutane

42. What is the generic name of Procardia?

    A. nifedipine
    B. propranolol
    C. diltiazem
    D. atenolol

43. Which suffix means "inflammation"?

    A. –*iasis*
    B. –*itis*
    C. –*osis*
    D. –*trophy*

44. What is the trade name of prednisone?

    A. Deltasone
    B. Decadron
    C. Trilafon
    D. Ultralente

45. What is the trade name of azithromycin?

    A. Zocor
    B. Zestril
    C. Relafen
    D. Zithromax

46. Herpes zoster is also called:

    A. warts
    B. shingles
    C. impetigo
    D. gangrene

47. Which term is used for the classification of temperatures between 15 degrees Celsius and 30 degrees Celsius?

    A. excessive heat
    B. room temperature
    C. cold
    D. cool

48. An inherited disorder characterized by the presence of abnormal hemoglobin (Hbs) is called:

    A. iron deficiency anemia
    B. hemolytic anemia
    C. sickle cell anemia
    D. septicemia

49. A 14-year-old girl weighs 85 lbs. Calculate the amount of medication that the child should receive by using Young's Rule (the adult dose is 40 mg).

    A. 11 mg
    B. 21 mg
    C. 26 mg
    D. 32 mg

50. What is the generic name of alprazolam?

    A. Xanax
    B. Xalatan
    C. Volmax
    D. Vasotec

51. Which law required all narcotics to be labeled "Warning: May Be Habit Forming"?

    A. Kefauver-Harris Amendment
    B. Durham-Humphrey Amendment
    C. Harrison Narcotics Act
    D. Comprehensive Drug Abuse Prevention and Control Act

52. What is the amount of medication in a 1-oz tube of 1% cream?

    A. 0.3 mcg
    B. 0.3 mg
    C. 0.3 g
    D. 3 g

53. Which gland releases glucagon?

    A. thyroid
    B. pancreas
    C. ovaries
    D. adrenal cortex

54. What is the generic name of Azmacort?

    A. losartan
    B. ranitidine
    C. glipizide
    D. triamcinolone

55. Which word is misspelled?

    A. venous
    B. prostate
    C. homostasis
    D. integumentary

56. Carbohydrate is stored in the liver as:

    A. starch
    B. sucrose
    C. disaccharides
    D. glycogen

57. According to the Controlled Substance Act, for how long is DEA Form 222 valid?

    A. 7 days
    B. 30 days
    C. 60 days
    D. 90 days

58. The junction between two neurons is called a:

    A. synapse
    B. axon
    C. bipolar
    D. hillock

59. Which type of formulary is a limited list of medications?

    A. open
    B. closed
    C. both
    D. neither

60. What is the concentration of heparin 15,000 units in 500 mL of D_5W?

    A. 15 units/mL
    B. 30 units/mL
    C. 50 units/mL
    D. 100 units/mL

61. Which term is misspelled?

    A. peristalsis
    B. salmonella
    C. disphagia
    D. repression

62. *Angioplasty* is defined as:

    A. surgical repair of a blood vessel
    B. surgical excision of a vein
    C. surgical excision of an artery
    D. surgical incision of the heart

63. Which law divided all drugs into two groups: prescription medications and over-the-counter (OTC) medications?

    A. Durham-Humphrey Act
    B. Poison Prevention Packaging Act
    C. Drug Listing Act
    D. Pure Food and Drug Act

64. Adrenergic synapses release the neurotransmitter:

    A. serotonin
    B. acetylcholine
    C. dopamine
    D. norepinephrine

65. Which of the following is NOT classified as an antihyperlipidemic?

    A. Welchol
    B. Folic acid
    C. Lopid
    D. Pravachol

66. When the dose of a medication is 250 mcg, how many doses can be prepared from 0.140 g?

    A. 6
    B. 56
    C. 336
    D. 560

67. Which abbreviation means "every day"?

    A. b.i.d.
    B. t.i.d.
    C. q.i.d.
    D. q.d.

68. What is the trade name of esomeprazole?

    A. Zyprexa
    B. Nexium
    C. Paxil
    D. Prozac

69. A male with type A blood has:

    A. B agglutinins in his plasma
    B. A agglutinins on his red blood cells
    C. A agglutinogens in his plasma
    D. B agglutinogens on his red blood cells

70. Which law prohibited all legend drugs from being dispensed without a prescription?

    A. Food, Drug, and Cosmetic Act
    B. Durham-Humphrey Amendment
    C. Poison Prevention Act
    D. Controlled Substance Act

71. Which type of insulin has the longest duration of action?

    A. regular
    B. Humalog
    C. Ultralente
    D. none of the above

72. The loss of the sense of smell is known as:

    A. aphonia
    B. anosmia
    C. amnesia
    D. anorexia

73. Which prefix means "bad, difficult, painful"?

    A. *ex-*
    B. *dis-*
    C. *dys-*
    D. *meta-*

74. What is the generic name of Plavix?

    A. clopidogrel
    B. glimepiride
    C. bupropion
    D. fexofenadine

75. Which category of drugs are contraindicated for the treatment of congestive heart failure?

    A. beta-adrenergic blockers
    B. antiarrhythmics
    C. ACE inhibitors
    D. angiotensin II antagonists

76. Which is the strongest dose of a medication?

    A. 1/50 gr
    B. 1/100 gr
    C. 1/150 gr
    D. 1/200 gr

77. Which law indicated that opium must be dispensed only with a prescription?

    A. Food, Drug, and Cosmetic Act
    B. Federal Food and Drug Act
    C. Harrison Narcotic Act
    D. Comprehensive Drug Abuse Prevention and Control Act

78. In which structure is blood pressure the highest?

    A. capillary
    B. vein
    C. artery
    D. arteriole

79. Which dietary supplement is used to treat depression?

    A. St. John's wort
    B. ginkgo biloba
    C. saw palmetto
    D. glucosamine

80. Hay fever, anaphylaxis, asthma, and eczema are examples of which type of hypersensitivities?

    A. Type I
    B. Type II
    C. Type III
    D. Type IV

81. Which antibiotic can discolor the urine, saliva, and sweat, causing each to become reddish-orange, and may also permanently discolor soft contact lenses?

    A. Vancomycin
    B. Rifampin
    C. Metronidazole
    D. Nystatin

82. How many Tbsp are equal to 6 fl oz?

    A. 8
    B. 12
    C. 16
    D. 22

83. Which disease can result from antidiuretic hormone deficiency?

    A. dwarfism
    B. diabetes mellitus
    C. diabetes insipidus
    D. myxedema

84. Which DEA form can be used to transfer scheduled medications from one pharmacy to another?

    A. Form 106
    B. Form 222
    C. Form 224
    D. Form 41

85. What is the trade name of atorvastatin?

    A. Lipitor
    B. Zocor
    C. Zantac
    D. Vasotec

86. The abbreviation "NS" for an IV admixture means:

    A. normal solution
    B. normal saline
    C. both A or B
    D. neither A nor B

87. A physician ordered 120 mg of a drug that comes only in 15 mg tablets. How many tablets constitute a dose?

    A. 4
    B. 8
    C. 10
    D. 12

88. What are the first line of cellular defense against pathogens?

    A. B cells
    B. T cells
    C. plasma cells
    D. phagocytes

89. If a pharmacist dispenses a partial Schedule II drug, how long does he or she have to provide the remaining medications?

    A. 24 hours
    B. 48 hours
    C. 72 hours
    D. 7 days

90. The underlined portion of the word *hypolipidemia* represents which word part?

    A. prefix
    B. root
    C. suffix
    D. combining form

91. The cost of 100 capsules is $3.50. What would the retail price be if there were a 25% gross profit?

    A. $2.30
    B. $2.50
    C. $3.35
    D. $4.38

92. The nonproprietary name of a drug is also called its:

    A. brand name
    B. generic name
    C. trade name
    D. none of the above

93. Which class of drugs is most appropriate for a patient with a persistent cough?

    A. antiemetics
    B. antipruritics
    C. antitussives
    D. antidotes

94. Immunoglobulins that are the first antibodies to be produced in response to infection are referred to as:

    A. IgG
    B. IgM
    C. IgD
    D. IgE

95. The abbreviation "b.i.d." means:

    A. every other day
    B. every 6 hours
    C. twice a day
    D. once a day

96. A total parenteral solution is what type of solution?

    A. isotonic
    B. hypertonic
    C. hypotonic
    D. none of the above

97. If a child must take a 5 mL suspension that contains 250 mg t.i.d. of amoxicillin, how many milligrams of the drug would be taken daily?

    A. 250 mg
    B. 500 mg
    C. 750 mg
    D. 900 mg

98. Accutane prescriptions must be filled within:

    A. 3 days
    B. 7 days
    C. 21 days
    D. 30 days

99. *Ung* is a Latin abbreviation meaning:

    A. lozenge
    B. emulsion
    C. plaster
    D. ointment

100. The portion of the nephron that attaches to the collecting duct is the:

    A. proximal convoluted tubule
    B. loop of Henle
    C. distal convoluted tubule
    D. minor calyx

Self-Evaluation: Test 5

1. Perpetual inventories of all Schedule II controlled drugs must be reconciled at least every:

   A. day
   B. 7 days
   C. 10 days
   D. 30 days

2. Which schedule of drugs must be counted or measured exactly?

   A. I
   B. II
   C. III
   D. IV

3. The dose of a drug is 500 mg for an adult. Based on Clark's Rule, how many milligrams should be given to a child weighing 55 lbs?

   A. 8.3 mg
   B. 18.3 mg
   C. 183.3 mg
   D. 225 mg

4. The drug name Paxil is considered to be a:

   A. generic name
   B. chemical name
   C. brand name
   D. national drug code

5. Which statement about H_1N_1 flu is false?

   A. It is caused by a virus.
   B. Patients receive either one or two vaccines for this type of flu.
   C. It first became an epidemic in New Mexico in 2009.
   D. Children must be the first people vaccinated against it.

6. A Class II drug recall is one in which:

   A. the use or exposure to the product will cause severe adverse reactions or death
   B. the use of or exposure to the product will cause temporary or medically reversible adverse effects
   C. the use of or exposure to the product is not likely to cause adverse health hazards
   D. none of the above is true

7. The abbreviation "O.U." means:

   A. left eye
   B. each eye
   C. right eye
   D. right ear

8. "Consigned inventory" means:

   A. products that are purchased outright by the pharmacy
   B. products that are sold in the pharmacy but are actually still owned by the manufacturer
   C. nonreusable drug products
   D. restricted formulary products

9. Consider two fractions with the same denominator. The fraction with the smallest numerator has:

   A. the lesser value
   B. the greater value
   C. equal value
   D. a value equal to 1

10. How many milligrams are in 1 gram?

    A. 10
    B. 100
    C. 1000
    D. 10,000

11. Which drug is not an ACE inhibitor?

    A. Capoten
    B. Atacand
    C. Vasotec
    D. Lotensin

12. Which governmental agency regulates compounding procedures in the hospital?

    A. Joint Commission
    B. DEA
    C. FDA
    D. both A and B

13. Which balance is NOT appropriate for prescription compounding?

    A. Class A prescription balance
    B. electronic balance
    C. counter balance
    D. both A and B

14. Which agency is deeply involved in the war against the human immunodeficiency virus (HIV) and acquired immunodeficiency syndrome (AIDS)?

    A. FDA
    B. CDC
    C. DEA
    D. HHS

15. A condition characterized by wasting of muscular tissue as a result of disease or poor nutrition is called:

    A. myalgia
    B. myopathy
    C. atrophy
    D. polyphagia

16. Which hormone is NOT produced by the anterior pituitary gland?

    A. thyroid-stimulating
    B. luteinizing
    C. antidiuretic
    D. adrenocorticotropic

17. What is the decimal equivalent of 6/1000?

    A. 0.06
    B. 0.006
    C. 0.6
    D. 0.0006

18. What is the advantage of a conical graduate?

    A. It is less expensive.
    B. It is calibrated in metric units only.
    C. It is easier to clean.
    D. It is easier to read.

19. How frequently are drug formularies revised?

    A. every day
    B. every week
    C. every month
    D. every year

20. A DEA number consists of a two-letter prefix followed by:

    A. three digits
    B. five digits
    C. seven digits
    D. nine digits

21. Which agency oversees controlled drugs and prosecutes individuals who illegally distribute them?

    A. FDA
    B. CDC
    C. DEA
    D. HIPAA

22. Which abbreviation refers to the left ear?

    A. OU
    B. AD
    C. AS
    D. OS

23. A patient presents to the pharmacy a prescription for Omnicef 125 mg/5 mL. Sig: 1¼ tsp PO daily for 10 days. Dispense: quantity sufficient for 10 days. Omnicef is available as an oral suspension containing 60 mL per bottle. How much Omnicef suspension would be required to fill this prescription?

    A. 6.2 mL
    B. 16.2 mL
    C. 32.5 mL
    D. 62.5 mL

24. Faxed prescriptions for Schedule II drugs must be followed up by a written prescription, which the pharmacy must receive within:

    A. 1 day
    B. 2 days
    C. 3 days
    D. 7 days

25. Orphan drugs are used for all of the following disorders or conditions, EXCEPT:

    A. snakebite
    B. cystic fibrosis
    C. peptic ulcer
    D. blepharospasm

26. Which piece of equipment is used to remove seals placed onto vials?

    A. decapper
    B. crimper
    C. hot plate
    D. heat gun

27. Baldness or hair loss is referred to as:

    A. boil
    B. purpura
    C. albinism
    D. alopecia

28. What is the maximum amount of items that may be ordered on DEA Form 222?

    A. 3
    B. 5
    C. 10
    D. 15

29. A label of a drug indicates 0.2 mcg/2 mL, and the patient receives 0.125 mcg. How many milliliters has the patient received?

    A. 0.5 mL
    B. 1 mL
    C. 1.25 mL
    D. 1.5 mL

30. When you are compounding a solution, which form of the drug should you use?

    A. salt form
    B. free-acid form
    C. free-base form
    D. none of the above

31. The pharmacy has an order to mix heparin 25,000 units in 500 mL of D5W. What is the final concentration in units per mL?

    A. 20 units per mL
    B. 30 units per mL
    C. 40 units per mL
    D. 50 units per mL

32. The suffix –ology, as in the word "hematology," means:

    A. blood
    B. below
    C. the study of
    D. laboratory

33. Garlic is an herb used for lowering cholesterol and modestly lowering blood pressure. Which types of drugs would you caution patients about taking concurrently with garlic?

    A. antilipidemics
    B. anti-inflammatories
    C. antihypertensives
    D. antidepressants

34. Which regulatory agency manages a national drug intelligence program?

    A. Food and Drug Administration
    B. Drug Enforcement Agency
    C. Environmental Protection Agency
    D. Centers for Medicare and Medicaid Services

35. Which statement is true about routine vaccinations with meningococcal vaccine in children younger than 2 years of age?

    A. They are very expensive.
    B. They are ineffective.
    C. They cause brain damage.
    D. They cause cardiac arrest.

36. Softening of the bones is referred to as:

    A. osteomyelitis
    B. osteome
    C. osteomalacia
    D. osteoarthritis

37. Which type of base is water-miscible and often used in vaginal and rectal suppositories?

    A. cocoa butter
    B. polyethylene glycol
    C. glycerinated gelatin
    D. carbowax

38. The labeling of a medication in a way that is false or misleading is referred to as:

    A. distribution
    B. adulteration
    C. fraud
    D. misbranding

39. Lotensin (benazepril) is classified as a(n):

    A. beta blocker
    B. ACE inhibitor
    C. alpha blocker
    D. calcium channel blocker

40. The pharmacy technician mixes a TPN stock solution containing 500 mL of 50% dextrose and 500 mL of amino acid for a total volume of 1 L. What is the final concentration of dextrose in each 1 L bag?

    A. 15%
    B. 20%
    C. 25%
    D. 30%

41. What does the word "hematuria" mean?

    A. excess urination
    B. excess salivation
    C. blood in the urine
    D. blood in the saliva

42. Pharmacy technicians must make sure that the prescription information in the computer matches the:

    A. printed labels
    B. fax numbers
    C. prescription
    D. USP

43. Unlike compounded solutions, suspensions:

    A. are difficult to compound
    B. should never be shaken
    C. always need to be filtered
    D. have problematic physical stability once compounded

44. What percent of 122 is 18?

    A. 22.3%
    B. 14.8%
    C. 21.5%
    D. 12.3%

45. Which form is required for all hazardous chemicals or substances used in the pharmacy?

    A. CMS-1500
    B. IRS Form 941
    C. TRICARE
    D. MSDS

46. The prefix *sub-* means:

    A. within
    B. above
    C. below
    D. outside of

47. What is the generic name of Prevacid?

    A. lansoprazole
    B. omeprazole
    C. esomeprazole
    D. pantoprazole

48. The normal dosage for amoxicillin is 45 mg/kg/24 hours, administered in divided doses. What would the dosage be for a 44-pound child if the dose is ordered b.i.d.?

    A. 45 mg
    B. 145 mg
    C. 245 mg
    D. 450 mg

49. The yellowish substance secreted by the glands in the external ear is called:

    A. eczema
    B. sebum
    C. keratitis
    D. cerumen

50. In a hospital, the external audit point system is used to show where:

    A. medications used are either generic or trade name
    B. medical record documentation is insufficient
    C. diagnoses of patient conditions are appropriate
    D. random audits are conducted

51. Standard precautions should be followed if the pharmacy technician is exposed to:

    A. chemical materials
    B. human body fluids
    C. dangerous gases
    D. radioactive substances

52. What is the percent equivalence of the ratio 1:20?

    A. 0.02%
    B. 0.2%
    C. 0.5%
    D. 5%

53. Alphabetic keys on a keyboard are also called:

    A. typing keys
    B. control keys
    C. shift keys
    D. page up keys

54. What is the basis of the computerized purchasing and control system?

    A. PDR
    B. medication database
    C. EOQ
    D. reorder point

55. Which is the smallest measurement used in the apothecary system for volume?

A. milliliter
B. minim
C. dram
D. ounce

56. A condition of imperfect dilation of the lungs is referred to as:

A. pneumonitis
B. atelectasis
C. bronchiectasis
D. hemoptysis

57. A nitroglycerin drip is ordered to be infused at 20 mcg/minute. The stock solution available has a concentration of 50 mg/250 mL. How many mL/hr of the IV should be administered?

A. 3 mL/hr
B. 6 mL/hr
C. 9 mL/hr
D. 15 mL/hr

58. What is the generic name for Depakote?

A. valproic acid
B. primidone
C. divalproex
D. gabapentin

59. According to federal law, who should accept new prescriptions by phone?

A. pharmacy technicians
B. pharmacy residents
C. pharmacists
D. any of the above

60. Inventory control is closely associated with the function of:

A. purchasing
B. compounding
C. discounting
D. product dating

61. Elixirs differ from tinctures in that they are:

A. colorless
B. tasteless
C. sweetened
D. bitter

62. What is the abbreviation for a "drop"?

A. gtt
B. pulv
C. disp
D. fl

63. What is the route of administration of a drug that is placed between the cheek and gum?

A. transdermal
B. sublingual
C. buccal
D. topical

64. Glucagon is released from the:

A. pancreas
B. liver
C. thyroid gland
D. adrenal cortex

65. Which drug is applied topically but is intended for systemic absorption into the body?

A. hydrocortisone
B. diphenhydramine
C. nitroglycerin
D. benzocaine

66. How long must a pharmacy keep logs of occupational injuries available for inspection?

A. 1 year
B. 3 years
C. 5 years
D. 10 years

67. What is one of the simplest and most widely used methods of inventory control?

A. notebook
B. want book
C. red book
D. orange book

68. What is the trade name for diphenhydramine?

A. Benadryl
B. Allegra
C. Biaxin
D. Proventil

69. Which DEA form is used as a receipt for Schedule II substances?

A. 224
B. 222
C. 106
D. 41

70. Concurrent use of alcoholic beverages and sedatives may result in:

A. excessive CNS depression
B. excitability
C. GI disturbances
D. headache

71. Which is NOT a live attenuated virus vaccine?

    A. yellow fever
    B. smallpox
    C. rabies
    D. measles, mumps, rubella

72. A document that authorizes items to be purchased from vendors is a(n):

    A. invoice
    B. purchase order
    C. inventory
    D. receiving report

73. Which organization has standards that are used for transfer of pharmaceutical care information?

    A. HIPAA
    B. NCPDP
    C. DEA
    D. CSA

74. An order is presented for 50 mg of medication to be given p.o. On hand are 20 mg tablets. How many tablets must you dispense to the patient?

    A. 1.5
    B. 2.5
    C. 3.5
    D. 4.5

75. What is the abbreviation for "nothing by mouth"?

    A. n.o.
    B. m.n.o.
    C. n.p.o.
    D. p.o.

76. Wholesale records (of purchases and sales) must be maintained for a minimum of:

    A. 2 months
    B. 6 months
    C. 12 months
    D. 2 years

77. A disease in which plaque builds up in the walls of large arteries is known as

    A. coronary artery disease
    B. atherosclerosis
    C. arteriosclerosis
    D. hyperlipidemia

78. A prescription order reads as follows: "Dispense 1 pound of triamcinolone 0.1%." How many grams should be dispensed?

    A. 100 grams
    B. 128 grams
    C. 455 grams
    D. 548 grams

79. Vitamin B_1 is used in the treatment of :

    A. pellagra
    B. scurvy
    C. beriberi
    D. iron deficiency anemia

80. The abbreviation "EDI" stands for:

    A. electronic details and information
    B. electronic data interchange
    C. emergency data interchange
    D. electronic detail interaction

81. In the hospital, when pharmacy technicians must look at patients' medical records, they must follow the guidelines of

    A. CDC
    B. TJC
    C. HD
    D. HIPAA

82. In which schedule are drugs with the highest potential for abuse and addiction classified?

    A. I
    B. II
    C. IV
    D. V

83. The suffix –emesis means:

    A. binding
    B. condition
    C. vomiting
    D. pertaining to

84. How many drops are there in 1 mL?

    A. 5
    B. 10
    C. 15
    D. 30

85. Which health-care program serves the families of veterans who have total, permanent service-connected disabilities?

    A. Medicaid
    B. TRICARE
    C. Medicare
    D. CHAMPVA

86. What is the most common psychiatric disorder in the United States?

    A. depression
    B. panic disorder
    C. Parkinson's disease
    D. epileptic disorder

87. Which class of drugs is NOT of use in achieving the treatment goals for angina pectoris?

    A. nitrates
    B. calcium channel blockers
    C. diuretics
    D. beta-adrenergic blockers

88. Which gland releases the hormone thymosin?

    A. thyroid gland
    B. thymus gland
    C. testes
    D. pancreas

89. In the retail pharmacy, each metal storage unit easily stores how many prescriptions?

    A. 100
    B. 200
    C. 500
    D. 1000

90. Which key is considered a "control key"?

    A. Num Lock
    B. Tab
    C. Shift
    D. Page Up

91. Excessive secretion of milk after the cessation of nursing is known as:

    A. gigantism
    B. galactorrhea
    C. dysmenorrheal
    D. amenorrhea

92. Violation of HIPAA can result in which of the following penalties?

    A. criminal penalties
    B. civil penalties
    C. both
    D. neither

93. The minimum amount you should measure with a 100 mL graduated cylinder is:

    A. 5 mL
    B. 10 mL
    C. 20 mL
    D. 50 mL

94. What is the largest single medical benefits program in the United States?

    A. Workers' compensation
    B. Medicaid
    C. Medicare
    D. Health Maintenance Organization

95. Patients who miss a dose of a scheduled medication should:

    A. double up when the next dose is due
    B. consult with the pharmacist or physician regarding the missed dose
    C. stop the medication and wait until their next office visit
    D. do none of the above

96. In most states, pharmacists are usually given certificates of registration that are granted for a period of:

    A. 10 to 12 years
    B. 10 to 12 months
    C. 1 to 3 years
    D. 3 to 5 years

97. Which DEA form is used to document the destruction of outdated or damaged controlled substances?

    A. 222
    B. 224
    C. 106
    D. 41

98. Drugs that are most often abused include:

    A. opioids
    B. antidepressants
    C. antihistamines
    D. antibiotics

99. Gentamicin 60 mg IM was prescribed. The drug is available in a dosage of 80 mg/2 mL per vial. How many mL of gentamicin should be administered?

    A. 0.5
    B. 1
    C. 1.5
    D. 2.5

100. Drugs in Schedules II, III, and IV must bear which of the following statements?

    A. Federal law prohibits the transfer of this drug to any person other than the patient for whom it was prescribed.
    B. Federal law allows partial refilling.
    C. May refill up to 10 times.
    D. May refill up to 5 times.

Self-Evaluation: Test 6

1. Which act offers federal financial incentives to commercial and nonprofit organizations for the development of drugs?

   A. Medical Device Amendment
   B. Drug Listing Act
   C. Orphan Drug Act
   D. Poison Prevention Packaging Act

2. The most effective vaccines are made from:

   A. inactivated pathogens
   B. living organisms
   C. toxins
   D. extracts

3. A useful agent in the treatment of schizophrenia is:

   A. lorazepam (Ativan)
   B. diazepam (Valium)
   C. phenytoin (Dilantin)
   D. perphenazine (Trilafon)

4. Hypersecretion of growth hormone before puberty is referred to as:

   A. myxedema
   B. gigantism
   C. dwarfism
   D. acromegaly

5. A liquid's lower surface in a container is called the:

   A. minim
   B. meniscus
   C. pastille
   D. paste

6. Which of the following is NOT required by HIPAA's Privacy Rule?

   A. The employee is obligated to promptly notify the employer of an injury.
   B. Covered entities must have a privacy official.
   C. Patients must be notified about the use of their private information.
   D. Employees must be educated about privacy practices.

7. Calculate one dose of the following: "Demerol syrup 75 mg p.o. q4h prn pain." On hand is Demerol syrup 50 mg/5 mL. One dose equals how many mL?

   A. 75 mL
   B. 7.5 mL
   C. 0.75 mL
   D. 750 mL

8. Which act was designed to protect the public health by forbidding the interstate distribution or sale of adulterated and misbranded food and drugs?

   A. Durham-Humphrey Amendment
   B. Kefauver-Harris Amendment
   C. Harrison Narcotics Tax Act
   D. Pure Food and Drug Act

9. Diabetes insipidus results from the lack or deficiency of:

   A. thyroxin
   B. thymosin
   C. aldosterone
   D. vasopressin

10. Which vitamin or mineral is an example of a soft gelatin capsule?

    A. vitamin E
    B. mineral oil
    C. A and B
    D. none of the above

11. If a dose of Maalox is 1 Tbsp, how many doses must be prepared from a pint bottle?

    A. 12
    B. 16
    C. 32
    D. 48

12. What is the deepest inner layer of the eyes?

    A. sclera
    B. red pulp
    C. retina
    D. choroid

13. Failure to use a reasonable amount of care to prevent injury or damage to a pharmacy's customers would result in a charge of:

    A. libel
    B. slander
    C. negligence
    D. abuse

14. Which drug is an HIV antiviral agent?

    A. zidovudine
    B. ketoconazole
    C. butenafine
    D. griseofulvin

15. Up to how many tablets per minute can the Baker Cells system, an automated dispensing system, count and dispense?

    A. 250
    B. 600
    C. 375
    D. 100

16. Which statement is NOT true regarding the maintenance of files for schedule drugs?

    A. One file is used for schedule drugs dispensed.
    B. One file is used for Schedule III, IV, and V drugs dispensed.
    C. One file is used for Schedule I and II drugs dispensed.
    D. One file is used for prescription orders for all other drugs.

17. Which suffix means "inflammation"?

    A. –tomy
    B. –algia
    C. –trophy
    D. –itis

18. Lanoxin 0.15 mg PO q12h is ordered for a child who weighs 31.8 kg. If the recommended dosage is 7 mcg/kg/day, how much should be given to this child over the course of 24 hours?

    A. 22 mg/day
    B. 1.22 mg/day
    C. 0.22 mg/day
    D. 2.2 mg/day

19. Inflammation and infection of the testes is called:

    A. orchitis
    B. epididymitis
    C. varicocele
    D. cryptorchidism

20. In the retail pharmacy, a record of the prescriptions that are dispensed is kept on hand via:

    A. computer files
    B. hard copy files
    C. floppy disc files
    D. hard copy and computer files

21. Which of the following is NOT a proton pump inhibitor?

    A. Prilosec
    B. Pepcid
    C. Prevacid
    D. AcipHex

22. Which health-care plan may conduct random audits of medical records before paying for patient charges?

    A. Blue Cross Blue Shield
    B. Medicare
    C. TRICARE
    D. CHAMPVA

23. The suffix –ose means:

    A. carbohydrate
    B. lip
    C. pain
    D. condition

24. The order is for V-Cillin K 300,000 U PO q.i.d. On hand is V-Cillin K 200,000 U/5 mL. What is one dose, in mL?

    A. 7 mL
    B. 17 mL
    C. 7.5 mL
    D. 7.75 mL

25. Which agency oversees the practice of pharmacy?

    A. State BOP
    B. DEA
    C. FDA
    D. APhA

26. Pharmacies must provide safety training to pharmacy technicians:

    A. upon firing them
    B. upon hiring them
    C. at least once a month
    D. if they are expectant mothers

27. Which organization represents the chain drug store's interests?

    A. NCPA
    B. NABP
    C. NACDS
    D. APHA

28. An agent used to treat fungal diseases is:

    A. didanosine
    B. amprenavir
    C. azidothymidine
    D. fluconazole

29. How many grams are equivalent to 0.0546 kg?

    A. 5.046 g
    B. 5.46 g
    C. 54.6 g
    D. 540.6 g

30. Cystalgia is pain in the:

    A. rectum
    B. vagina
    C. stomach
    D. bladder

31. Which part of Medicare covers prescriptions for senior citizens?

    A. Part A
    B. Part B
    C. Part C
    D. Part D

32. Automated systems for oral liquid repackaging exclusively use which type of container?

    A. plastic
    B. glass
    C. either plastic or glass
    D. neither plastic or glass

33. Adalat and Procardia are the trade names of:

    A. nadolol
    B. propranolol
    C. verapamil
    D. nifedipine

34. Home infusion pharmacy typically includes:

    A. durable medical equipment
    B. enteral nutrition therapy
    C. compounded topical therapy
    D. compounded radiopharmaceuticals

35. What is the trade name of salmeterol?

    A. Serevent
    B. Ventolin
    C. Alupent
    D. Proventil

36. Which duty is NOT a responsibility of technicians in the hospital setting?

    A. delivering medication to nurses
    B. preparing, packaging, and labeling drugs
    C. providing advice to nurses and patients
    D. checking patient charts in conjunction with prescriptions

37. How many Tbsp are equivalent to 6 oz?

    A. 6
    B. 9
    C. 12
    D. 15

38. Which of the following comprises the proximal portion of the small intestine?

    A. sigmoid
    B. ilium
    C. jejunum
    D. duodenum

39. Which agency oversees Medicare and Medicaid services?

    A. TJC
    B. FDA
    C. BOP
    D. CMS

40. The sense of smell is controlled by the:

    A. olfactory organs
    B. soft palate
    C. vestibular nuclei
    D. gustatory receptors

41. How many amoxicillin capsules, each containing 250 mg of amoxicillin, are required for providing 60 mg/kg of body weight for 10 days for a person weighing 165 lb?

    A. 18
    B. 92
    C. 180
    D. 224

42. Which drug is NOT an antihistamine?

    A. brompheniramine (Dimetane)
    B. cetirizine (Zyrtec)
    C. hydrocodone (Histussin)
    D. loratadine (Claritin)

43. Which part of a needle refers to the diameter of its shaft?

    A. hub
    B. tip
    C. bevel
    D. gauge

44. Diluents used in tablet compounding are usually mixtures of:

    A. lactose, sucrose, ethyl alcohol, and water
    B. glycogen, glucose, and water
    C. maltose, sucrose, and ethyl alcohol
    D. lactose, maltose, methyl alcohol, and water

45. An order is presented for 10 mg of a medication. On hand are vials containing 20 mg/mL. How many milliliters must you dispense to the patient?

    A. 5 mL
    B. 2.5 mL
    C. 1.5 mL
    D. 0.5 mL

46. Which set of letters would begin the valid DEA number of "Dr. Amanda Sabet," a sole practitioner?

    A. CA
    B. CS
    C. JS
    D. JC

47. Bipolar disorder is characterized by:

    A. euphoric and depressed moods
    B. fever and eating disorders
    C. autism and amnesia
    D. obsessions and narcolepsy

48. Outdated tetracycline has been shown to cause damage to which body organs?

    A. bones
    B. lungs
    C. kidneys
    D. liver and gallbladder

49. What is the most important thing a pharmacy technician should do regarding expired drugs and their disposal?

    A. Return them to the manufacturer.
    B. Ship them to Red Cross.
    C. Flush them down a drain.
    D. Document what is done with them.

50. The "brain" of the computer is the:

    A. memory
    B. CPU
    C. hard drive
    D. mouse

51. Which disease is transmitted from animals to people by saliva?

    A. rabies
    B. pneumonia
    C. meningitis
    D. tuberculosis

52. Which drug is NOT a primary antitubercular drug?

    A. ethambutol
    B. imipramine
    C. isoniazid
    D. rifampin

53. Which endocrine gland releases aldosterone?

    A. thymus
    B. adrenal
    C. thyroid
    D. pituitary

54. What is the generic name of Axid?

    A. ranitidine
    B. cimetidine
    C. famotidine
    D. nizatidine

55. The combining form *cutane/o* means:

    A. sweat
    B. skin
    C. tissue
    D. white

56. Which amount is equivalent to 2 cc?

    A. 0.02 L
    B. 0.002 L
    C. 0.0002 L
    D. 2 L

57. Which diuretic requires a potassium supplement?

    A. Lasix
    B. Aldactone
    C. Dyrenium
    D. Dyazide

58. Which base component must be mixed last into a TPN bag?

    A. dextrose
    B. lipids
    C. sterile water
    D. amino acids

59. Which law allowed pharmacists to accept prescriptions over the telephone from a practitioner?

    A. Comprehensive Drug Abuse Prevention and Control Act
    B. Food, Drug, and Cosmetic Act
    C. Durham-Humphrey Amendment
    D. Prescription Drug Marketing Act

60. Medical records should be correctly documented by using guidelines of the:

    A. Centers for Medicaid and Medicare Services
    B. Centers for Disease Control and Prevention
    C. Diagnostic and Statistical Manual
    D. Federal Trade Commission

61. Which statement is TRUE about the Poison Prevention Packaging Act?

    A. Fifty percent of adults can open a child-resistant container.
    B. Ninety-nine percent of children younger than age 5 cannot open a child-resistant container.
    C. Eighty percent of children younger than age 5 cannot open a child-resistant container.
    D. None of the above is true.

62. Iodine deficiency may cause:

    A. hypertension
    B. anemia
    C. impaired growth
    D. goiter

63. The abbreviation "FDA" means:

    A. Food and Drug Association
    B. Food and Drug Assistance
    C. Food and Drug Administration
    D. Food and Drug Abuse

64. An example of patient information that must be kept confidential is a patient's:

    A. list of medications
    B. hospital room number
    C. medical record number
    D. initials

65. A pharmacy technician must prepare 65 mL of a 24% medication solution. He has in stock 46 g/mL solution. How many milliliters of the 46 g/mL solution will he use?

    A. 0.31 mL
    B. 0.34 mL
    C. 0.36 mL
    D. 0.39 mL

66. What is most commonly used for the compounding of IV antibiotics?

    A. intravenous piggybacks
    B. large-volume bags
    C. irrigations
    D. none of the above

67. What is the most suitable, flexible, and open-ended dispensing system on the market?

    A. unit-of-use system
    B. point-of-sale master
    C. repackaging system
    D. batch repackaging system

68. Which suffix means "flow" or "discharge"?

    A. –rrhexis
    B. –rrho
    C. –rrhaphy
    D. –rrhea

69. A physician orders 1500 mg of a medication. On hand are 500 mg tablets. How many tablets must you dispense to the patient?

    A. 2
    B. 3
    C. 5
    D. 6

70. What is the most common type of reaction to a vaccine?

    A. local
    B. systemic
    C. allergic
    D. anaphylaxis

71. Which portion of the brain controls and coordinates skeletal activity?

    A. pons
    B. hypothalamus
    C. medulla oblongata
    D. cerebellum

72. In 1 L of D$_{10}$W, how much dextrose is contained?

    A. 100 mg
    B. 500 mg
    C. 100 g
    D. 500 g

73. Robots differ from the carousel (cassette) type of automated systems in that they do not require:

    A. electricity
    B. computers
    C. space
    D. staff members to intervene with their actions

74. The abbreviation meaning "right eye" is:

    A. OS
    B. OD
    C. AD
    D. AU

75. What is the markup rate for a medication that costs $23.65 and retails for $31.15?

    A. 28.2%
    B. 31.7%
    C. 35%
    D. 38%

76. Sterile irrigations are used for:

    A. intravenous injections
    B. rehydration
    C. surgical sites
    D. all of the above

77. An example of an emulsion is:

    A. cod liver oil
    B. Tylenol elixir
    C. Nutraderm lotion
    D. aromatic spirits of ammonia

78. NRC is the abbreviation for:

    A. Nuclear Regulatory Commission
    B. Nuclear Registry Center
    C. Nuclear Remission Cancer
    D. Nuclear Register Consulting

79. How many mL are equivalent to 4 cups?

    A. 240
    B. 360
    C. 480
    D. 960

80. Which drug is an example of a Schedule V drug?

    A. diazepam
    B. Lomotil
    C. amphetamine
    D. Talwin

81. Cyclooxygenase-2 inhibitors are contraindicated in which of the following?

    A. osteoarthritis
    B. menstrual cramps
    C. acute pain
    D. congestive heart failure

82. What is typically a pharmacy's largest asset?

    A. pharmacist
    B. location
    C. inventory
    D. customer base

83. A pharmacy technician was asked to mix alcohols of 95% and 50% strengths to prepare 200 mL of a 70% alcohol solution. Which are the correct amounts of each to use?

    A. 95% - 5 : 9 50% - 4 : 9
    B. 95% - 4 : 9 50% - 5 : 9
    C. 95% - 4 : 5 50% - 9 : 4
    D. none of the above

84. Clinical services that pharmacists provide to hospice patients usually include:

    A. pharmacokinetic monitoring
    B. anticoagulation monitoring
    C. diabetes education
    D. pain management

85. What Celsius temperature is equivalent to 102.4° Fahrenheit?

    A. 37°
    B. 38°
    C. 39.11°
    D. 41.06°

86. Contaminated multidose vials may cause:

    A. turbidity
    B. infestation
    C. infection
    D. infarction

87. Which vitamin deficiency may cause night blindness?

    A. A
    B. B$_{12}$
    C. C
    D. D

88. Most dispensed medications in the community pharmacy are:

    A. compounded medications
    B. sterile medications
    C. prefabricated into dosage forms
    D. none of the above

89. Dating the prescription on the date it is filled determines:

    A. appropriate refill frequency
    B. physician prescribing habits
    C. pharmacy inventory control
    D. drug expiration

90. In which drug schedule is Ritalin classified?

    A. I
    B. II
    C. III
    D. V

91. Examinations or verifications conducted to assure effectiveness and correctness are known as:

    A. enforcement
    B. audits
    C. attuning
    D. attendance

92. The antagonist (antidote) to heparin is derived from:

    A. liver
    B. fish sperm
    C. basophils
    D. monocytes

93. Deep thrombophlebitis occurs most commonly in the:

    A. lower legs
    B. lower arms
    C. lungs
    D. lower abdomen

94. What is the brand name of tobramycin?

    A. Garamycin
    B. Mycifradin
    C. Streptomycin
    D. Nebcin

95. What does the abbreviation "w/v" mean?

    A. number of grams per 1 L
    B. number of grams per 500 mL
    C. number of grams per 100 mL
    D. number of milligrams per 100 mL

96. Master formula sheets are also referred to as:

    A. insurance records
    B. medical order records
    C. bulk compounding formulary records
    D. none of the above

97. What is the brand name of carvedilol?

    A. Coreg
    B. Calan
    C. Micronase
    D. Fosamax

98. Pertussis is also called:

    A. mumps
    B. chickenpox
    C. measles
    D. whooping cough

99. How many refills are allowed for noncontrolled medications?

    A. 1
    B. 5 times in 6 months
    C. 11 times within a year
    D. an unlimited number within a year

100. Which agency oversees quality compounding of sterile products?

    A. FDA
    B. ASHP
    C. CMS
    D. CDER

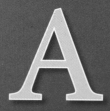

APPENDIX A

Pharmacy Technician Certification Examinations

Several national pharmacy technician certification examinations are available. Table A–1 summarizes important information about each of these exams and the organizations that offer them.

TABLE A–1 Pharmacy Technician Certification Examinations

Examination	Organization	Format	Requirements
Pharmacy Technician Certification Examination (PTCE)—anyone who successfully passes the test is designated as a "Certified Pharmacy Technician (CPhT)"	Pharmacy Technician Certification Board (www.ptcb.org) via the Professional Examination Service	90 (plus 10 unscored) multiple-choice questions divided into three sections: 1. Assisting the pharmacist in serving patients 2. Maintaining medication and inventory control systems 3. Participating in the administration and management of pharmacy practice	Certification must be renewed every two years, and PTCB certified pharmacy technicians must complete 20 hours of continuing education, with at least one hour of education focused on pharmacy law.
Exam for the Certification of Pharmacy Technicians (ExCPT)	National Community Pharmacists Association (NCPA) and the National Association of Chain Drug Stores (NACDS), administered by the Institute for the Certification of Pharmacy Technicians (ICPT)—see www.nationaltechexam.org—which is a part of the National Healthcareer Association (NHA)	110 (10 unscored) multiple choice questions, divided into nine sections: 1. Overview of technician duties and general information 2. Controlled substances 3. Other laws and regulations 4. Drug classification 5. Most frequently prescribed medications 6. Prescription information 7. Preparing / dispensing prescriptions 8. Calculations 9. Sterile products, unit dose, and repackaging	Certification is renewable every two years, plus a continuing education requirement of 20 hours for each certification cycle; accepted in nearly every state.

TABLE A–1 (continued)

Examination	Organization	Format	Requirements
NCCT Pharmacy Technician Certification Exam	National Center for Competency Testing (NCCT)—see www.ncctinc.com	Exam is divided into six sections, with questions being reduced by 10–20% currently in an attempt to streamline this test along with all of the other exams they offer: 1. Naming and abbreviations 2. Common drugs and uses 3. Pharmacy procedures 4. Pharmacy regulations 5. Prescription drug dosage and preparation 6. Substance abuse 7. Systems of measurement / pharmacy math	Must already be employed as a pharmacy technician for at least one year prior to taking this exam; not yet recognized in all states.

State Boards of Pharmacy

National Association of Boards of Pharmacy

Carmen A. Catizone, Executive Director/Secretary
1600 Feehanville Drive
Mount Prospect, IL 60056
Phone: 847/391-4406
Web site: http://www.nabp.net
E-mail: exec-office@nabp.net

Alabama

Herbert "Herb" Bobo, Executive Director
10 Inverness Center, Suite 110
Birmingham, AL 35242
Phone: 205/981-2280
Web site: www.albop.com
Email: hbobo@albop.com

Alaska

Sher Zinn, Licensing Examiner
PO Box 110806
Juneau, AK 99811-0806
Phone: 907/465-2589
Web site: http://www.commerce.state.ak.us/occ/ppha.htm
E-mail: sher.zinn@alaska.gov

Arizona

Hal Wand, Executive Director
1700 W Washington St., Suite 250
Phoenix, AZ 85007
Phone: 602/771-2727
Web site: www.azpharmacy.gov
E-mail: chunter@azpharmacy.gov

Arkansas

Charles S. Campbell, Executive Director
101 E Capitol, Suite 218
Little Rock, AR 72201

Phone: 501/682-0190
Web site: http://www.arkansas.gov/asbp
E-mail: Charlie.Campbell@arkansas.gov

California

Virginia "Giny" Herold, Executive Officer
1625 N Market Blvd., Suite N219
Sacramento, CA 95834
Phone: 916/574-7912
Web site: http://www.pharmacy.ca.gov
E-mail: Virginia_herold@dca.ca.gov

Colorado

Wendy Anderson, Program Director
1560 Broadway, Suite 1300
Denver, CO 80202-5143
Phone: 303/894-7800
Web site: http://www.dora.state.co.us/pharmacy
E-mail: pharmacy@dora.state.co.us

Connecticut

Delinda Brown-Jagne, Board Administrator
165 Capital Avenue, Room 147
Hartford, CT 06106
Phone: 860/713-6070
Web site: http://www.ct.gov/dcp/site/default.asp
E-mail: delina.brown-jagne@ct.gov

Delaware

David W. Dryden, Executive Secretary
861 Silver Lake Blvd., Suite 203
Dover, DE 19904
Phone: 302/744-4526
Web site: http://dpr.delaware.gov/boards/pharmacy/newpharmacy.shtml
E-mail: debop@state.de.us

District of Columbia

Marcia B. Wooden, Executive Director
717 – 14th St NW, Suite 600
Washington, DC 20005
Phone: 202/442-4762
Web site: http://hpla.doh.dc.gov/hpla/cwp
E-mail: Marcia.wooden@dc.gov

Florida

Rebecca Poston, Executive Director
4052 Bald Cypress Way, Bin #C04
Tallahassee, FL 32399-3254
Phone: 850/245-4292
Web site: http://www.doh.state.fl.us/mqa/
pharmacy
E-mail: MQA_Pharmacy@doh.state.fl.us

Georgia

Lisa Durden, Executive Director
237 Coliseum Dr
Macon, GA 31217-3858
Phone: 478/207-2440
Web site: www.sos.ga.gov/plb/pharmacy
E-mail: http://sos.georgia.gov/cgi-bin/email.asp

Guam

Jane M. Diego, Secretary for the Board
PO Box 2816
Hagatna, GU 96932
Phone: 671/735-7406 ext 11
Website: http://www.dphss.guam.gov
E-mail: jane.diego@dphss.guam.gov

Hawaii

Lee Ann Teshima, Executive Officer
PO Box 3469
Honolulu, HI 96801
Phone: 808/586-2694
Web site: www.hawaii.gov/dcca/areas/pvl/boards/
pharmacy
E-mail: pharmacy@dcca.hawaii.gov

Idaho

Mark D. Johnston, Executive Director
3380 Americana Terrace, Suite 320
Boise, ID 83706
Phone: 208/334-2356
Web site: www.accessidaho.org/bop
E-mail: info@bop.idaho.gov

Illinois

Kim Scott, Pharmacy Board Liaison
320 W Washington, 3rd Floor
Springfield, IL 62786
Phone: 217/782-8556
Web site: www.idfpr.com
E-mail: fpr.prfgroup10@illinois.gov

Indiana

Marty Allain, Director
402 W Washington St, Room W072
Indianapolis, IN 46204-2739
Phone: 317/234-2067
Web site: http://www.in.gov/pla/2361.htm
E-mail: pla4@pla.IN.gov

Iowa

Lloyd K. Jessen, Executive Director/Secretary
400 SW 8th St, Suite E
Des Moines, IA 50309-4688
Phone: 515/281-5944
Web site: www.state.ia.us/ibpe
E-mail: lloyd.jessen@iowa.gov

Kansas

Debra L. Billingsley, Executive Secretary
Landon State Office Building, 900 SW Jackson,
Room 560
Topeka, KS 66612-1231
Phone: 785/296-4056
Web site: www.kansas.gov/pharmacy
E-mail: dbillingsley@pharmacy.ks.gov

Kentucky

Michael A. Burleson, Executive Director
Spindletop Administration Bldg., Suite 302,
2624 Research Park Dr,
Lexington, KY 40511
Phone: 859/246-2820
Web site: http://pharmacy.ky.gov
E-mail: pharmacy.board@ky.gov

Louisiana

Malcolm J. Broussard, Executive Director
5615 Corporate Blvd., Suite 8E
Baton Rouge, LA 70808-2537
Phone: 225/925-6496
Web site: www.labp.com
E-mail: exec@labp.com

Maine

Geraldine L. "Jeri" Betts, Board Administrator
35 State House Station
Augusta, ME 04333
Phone: 207/624-8603
Web site: www.maine.gov/professionallicensing
E-mail: geraldine.l.betts@maine.gov

Maryland

La Verne George Naesea, Executive Director
4201 Patterson Ave
Baltimore, MD 21215-2299
Phone: 410/764-4755
Web site: www.dhmh.state.md.us/pharmacyboard
E-mail: mdbop@dhmh.state.md.us

Massachusetts

James D. Coffey, Director
239 Causeway St, 2nd Floor, Suite 200
Boston, MA 02114
Phone: 617/973-0950
Web site: www.mass.gov/reg/boards/ph
E-mail: James.d.coffey@state.ma.us

Michigan

Rae Ramsdell, Director, Licensing Division
611 W Ottawa, First Floor
PO Box 30670
Lansing, MI 48909-8170
Phone: 517/335-0918
Web site: http://www.michigan.gov/
healthlicense
E-mail: rhramsd@michigan.gov

Minnesota

Cody C. Wiberg, Executive Director
2829 University Ave SE, Suite 530
Minneapolis, MN 55414-3251
Phone: 651/201-2825
Web site: http://www.phcybrd.state.mn.us
E-mail: pharmacy.board@state.mn.us

Mississippi

Leland "Mac" McDivitt, Executive Director
204 Key Dr, Suite D
Madison, MS 39110
Phone: 601/605-5388
Web site: www.mbp.state.ms.us
E-mail: lmcdivitt@mbp.state.ms.us

Missouri

Debra C. Ringgenberg, Executive Director
PO Box 625
Jefferson City, MO 65102
Phone: 573/751-0091
Web site: http://www.pr.mo.gov/pharmacists.asp
E-mail: pharmacy@pr.mo.gov

Montana

Ronald J. Klein, Executive Director
PO Box 200513
301 S Park Ave, 4th Floor
Helena, MT 59620-0513
Phone: 406/841-2371
Web site: http://mt.gov/dli/bsd/license/bsd_boards/
pha_board/board_page.asp
E-mail: roklein@mt.gov

Nebraska

Becky Wisell, Administrator
PO Box 94986
Lincoln, NE 68509-4986
Phone: 402/471-2118
Web site: www.hhs.state.ne.us
E-mail: becky.wisell@dhhs.ne.gov

Nevada

Larry L. Pinson, Executive Secretary
431 W Plumb Lane
Reno, NV 89509
Phone: 775/850-1440
Web site: http://bop.nv.gov
E-mail: pharmacy@pharmacy.nv.gov

New Hampshire

Paul G. Boisseau, Executive Secretary
57 Regional Dr
Concord, NH 03301-8518
Phone: 603/271-2350
Web site: www.nh.gov/pharmacy
E-mail: pharmacy.board@nh.gov

New Jersey

Joanne Boyer, Executive Director
PO Box 45013
Newark, NJ 07101
Phone: 973/504-6450
Web site: http://www.state.nj.us/lps/ca/boards.htm
E-mail: boyerj@dca.lps.state.nj.us

New Mexico

William Harvey, Executive Director/Chief Drug
Inspector
5200 Oakland NE, Suite A
Albuquerque, NM 87113
Phone: 505/222-9830
Web site: http://www.rld.state.nm.us/Pharmacy
E-mail: pharmacy.board@state.nm.us

New York

Lawrence H. Mokhiber, Executive Secretary
89 Washington Ave, 2nd Floor W
Albany, NY 12234-1000
Phone: 518/474-3817 ext. 130
Web site: www.op.nysed.gov
E-mail: pharmbd@mail.nysed.gov

North Carolina

Jack W. "Jay" Campbell IV, Executive Director
PO Box 4560
Chapel Hill, NC 27515-4560
Phone: 919/246-1050
Web site: www.ncbop.org
E-mail: jcampbell@ncbop.org

North Dakota

Howard C. Anderson, Jr., Executive Director
1906 E Broadway Ave
Bismarck, ND 58501-1354
Phone: 701/328-9535
Web site: www.nodakpharmacy.com
E-mail: ndboph@btinet.net

Ohio

William T. Winsley, Executive Director
77 S High St, Room 1702
Columbus, OH 43215-6126
Phone: 614/466-4143
Web site: www.pharmacy.ohio.gov
E-mail: exec@bop.state.oh.us

Oklahoma

Bryan H. Potter, Executive Director
4545 Lincoln Blvd., Suite 112
Oklahoma City, OK 73105-3488
Phone: 405/521-3815
Web site: www.pharmacy.ok.gov
E-mail: pharmacy@pharmacy.ok.gov

Oregon

Gary A. Schnabel, Executive Director
800 NE Oregon St, Suite 150
Portland, OR 97232
Phone: 971/673-0001
Web site: www.pharmacy.state.or.us
E-mail: pharmacy.board@state.or.us

Pennsylvania

Melanie Zimmerman, Executive Secretary
PO Box 2649
Harrisburg, PA 17105-2649
Phone: 717/783-7156
Web site: www.dos.state.pa.us/pharm
E-mail: st-pharmacy@state.pa.us

Puerto Rico

Magda Bouet, Executive Director, Department
of Health
Call Box 10200
Santurce, PR 00908
Phone: 787/725-7506
E-mail: mbouet@salud.gov.pr

Rhode Island

Catherine A. Cordy, Executive Director
3 Capitol Hill, Room 205
Providence, RI 02908-5097
Phone: 401/222-2840
Web site: http://www.health.ri.gov/hsr/professions/
pharmacy.php
E-mail: cathyc@doh.state.ri.us

South Carolina

Lee Ann Bundrick, Administrator
110 Centerview Dr, Suite 306
Columbia, SC 29210
Phone: 803/896-4700
Web site: www.llronline.com/POL/pharmacy
E-mail: bundricl@llr.sc.gov

South Dakota

Ronald J. Huether, Executive Secretary
4305 S Louise Ave, Suite 104
Sioux Falls, SD 57106
Phone: 605/362-2737
Web site: www.pharmacy.sd.gov
E-mail: ronald.huether@state.sd.us

Tennessee

Kevin K. Eidson, Executive Director
227 French Landing, Suite 300
Nashville, TN 37243
Phone: 615/741-2718
Web site: http://health.state.tn.us/Boards/Pharmacy/index.shtml
E-mail: kevin.eidson@state.tn.us

Texas

Gay Dodson, Executive Director/Secretary
333 Guadalupe, Tower 3, Suite 600
Austin, TX 78701-3943
Phone: 512/305-8000
Web site: www.tsbp.state.tx.us
E-mail: gay.dodson@tsbp.state.tx.us

Utah

Noel Taxin, Bureau Manager
PO Box 146741
Salt Lake City, UT 84114-6741
Phone: 801/530-6621
Web site: http://www.dopl.utah.gov
E-mail: ntaxin@utah.gov

Vermont

Peggy Atkins, Board Administrator
National Life Bldg., North FL2
Montpelier, VT 05620-3402
Phone: 802/828-2373
Web site: www.vtprofessionals.org
E-mail: patkins@sec.state.vt.us

Virgin Islands

Lydia T. Scott, Executive Assistant
48 Sugar Estate
St Thomas, VI 00802
Phone: 340/774-0117
E-mail: lydia.scott@usvi-doh.org

Virginia

Elizabeth Scott Russell, Executive Director
9960 Mayland Drive, Suite 300
Richmond, VA 23233-1463
Phone: 804/367-4456
Web site: www.dhp.virginia.gov/pharmacy
E-mail: pharmbd@dhp.virginia.gov

Washington

Steven M. Saxe, Executive Director
PO Box 47863
Olympia, WA 98504-7863
Phone: 360/236-4825
Web site: https://fortress.wa.gov/doh/hpqa1/hps4/pharmacy/default.htm
E-mail: steven.saxe@doh.wa.gov

West Virginia

David E. Potters, Executive Director and General Counsel
232 Capitol St
Charleston, WV 25301
Phone: 304/558-0558
Web site: http://www.wvbop.com
E-mail: dpotters@wvbop.com

Wisconsin

Thomas Ryan, Bureau Director
PO Box 8935
Madison, WI 53708-8935
Phone: 608/266-2112
Web site: http://www.drl.state.wi.us
E-mail: thomas.ryan@drl.state.wi.us

Wyoming

Mary K. Walker, Executive Director
632 S David St
Casper, WY 82601
Phone: 307/234-0294
Web site: http://pharmacyboard.state.wy.us
E-mail: wybop@state.wy.us

Source: www.nabp.net

Professional Organizations

American Association of Colleges of Pharmacy (AACP)

1727 King Street
Alexandria, VA 22314
(703) 739-2330
http://www.aacp.org
Established in 1900, the AACP represents all 105 pharmacy colleges and schools in the United States.

American Association of Pharmaceutical Scientists (AAPS)

2107 Wilson Blvd., Suite 700
Arlington, VA 22201-3042
(703) 243-2800
http://www.aaps.org
Established in 1986, the AAPS provides an international forum for the exchange of knowledge among scientists to enhance their contributions to public health. The AAPS publishes the following journals: *Pharmaceutical Research, Pharmaceutical Development and Technology, AAPSPharmSciTech,* and *The AAPS Journal.*

American Association of Pharmacy Technicians (AAPT)

PO Box 1447
Greensboro, NC 27402
(877) 368-4771
http://www.pharmacytechnician.com
Established in 1979, the AAPT promotes the safe, efficacious, and cost-effective dispensing, distribution, and use of medicines.

American College of Clinical Pharmacy (ACCP)

13000 W 87th St Parkway
Lenexa, KS 66215-4530
(913) 492-3311
http://www.accp.com
Established in 1979, the ACCP is a professional, scientific society that provides leadership, education, advocacy, and resources that enable clinical pharmacists to achieve excellence in practice and research.

American Council on Pharmaceutical Education (ACPE)

20 North Clark Street, Suite 2500
Chicago, IL 60602-5109
(312) 664-3575
http://www.acpe-accredit.org
Also referred to as the "Accreditation Council on Pharmaceutical Education," the ACPE was established in 1932 and is the national agency for the accreditation of professional degree programs in pharmacy and of providers of continuing pharmacy education.

American Pharmacists Association (APhA)

1100 15th Street NW, Suite 400
Washington, DC 20005-1707
(202) 628-4410
http://www.aphanet.org
Established in 1852 as the American Pharmaceutical Association, the APhA is a leader in providing professional education and information for pharmacists and is an advocate for improved health of the American public through the provision of comprehensive

pharmaceutical care. The APhA consists of three academies:

- The Academy of Pharmacy Practice and Management (APhA-APPM)
- The Academy of Pharmaceutical Research and Science (APhA-APRS)
- The Academy of Students of Pharmacy (APhA-APS)

American Society of Health-System Pharmacists (ASHP)

7272 Wisconsin Avenue
Bethesda, MD 20814
(301) 657-3000
http://www.ashp.org
Established in 1942, the ASHP believes that the mission of pharmacists is to help people make the best use of medications. They strive to assist pharmacists in fulfilling this mission. The ASHP represents pharmacists who practice in:

- Health maintenance organizations (HMOs)
- Hospitals
- Home care agencies
- Long-term care facilities
- Other institutions

Pharmacy Technician Certification Board (PTCB)

1100 15th St NW, Suite 730
Washington, DC 20005-1707
(800) 363-8012
http://www.ptcb.org

Established in 1941, the PTCB develops, maintains, promotes, and administers a high-quality certification and recertification program for pharmacy technicians.

Pharmacy Technician Educators Council (PTEC)

6144 Knyghton Road
Indianapolis, IN 46220
(317) 962-0919
http://www.rxptec.org
Established in 1991, the PTEC strives to assist the profession of pharmacy in preparing high-quality, well-trained personnel through education and practical training.

United States Pharmacopeia (USP)

12601 Twinbrook Parkway
Rockville, MD 20852-1790
(800) 227-8772
http://www.usp.org
Established in 1820, the USP is the official public standards-setting authority for all prescription and over-the-counter medications, dietary supplements, and other health-care products manufactured and sold in the United States.

National Pharmacy Technicians Association (NPTA)

PO Box 683148
Houston, TX 72268
(888) 247-8700
http://www.pharmacytechnician.org
Established in 1991, the NPTA serves to provide education, advocacy, and support to pharmacy technicians.

Top 200 Prescription Drugs

Table D-1 lists the top 200 drugs by prescription.

TABLE D–1 Top 200 Drugs by Prescription

Number	Generic Name	Trade Name
1	hydrocodone w/APAP	Lortab
2	atorvastatin	Lipitor
3	amoxicillin	Trimox
4	lisinopril	Prinivil, Zestril
5	hydrochlorothiazide	Diaqua, Esidrix
6	atenolol	Tenormin
7	azithromycin	Zithromax
8	furosemide	Lasix
9	alprazolam	Xanax
10	metoprolol	Toprol XL
11	albuterol	Proventil
12	amlodipine	Norvasc
13	levothyroxine	Synthroid
14	metformin	Glucophage, Glucophage XR
15	sertraline	Zoloft
16	escitalopram	Lexapro
17	ibuprofen	Motrin
18	cephalexin	Keflex
19	zolpidem	Ambien
20	prednisone	Deltasone
21	esomeprazole magnesium	Nexium

Number	Generic Name	Trade Name
22	triamterene	Dyrenium
23	propoxyphene	Darvon-N
24	simvastatin	Zocor
25	montelukast	Singulair
26	lansoprazole	Prevacid
27	metoprolol tartrate	Lopressor
28	fluoxetine	Prozac
29	lorazepam	Ativan
30	clopidogrel	Plavix
31	oxycodone w/APAP	Percocet
32	salmeterol	Serevent
33	alendronate	Fosamax
34	venlafaxine	Effexor, Effexor XR
35	warfarin	Coumadin
36	paroxetine hydrochloride	Paxil
37	clonazepam	Klonopin
38	cetirizine	Zyrtec
39	pantoprazole	Protonix
40	potassium chloride	K-Lor
41	acetaminophen/codeine	Tylenol-Codeine
42	trimethoprim/ sulfamethoxazole	Septra, Bactrim
43	gabapentin	Neurontin
44	conjugated estrogens	Premarin

(continued)

TABLE D-1 (continued)

Number	Generic Name	Trade Name
45	fluticasone	Flonase
46	trazodone	Desyrel
47	cyclobenzaprine	Flexeril
48	amitriptyline	Elavil, Enovil
49	levofloxacin	Levaquin
50	tramadol	Ultram
51	ciprofloxacin	Cipro
52	amlodipine/benazepril	Lotrel
53	ranitidine	Zantac
54	fexofenadine	Allegra
55	levothyroxine	Levoxyl
56	valsartan	Diovan
57	enalapril	Vasotec
58	diazepam	Valium
59	naproxen	Anaprox, Naprosyn
60	fluconazole	Diflucan
61	lisinopril/HCTZ	Zestoretic
62	potassium chloride	Klor-Con
63	ramipril	Altace
64	bupropion	Wellbutrin, Wellbutrin XL
65	celecoxib	Celebrex
66	sildenafil citrate	Viagra
67	doxycycline hyclate	Vibra-Tabs
68	ezetimibe	Zetia
69	rosiglitazone maleate	Avandia
70	lovastatin	Mevacor
71	valsartan/ hydrochlorothiazide	Diovan HCT
72	carisoprodol	Soma, Rela
73	drospirenone/ethinyl estradiol	Yasmin 28
74	allopurinol	Alloprin
75	clonidine	Catapres
76	methylprednisolone	Medrol
77	pioglitazone hydrochloride	Actos

Number	Generic Name	Trade Name
78	pravastatin	Pravachol
79	risedronate sodium	Actonel
80	norelgestromin/ethinyl estradiol	Ortho Evra
81	citalopram hydrobromide	Celexa
82	verapamil	Calan
83	isosorbide mononitrate	Ismotic
84	penicillin V	Penicillin VK
85	glyburide	Micronase
86	amphetamine sulfate	Adderall
87	mometasone furoate	Nasonex
88	folic acid	Folacin
89	quetiapine fumarate	Seroquel
90	losartan potassium	Cozaar
91	fenofibrate	Tricor
92	carvedilol	Coreg
93	methylphenidate hydrochloride	Concerta
94	ezetimibe	Vytorin
95	insulin glargine	Lantus
96	promethazine hydrochloride	Phenergan
97	meloxicam	Mobic
98	tamsulosin hydrochloride	Flomax
99	rosuvastatin	Crestor
100	glipizide	Glucotrol XL
101	norgestimate/ethinyl estradiol	Ortho Tri-Cyclen Lo
102	temazepam	Restoril
103	omeprazole	Prilosec
104	cefdinir	Omnicef
105	albuterol	Ventolin
106	risperidone	Risperdal
107	rabeprazole sodium	AcipHex
108	digoxin	Digitek
109	spironolactone	Aldactone

(continued)

TABLE D-1 (continued)

Number	Generic Name	Trade Name
110	valacyclovir hydrochloride	Valtrex
111	latanoprost	Xalatan
112	metformin	Fortamet
113	losartan potassium/ hydrochlorothiazide	Hyzaar
114	quinapril	Accupril
115	clindamycin	Cleocin
116	metronidazole	Flagyl
117	triamcinolone	Atolone
118	topiramate	Topamax
119	ipratropium bromide/ albuterol sulfate	Combivent
120	benazepril	Lotensin
121	gemfibrozil	Lopid
122	irbesartan	Avapro
123	glimepiride	Amaryl
124	norgestimate/ethinyl estradiol	Trinessa
125	estradiol	Alora, Climara
126	hydroxyzine	Atarax
127	metoclopramide	Maxolon, Reglan
128	fexofenadine/ pseudoephedrine	Allegra-D 12 Hour
129	doxazosin mesylate	Cardura
130	warfarin	Jantoven
131	glipizide	Glucotrol
132	diclofenac sodium	Voltaren
133	raloxifene hydrochloride	Evista
134	diltiazem	Cardizem, Tiazac
135	tolterodine tartrate	Detrol, Detrol LA
136	meclizine	Antivert, Bonamine
137	glyburide/metformin	Glucovance
138	atomoxetine	Strattera
139	duloxetine hydrochloride	Cymbalta
140	nitrofurantoin	Furadantin

Number	Generic Name	Trade Name
141	promethazine/codeine	Phenergan with Codeine
142	olmesartan medoxomil	Benicar
143	mirtazapine	Remeron
144	bisoprolol/HCTZ	Ziac
145	desloratadine	Clarinex
146	oxycodone	OxyContin
147	minocycline	Arestin, Minocin
148	sumatriptan	Imitrex
149	nabumetone	Relafen
150	olanzapine	Zyprexa
151	lamotrigine	Lamictal
152	cetirizine/ pseudoephedrine	Zyrtec-D
153	polyethylene glycol	Glycolax
154	acyclovir	Zovirax
155	propranolol	Inderal
156	triamcinolone acetonide	Nasacort AQ
157	donepezil hydrochloride	Aricept
158	butalbital/ acetaminophen/caffeine	Fioricet
159	niacin	Niaspan
160	azithromycin	Zmax
161	divalproex sodium	Depakote
162	buspirone	Buspar
163	norgestimate/ethinyl estradiol	Tri-Sprintec
164	methotrexate	Amethopterin, MTX
165	oxycodone	Roxicodone
166	budesonide	Rhinocort Aqua
167	olmesartan medoxomil hydrochlorothiazide	Benicar HCT
168	terazosin	Hytrin
169	metaxalone	Skelaxin
170	clotrimazole/ betamethasone	Lotrisone
171	tadalafil	Cialis
172	irbesartan/ hydrochlorothiazide	Avalide

(continued)

TABLE D-1 (continued)

Number	Generic Name	Trade Name
173	fexofenadine	Telfast®
174	norgestimate/ethinyl estradiol	Ortho Tri-Cyclen
175	bupropion hydrochloride	Wellbutrin, Zyban
176	benzonatate	Tessalon
177	olopatadine hydrochloride	Patanol
178	quinine	Quinamm, Quiphile
179	diltiazem hydrochloride	Cartia XT
180	insulin lispro, rDNA origin	Humalog
181	paroxetine	Paxil CR
182	levonorgestrel and ethinyl estradiol	Aviane
183	digoxin	Lanoxin
184	amphetamine	Adderall XR
185	famotidine	Pepcid, Pepcid AC
186	digoxin	Lanoxicaps

Number	Generic Name	Trade Name
187	levothyroxine	Levothroid
188	nifedipine	Adalat, Procardia
189	nortriptyline	Aventyl
190	hydrocodone polistirex/ chlorpheniramine polistirex	Tussionex
191	nitroglycerin	NitroQuick
192	phenytoin	Dilantin
193	budesonide	Endocet
194	etodolac	Lodine, Lodine XL
195	atenolol/chlorthalidone	Tenoretic
196	phentermine	Fastin
197	tramadol/ acetaminophen	Ultracet
198	tizanidine	Zanaflex
199	cetirizine hydrochloride/ pseudoephedrine	Virlix-D
200	divalproex sodium	Depakote ER

Vitamins

Table E–1 lists the common vitamins and covers their main actions and the deficiency symptoms.

TABLE E–1   Vitamins

Vitamin	Main Actions	Deficiency Symptoms
Water-Soluble		
B_1 (thiamine or thiamin)	Plays a role in carbohydrate metabolism and is essential for normal metabolism of the nervous system, heart, and muscles.	Loss of appetite, irritability, tiredness, nervous disorders, sleep disturbance, beriberi, loss of coordination, and paralysis.
B_2 (riboflavin)	Is essential for certain enzyme systems in the metabolism of fats and proteins.	Impaired growth, weakness, lip sores, cracks at corners of mouth, cheilosis, photophobia, cataracts, anemia, and glossitis.
B_3 (niacin or nicotinic acid)	Part of two enzymes that regulate energy metabolism.	Pellagra (dermatitis, diarrhea, dementia, and death), gastrointestinal and mental disturbances.
B_4 (adenine)	Important for cellular respiration and protein synthesis.	Retarded growth rate, blood and skin disorders, constipation, nausea, GI disturbances, etc.
B_5 (pantothenic acid or calcium panthothenate)	Is essential for fatty acid metabolism, manufacture of sex hormones, utilization of other vitamins, functioning of the nervous system and adrenal glands, and normal growth and development.	Fatigue, headaches, nausea, abdominal pain, numbness, tingling, muscle cramps, respiratory infection susceptibility, peptic ulcers.
B_6 (pyridoxine)	Aids enzymes in the synthesis of amino acids and is essential for proper growth and maintenance of body functions.	Anemia, neuritis, anorexia, nausea, depressed immunity, and dermatitis.
B_7 (biotin, formerly "Vitamin H")	Is essential for the breakdown of fatty acids and carbohydrates, and for the excretion of the waste products of protein breakdown.	Not common, but may involve the intestinal tract, skin, hair, CNS, and PNS.
B_8 (inositol)	Plays an important role as the structural basis of secondary messengers in eukaryotic cells.	Eczema, hair loss, constipation, eye abnormalities, and raised cholesterol.

(continued)

TABLE E–1 (continued)

Vitamin	Main Actions	Deficiency Symptoms
B_9 (folic acid or folacin)	Is essential for cell growth and the reproduction of red blood cells.	Anemia, and spina bifida in fetal development.
B_{10} [betaine or para-aminobenzoic acid (PABA)]	Is an intermediate in the bacterial synthesis of folate.	GI disturbances, premature graying of hair, pancreatic enzyme deficiencies, and rickettsial infections.
B_{11} (choline, a form of folic acid)	Needed for structural integrity and signaling roles for cell membranes, synthesis of acetylcholine, and as a major source for methyl groups.	Retarded growth and various anemias.
B_{12} (cobalamin or cyanocobalamin)	Aids in hemoglobin synthesis, is essential for normal functioning of all cells, and is important in energy metabolism.	Pernicious anemia and neurological disorders.
C (ascorbic acid or L-ascorbate)	It protects the body against infections and helps heal wounds.	Scurvy (gingivitis, loose teeth, slow wound healing), decreased resistance to infections, joint tenderness, dental caries, bleeding gums, bruising, hemorrhage, and anemia.
Fat-Soluble		
A (retinol or carotene)	Contributes to the maintenance of epithelial cells and mucous membranes, is important for night vision, and also necessary for normal growth, development, reproduction, and adequate immune response.	Retarded growth, susceptibility to infection, dry skin, night blindness, xerophthalmia, abnormal GI function, dry mucous membranes, degeneration of spinal cord and peripheral nerves.
D (cholecalciferol or calcitriol)	Essential for the normal formation of bones and teeth, aids in reabsorption of calcium and phosphorus, and regulates blood levels of calcium.	Rickets and osteomalacia.
E (tocopherol)	It prevents oxidative destruction of vitamin A in the intestine, and is essential for normal reproduction, muscle development, and resistance of RBCs to hemolysis; also helps to maintain normal cell membranes.	Neurological problems as a result of poor nerve conduction and anemia.
K (phylloquinone or phytomenadione)	Essential to blood-clotting.	Hemorrhage.

Self Evaluation Tests Answer Keys

Self-Evaluation

Test 1

1. C	35. D	68. D
2. B	36. B	69. A
3. A	37. A	70. B
4. C	38. D	71. D
5. B	39. A	72. D
6. D	40. B	73. C
7. C	41. C	74. C
8. A	42. B	75. C
9. A	43. A	76. C
10. A	44. C	77. D
11. C	45. B	78. B
12. D	46. B	79. A
13. D	47. D	80. C
14. B	48. D	81. C
15. A	49. C	82. D
16. C	50. C	83. B
17. A	51. D	84. B
18. C	52. C	85. B
19. A	53. A	86. A
20. D	54. B	87. D
21. B	55. B	88. D
22. C	56. B	89. B
23. C	57. D	90. B
24. A	58. C	91. C
25. C	59. C	92. C
26. B	60. D	93. A
27. D	61. B	94. D
28. B	62. A	95. D
29. A	63. B	96. C
30. D	64. C	97. D
31. C	65. D	98. B
32. C	66. D	99. B
33. B	67. B	100. A
34. A		

Test 2

1. D	35. D	68. D
2. A	36. D	69. B
3. A	37. A	70. B
4. D	38. D	71. B
5. B	39. C	72. D
6. D	40. C	73. D
7. C	41. C	74. B
8. C	42. C	75. A
9. D	43. C	76. B
10. A	44. B	77. A
11. C	45. A	78. D
12. B	46. D	79. B
13. C	47. B	80. A
14. A	48. C	81. C
15. D	49. B	82. A
16. D	50. C	83. A
17. A	51. C	84. D
18. C	52. C	85. B
19. B	53. A	86. C
20. D	54. B	87. D
21. A	55. D	88. A
22. D	56. C	89. C
23. D	57. C	90. D
24. B	58. A	91. A
25. B	59. C	92. D
26. C	60. B	93. B
27. D	61. C	94. C
28. C	62. B	95. D
29. D	63. C	96. B
30. C	64. B	97. C
31. C	65. A	98. A
32. B	66. C	99. B
33. C	67. D	100. A
34. D		

Test 3

1. B	35. A	68. D
2. C	36. B	69. B
3. B	37. A	70. C
4. D	38. C	71. C
5. C	39. A	72. A
6. B	40. B	73. B
7. A	41. D	74. B
8. D	42. C	75. D
9. A	43. B	76. A
10. C	44. B	77. B
11. C	45. D	78. D
12. C	46. C	79. A
13. D	47. C	80. C
14. A	48. D	81. D
15. C	49. B	82. A
16. A	50. C	83. D
17. D	51. C	84. B
18. D	52. C	85. A
19. C	53. D	86. C
20. C	54. B	87. A
21. A	55. C	88. B
22. B	56. D	89. D
23. C	57. A	90. C
24. D	58. C	91. B
25. A	59. B	92. C
26. C	60. A	93. D
27. B	61. C	94. A
28. B	62. B	95. B
29. D	63. B	96. A
30. A	64. C	97. B
31. B	65. D	98. C
32. D	66. D	99. C
33. D	67. B	100. D
34. C		

Test 5

1. D	19. B	37. B
2. B	20. D	38. D
3. A	21. A	39. B
4. C	22. A	40. A
5. B	23. D	41. C
6. D	24. B	42. A
7. A	25. D	43. B
8. B	26. C	44. A
9. C	27. C	45. D
10. B	28. C	46. B
11. B	29. A	47. B
12. D	30. A	48. C
13. D	31. B	49. B
14. A	32. C	50. A
15. A	33. C	51. D
16. C	34. D	52. C
17. D	35. A	53. B
18. C	36. C	54. D

55. C	71. C	86. B
56. D	72. B	87. B
57. C	73. C	88. D
58. A	74. A	89. C
59. B	75. A	90. A
60. B	76. A	91. D
61. C	77. C	92. B
62. A	78. C	93. C
63. A	79. A	94. B
64. D	80. A	95. C
65. B	81. B	96. A
66. D	82. B	97. C
67. D	83. C	98. B
68. B	84. B	99. D
69. A	85. A	100. C
70. B		

Test 5

1. C	35. B	68. A
2. B	36. C	69. B
3. C	37. C	70. A
4. C	38. D	71. C
5. C	39. B	72. B
6. B	40. C	73. B
7. B	41. C	74. B
8. B	42. A	75. C
9. A	43. D	76. D
10. C	44. B	77. B
11. B	45. D	78. C
12. D	46. C	79. C
13. C	47. A	80. B
14. B	48. D	81. D
15. C	49. D	82. A
16. C	50. B	83. C
17. B	51. B	84. C
18. C	52. D	85. D
19. D	53. A	86. A
20. C	54. B	87. C
21. C	55. B	88. B
22. C	56. B	89. D
23. D	57. B	90. D
24. D	58. A	91. B
25. C	59. C	92. C
26. A	60. A	93. C
27. D	61. C	94. C
28. C	62. A	95. B
29. C	63. C	96. C
30. A	64. A	97. D
31. D	65. C	98. A
32. C	66. C	99. C
33. C	67. B	100. A
34. B		

Test 6

1. C	35. A	68. D
2. B	36. C	69. B
3. D	37. C	70. A
4. B	38. D	71. D
5. B	39. D	72. C
6. A	40. A	73. D
7. B	41. C	74. B
8. D	42. C	75. B
9. D	43. D	76. C
10. A	44. A	77. A
11. C	45. D	78. A
12. C	46. B	79. D
13. C	47. A	80. B
14. A	48. C	81. B
15. B	49. D	82. C
16. C	50. B	83. B
17. D	51. A	84. D
18. C	52. B	85. C
19. A	53. B	86. C
20. D	54. D	87. A
21. B	55. B	88. C
22. B	56. B	89. A
23. A	57. A	90. B
24. C	58. B	91. B
25. A	59. C	92. B
26. B	60. A	93. A
27. C	61. C	94. D
28. D	62. D	95. C
29. C	63. C	96. C
30. D	64. A	97. A
31. D	65. B	98. D
32. A	66. A	99. D
33. D	67. B	100. A
34. B		

ANSWER KEYS

Review Questions

Chapter 1

1. C	5. D	8. D
2. C	6. B	9. C
3. A	7. B	10. A
4. B		

Chapter 2

1. D	5. D	8. D
2. B	6. D	9. B
3. B	7. D	10. A
4. B		

Chapter 3

1. D	5. B	8. A
2. C	6. D	9. D
3. D	7. B	10. C
4. B		

Chapter 4

1. A	5. A	8. C
2. C	6. D	9. C
3. D	7. C	10. B
4. D		

Chapter 5

1. C	5. C	8. D
2. D	6. D	9. C
3. D	7. B	10. B
4. A		

Chapter 6

1. B	5. A	8. B
2. C	6. C	9. C
3. D	7. A	10. C
4. C		

Chapter 7

Calculations

1. 0.901	7. −0.206	13. 22.1
2. 6.39	8. 18.373	14. 2.046
3. 21.809	9. 41.87	(rounded)
4. 21.56	10. 0.00268	15. 40
5. 5.08	11. 8.928	16. 20
6. 2.95	12. 12.19881	

Conversions

1. 1:5	3. 1:3	5. 1:200
2. 3:4	4. 1:20	

Proportions

1. X = 13.5	3. X = 16	5. X = 125
2. X = 57.86	4. X = 45	
(rounded)		

Percentages

1. 12	3. 7.5	5. 60
2. 500	4. 10.8	

Equivalents

1. 1	3. 1 ½	5. 2 ⅔
2. 3	4. 32	

Metric Conversions

1. 9,000	3. 1.5	5. 8.010
2. 20	4. 16	

Apothecary Conversions

1. 3	3. 2	5. 24
2. 2	4. 0.00	

Temperature Conversions

1. 98.6	3. 16.7 (rounded)	5. 40
2. 33.9 (rounded)	4. 108.9 (rounded)	6. 212

Multiple Choice

1. A	15. A	29. C
2. A	16. B	30. C
3. D	17. D	31. D
4. B	18. D	32. D
5. D	19. D	33. C
6. B	20. D	34. B
7. C	21. A	35. B
8. A	22. B	36. D
9. C	23. D	37. C
10. D	24. C	38. C
11. B	25. C	39. B
12. C	26. A	40. D
13. D	27. D	
14. B	28. A	

Chapter 8

1. D	5. A	8. C
2. B	6. D	9. D
3. B	7. C	10. B
4. C		

Chapter 9

1. B	6. B	11. B
2. D	7. C	12. D
3. D	8. D	13. A
4. A	9. A	14. D
5. A	10. C	15. C

Chapter 10

1. A	5. D	8. D
2. A	6. C	9. B
3. D	7. C	10. D
4. B		

Chapter 11

1. D	5. A	8. D
2. A	6. B	9. C
3. B	7. B	10. A
4. B		

Chapter 12

1. D	5. A	8. C
2. B	6. B	9. B
3. C	7. A	10. D
4. D		

Chapter 13

1. A	5. C	8. D
2. D	6. B	9. B
3. C	7. B	10. C
4. C		

Chapter 14

1. A	5. A	8. D
2. D	6. B	9. B
3. C	7. C	10. C
4. B		

Chapter 15

1. A	5. C	8. A
2. D	6. D	9. D
3. D	7. B	10. D
4. B		

Chapter 16

1. D	5. B	8. B
2. A	6. D	9. A
3. D	7. D	10. D
4. C		

Chapter 17

1. B	5. B	8. C
2. C	6. C	9. A
3. B	7. C	10. C
4. A		

Chapter 18

1. B	5. B	8. A
2. C	6. D	9. C
3. D	7. C	10. B
4. C		

Chapter 19

1. D	5. D	8. C
2. B	6. B	9. C
3. C	7. D	10. B
4. A		

Chapter 20

1. B	5. C	8. A
2. A	6. D	9. C
3. B	7. B	10. B
4. A		

Glossary

A

Abbreviations – shortened forms of words

Absorption – the movement of a drug from its site of administration into the bloodstream

Accounting – a system of recording, classifying, and summarizing financial transactions for preparing a pharmacy budget

Acetylcholine (ACh) – a neurotransmitter

Acromegaly – abnormal growth of the bones of the face, hands, feet, and soft tissue that occurs after puberty; it is caused by hypersecretion of human growth hormone (hGH)

Addition – the combined effect of two agents, which is equal to the sum of the effects of each drug taken alone

Aerosol – a liquid or fine powder that is sprayed in a fine mist

Agonist – a drug or other agent that mimics the effects of another substance or function; it may do this by interacting at a cellular receptor

Agranulocyte – a type of white blood cell, including monocytes and lymphocytes, that is characterized by an absence of granules in its cytoplasm (cellular fluid)

Allergens – nonparasitic antigens that can stimulate a hypersensitivity reaction in certain individuals; common allergens include dust, pollen, and pet dander

Alveolar sacs (alveoli) – the cluster-like air sacs located at the end of each alveolar duct in the lungs

Ambulatory care – medical care given on an outpatient basis where patients can come and go to an office or clinic for diagnostic tests or treatments

Amortize – to spread the cost of services out over a period of several years

Ampule – a sealed glass container that usually contains a single dose of medicine; the top of the ampule must be broken off to open the container

Anaphylactic reaction – a life-threatening allergic reaction that is characterized by a drop in blood pressure and with difficulty in breathing

Anatomy – the branch of science that deals with the structure of body parts, their forms, and their organization

Angina pectoris – also called *angina*, this condition describes chest pain as a result of lack of blood and oxygen supply to the heart muscle, usually because of vessel obstruction or spasm

Antagonism – the combined effect of two drugs that is less than the effect of either drug taken alone

Antagonists – drugs or other agents that block the effects of other substances or functions

Antibiotics – drugs or therapeutic agents used to treat infections caused by bacteria and other microorganisms, slowing or stopping their growth

Antihistamines – drugs that counteract the action of histamine

Antitussive – a drug that reduces coughing, also called a *cough suppressant*

Anxiety – a physiological state consisting of fear, apprehension, or worry

Apothecary system – a very old English system of measurement that has been slowly replaced by the metric system; its basic units of measurement are the grain, dram, and minim

Arabic numbers – standard numerical numbers

Arrhythmias – various conditions of abnormal electrical heart activity; the heart may beat too fast, too slow, or irregularly

Arthus reaction – an acute local inflammatory reaction that occurs at the site of injection

Aseptic technique – preparing and handling sterile products in a manner that prevents microbial contamination

Assignment of benefits – an authorization to an insurance company to make payment directly to the pharmacy or physician

Autoclave – a sterilizing machine that uses a combination of heat, steam, and pressure to sterilize equipment

Automation – the automatic control or operation of equipment, processes, or systems that often involves robotic machinery controlled by computers; machinery controlled by computers that completes many tasks involved in prescription compounding and dispensing

Auxiliary labels – extra labels applied to products in the pharmacy that may contain warnings, cautions, directions for use, and dietary or other information

B

Bacteria – single-celled microorganisms that can exist either as independent organisms or as parasites

Bactericidal – capable of killing bacteria; a term that is typically used in reference to antiseptics, disinfectants, or antibiotics

Bacteriostatic – capable of stopping the growth and reproduction of bacteria; a term that is typically used to describe antibiotics that inhibit bacterial growth without killing the bacteria

Barrier precautions – types of personal protective equipment (PPE) used to minimize risk of exposure

Batch repackaging – the reassembling of a specific dosage and dosage form of medication at a given time

Beyond-use date – a date after which a product is no longer effective and should not be used

Bioavailability – measurement of the rate of absorption and total amount of drug that reaches systemic circulation

Bioethics – a discipline dealing with the ethical and moral implications of biological research and applications

Biohazard symbol – an image or object that serves as an alert that there is a risk such as ionizing radiation or harmful bacteria or viruses to organisms

Biometrics – a system of computerized identification that involves the use of hardware devices that read users' fingerprints

Biotransformation (metabolism) – the conversion of a drug within the body

Bowman's glomerular capsule – a sac that collects fluids from the blood in the glomerulus of the kidney and, through a process called *ultrafiltration*, processes the fluids to form urine

Bronchodilators – agents that relax the smooth muscle of the bronchial tubes

Buccal – pertaining to the inside of the cheek

C

Caplet – a tablet shaped like a capsule

Capsule – a solid dosage form in which the drug is enclosed in either a hard or soft shell of soluble material

Cassette system – the most common type of prescription filling robot; it can hold hundreds or thousands of dosage units

Cation – a positively charged atom

Cellular hypersensitivity reaction – the result of the activity of many leukocyte actions; the T1 lymphocytes become sensitized by their first contact with a specific antigen; subsequent exposure to an antigen stimulates multiple reactions aimed at destroying or inactivating the offending antigen

Centers for Medicare and Medicaid Services (CMS) – the federal organization that administers Medicare and Medicaid; its official Web site offers information about programs, statistical highlights, and the full text of laws and regulations affecting the agency; formerly known as the Health Care Financing Administration (HCFA)

Centrally acting skeletal muscle relaxants – also known as *spasmolytics*, these agents alleviate musculoskeletal pain and spasms to reduce spasticity (continual muscular contraction)

CHAMPVA – Civilian Health and Medical Program of the Veterans Administration; a program to cover medical expenses of the dependent spouse and children of veterans with total, permanent service-connected disabilities

Chancre – a painless, highly contagious lesion or ulceration that may form during the primary stage of syphilis

Chemical sterilization – a method of cleaning equipment used for instruments that cannot be exposed to the high temperatures of steam sterilization

Class A prescription balance (electronic balance) –a two-pan device that may be used for weighing small amounts of drugs (not more than 120 g)

Compounding – mixing drugs or other substances specifically for a certain patient

Compounding slab – made of ground glass, a plate with a hard, flat, and nonabsorbent surface for mixing compounds

Computerized physician order entry system (CPOE) – a computerized system in which the physician inputs the medication order directly for electronic receipt in the pharmacy

Conical graduates –used for measuring liquids, devices that have wide tops and wide bases and taper from the top to the bottom

Conjunctiva – mucous membranes of the eyes

Conjunctivitis – an inflammation of the outermost layer of the eye and inner surface of the eyelid, usually due to an allergic reaction or an infection; commonly called "pink eye"

Controlled substance medication order – an order for medication (generally narcotics) that requires monitored documentation of procurement, dispensation, and administration

Convulsion – an intense, involuntary muscle contraction or spasm, as is commonly seen during a seizure condition

Coordination of benefits – the prevention of duplicate payment for the same service

Copayment – most policies have a coinsurance, or cost-sharing requirement, that is the responsibility of the insured

Corpus callosum – a structure in the longitudinal fissure of the brain that connects the left and right cerebral hemispheres

Corticosteroids – the most potent and consistently effective anti-inflammatory agents that are currently available for relief of respiratory conditions

Cost control – the implementation of managerial efforts to achieve cost objectives

Counter balance – a device, a double-pan balance, capable of weighing much larger quantities, up to about 5 kg

Cream – a semisolid emulsion of either the oil-in-water or the water-in-oil type, ordinarily intended for topical use

Cylindrical graduates – used for measuring liquids, devices that have narrow diameters that are the same from top to base

Cytotoxic reaction – severe damage to or destruction of cells by a substance

D

Data – the raw facts the computer can manipulate

Deductible – a specific amount of money that a policyholder must pay each year before the policy benefits begin (e.g., $50, $100, $300, or $500)

Denominator – the total number of parts of the whole

Dependence – the total psychophysical state of one addicted to drugs or alcohol who must receive an increasing amount of the substance to prevent the onset of withdrawal symptoms

Demand/stat medication order – an order for medication to be given in rapid response to a specific medical condition

Department of Public Health (DPH) – an organization in which sciences, skills, and beliefs are combined and directed to the maintenance and improvement of the health of all the people

Dependents – the insured's spouse and children under the terms of the policy

Diaphragm – a sheet of muscle, important in the process of respiration, that extends across the bottom part of the rib cage

Disinfection – ability to kill microorganisms on the surfaces of various items

Dispensing fee – a pricing mechanism calculated by adding the operating expenses and profit margin and dividing by the total work units, either unit doses or inpatient prescriptions

Distal convoluted tubule – a portion of the nephron of the kidney, located between the loop of Henle and the collecting ducts, that is partly responsible for regulating potassium, sodium, calcium, and pH

Distribution – the process by which blood leaves the bloodstream and enters the tissues of the body

Diverticulum – a hollow or fluid-filled sac, many of which exist in the walls of the colon

Dividend – the number that is being divided; in 6 ÷ 3, the dividend is 6

Divisor – a number that is used to divide another; in 6 ÷ 3, the divisor is 3

Dram – a unit of weight in the apothecary system; 1 dram = 60 grains

Drip rate – the speed at which intravenous fluids are infused

Drive-through – an external site at a pharmacy that can be accessed by driving up in a vehicle

Drug control – a method of ensuring optimal safety in the distribution and use of medications by providing knowledge, procedures, controls, ethics, and other standards

Drug Enforcement Agency (DEA) – the government agency responsible for enforcing the controlled substance laws and regulations of the United States

Dry heat sterilization – a method of sterilization that uses heated dry air at a temperature of 320°F to 365°F (160°C to 180°C) for 90 minutes to 3 hours

Dry powder inhaler (DPI) – a device used to deliver medication in the form of micronized powder into the lungs

Dwarfism – the abnormal underdevelopment of the body that occurs during childhood commonly because of hyposecretion of growth hormone; it may be caused by many other conditions, including kidney disease and metabolic disorders

Dysuria – painful or difficult urination, often with a burning or stinging sensation

E

Edema – swelling of any tissue with the interstitial fluid surrounding the cells

Eligibility – the specific terms of coverage under a policy

Elixir – a clear, sweetened, hydroalcoholic liquid intended for oral use

Emergency medication order – an order for a medication to be given in response to a medical emergency

Emphysema – a chronic pulmonary disease characterized by loss of elasticity of the lung tissue often caused by exposure to toxic chemicals and smoke from tobacco products

Emulsion – a preparation containing two liquids that cannot be mixed; one liquid is dispersed, in the form of very small globules, throughout the other; a suspension containing two different liquids and an agent that holds them together

Endorphins – naturally occurring substances that, as part of the body's pain control system, mimic many of the effects of narcotics

Enteral – passing through the gastrointestinal tract to be absorbed by the body

Enteral nutrition – feedings, other than normal eating, given into the gastrointestinal system; usually applied to specially prepared liquid feedings

Ethics – the branch of philosophy that deals with the distinction between right and wrong and with the moral consequences of human actions

Exposure control plan – a written procedure for the treatment of persons exposed to biohazardous or similar chemically harmful materials

Extemporaneous – a medication that is made based upon a particular set of circumstances or criteria

Extemporaneous compounding – the preparation, mixing, assembling, packaging, and labeling of a drug product based on a prescription order from a licensed practitioner for the individual patient

Extremes – the two outside terms in a proportion

F

Fire safety plan – a written procedure that includes fire extinguisher locations, fire alarm pull-box locations, sprinkler system location, exit signs, and clear directions to the quickest and safest way to exit a building during an emergency

First-pass metabolism – the degree to which a drug is chemically altered as it circulates through the liver for the first time

Floor stock system – a system of drug distribution in which drugs are issued in bulk form and stored in medication rooms on patient care units

Fraction – an expression of division of a whole into parts

G

Gas sterilization – the use of a gas such as ethylene oxide to sterilize medical equipment

Gel – a jelly or the solid or semisolid phase of a colloidal solution

Gelcap – an oil-based medication that is enclosed in a soft gelatin capsule

Genitourinary – referring to the reproductive organs and the urinary system

Geometric dilution – when mixing agents, the medicament is first mixed with an equal weight of diluent; a further quantity of diluent equal in weight to the mixture is then incorporated; this process is repeated until all the diluent has been mixed in

Gigantism – abnormally large growth of body tissue as a result of an excess of growth hormone during childhood

Glomerulus – a knot of capillaries, surrounded by the Bowman's glomerular capsule, that receives blood from the renal circulation; each glomerulus and its surrounding capsule make up a renal corpuscle

Glucagon – an important hormone, antagonistic to insulin, involved in carbohydrate metabolism

Grain – the basic unit of weight in the apothecary system

Gram – the basic unit of weight in the metric system

Granule – a very small pill, usually gelatin- or sugar-coated, containing a drug to be given in a small dose

Granulocyte – a type of white blood cell, having granules in its cytoplasm, that includes neutrophils, eosinophils, and basophils

Group purchasing – many hospitals working together to negotiate with pharmaceutical manufacturers to get better prices and benefits based on the ability to promise high-committed volumes

H

Half-life – the time it takes for the plasma concentration to be reduced by 50%

Hardware – the parts of the computer that you can touch

Hazard communication plan – a plan that informs employees about all hazardous materials found in the workplace; it should outline employee training and an exposure control plan, should list locations of any existing hazards, and should explain hazard signs and chemical labels, especially the use and location of personal protective equipment and how to handle various types of spills

Health insurance – a contract between a policyholder and an insurance carrier or government program to reimburse the policyholder for all or a portion of the cost of medical care that health-care professionals render

Hormones – regulating and controlling organ and tissue activity, natural chemical substances secreted into the bloodstream from the endocrine glands; chemical messengers that move through the blood or through cells that carry signals; examples include estrogen, testosterone, melatonin, epinephrine, dopamine, and insulin

Hospice – originally a facility, usually within a hospital, intended to care for the terminally ill, in particular, by providing physical comfort to the patient and emotional support and counseling to the patient and the family

Hospital pharmacy – the provision of pharmaceutical services within an institutional or hospital setting

Hyperlipidemia – the presence of raised or abnormal levels of lipids (fatty molecules) or lipoproteins (biochemicals containing proteins and lipids) in the blood

Hyperpyrexia – extremely high temperature, which is considered a medical emergency

Hypersensitivity – an unpredictable reaction to a drug due to the development of antibodies against it; also known as an allergy

Hypertension – an abnormal increase in arterial blood pressure; high blood pressure; a chronic elevation of the blood pressure equivalent to or greater than 140/90

Hypnosis – a trance-like state, resembling sleep, or an increased tendency to sleep

Hypnotic – a drug that induces sleep; often used to treat insomnia and in surgical anesthesia

I

Idiosyncratic reaction – experience of a unique, strange, or unpredicted reaction to a drug

Implants (pellets) – implants or pellets are dosage forms that are placed intradermally, or under the skin, by means of minor surgery or special injections; the term *implant* may also mean a device inserted surgically under the skin for delivery of medications

Independent practice association (IPA) – a type of health maintenance organization (HMO) in which the HMO contracts directly with physicians, who continue in their existing practices

Independent purchasing – the director of the pharmacy or buyer directly contacts and negotiates pricing with pharmaceutical manufacturers

Inscription – the main part of a prescription, which indicates the drugs and quantities of each to be used in the mixture

Insulin – a hormone, secreted when the blood glucose level rises, that extensively affects metabolism and many other body systems

Intradermal injection – an injection that is given between the layers of the skin; a dose of an agent administered between the layers of the skin

Intramuscular injection – an injection that is given inside a muscle; normally used in the context of an injection given into a muscle

Intravenous injection – an injection that is given into a vein; most commonly used in the context of an injection given directly into a vein

Intrinsic factor – a glycoprotein produced by the parietal cells of the stomach; it is required for the body's absorption of vitamin B_{12}

Inventory – the stock of medications a pharmacy keeps immediately on hand

Inventory control – controlling the amount of product on hand to maximize the return on investment

Inventory turnover rate – a mathematical calculation of the number of times the average inventory is replaced over a period of time (usually annually)

Investigational medication order – an order for a medication given under direction of research protocols that also require strict documentation of procurement, dispensing, and administration

Invoice – a form describing a purchase and the amount due

J

Joint Commission – a not-for-profit organization that sets standards to ensure effective quality services (e.g., optimal standards for the operation of hospitals)

Just-in-time (JIT) inventory system – an inventory control system in which stock arrives just before it is needed

L

Laminar airflow hood – a system of circulating filtered air in parallel-flowing planes in hospitals or other health-care facilities; reduces the risk of airborne contamination and exposure to chemical pollutants in surgical theaters, food preparation areas, hospital pharmacies, and laboratories

Law – a principle or rule that is advisable or obligatory to observe

Legend drug – a medication that may be dispensed only with a prescription; also known as a *prescription drug*

Levigate – to grind into a smooth substance with moisture

Liter – the basic unit of volume in the metric system

Liver – one of the largest organs in the digestive system; among its many functions are manufacture of plasma proteins, storage of starch and vitamins, and the production of bile salts

Long-term care – a wide range of health and health-related support services

Long-term care pharmacy organization – an organization involving a licensed professional pharmacy or practice that provides medications and clinical services to long-term care facilities and their residents

Loop of Henle – a U-shaped structure, whose function is to reabsorb water and ions from the urine, that is located in the proximal convoluted tubule of the kidney

Lozenge (troche) – a small, disk-shaped tablet composed of solidifying paste containing an astringent, an antiseptic, or an oil-based drug used for local treatment of the mouth or throat; held in the mouth until dissolved

M

Mail-order pharmacy – a licensed pharmacy that uses the mail or other carriers (e.g., overnight carriers or parcel services) to deliver prescriptions to patients

Markup fee system – a pricing mechanism in which the price charged to the patient is calculated by adding a percentage markup, in addition to a dispensing fee, to the drug's acquisition cost

Means – the two inside terms in a proportion

Mechanical digestion – the breakdown of large food particles into smaller pieces by chewing and the mashing actions of muscles in the digestive tract

Mediastinum – the central compartment of the thoracic cavity within the chest

Medicaid – a federal/state medical assistance program to provide health insurance for specific populations

Medical asepsis – complete destruction of organisms after they leave the body

Medicare – a federal health insurance program created as part of the Social Security Act

Medication – a substance used in the treatment or maintenance of an illness

Medication order – the written order for particular medications and services to be provided to a patient within an institutional setting; physicians, nurse practitioners, or physician's assistants write medication orders

Melanin – a dark pigment that provides skin color and absorbs ultraviolet radiation in sunlight

Melanoma – malignant tumor of bottom-layer skin cells (melanocytes), which may also affect the eyes or bowels

Meningitis – inflammation of the meninges that cover the brain and spinal cord

Meniscus – the crescent-shaped curvature of the surface of a liquid standing in a narrow vessel such as a graduate; meaning "moon-shaped body"; indicates that the level of the liquid will be slightly higher at the edges

Metastatic – relating to the spread of cancer from one body part to another

Metastasis – the process by which cancer spreads from one part of the body to a distant site or sites

Meter – the basic unit of length in the metric system

Metered dose inhaler (MDI) – a hand-held pressurized device used to deliver medications for inhalation

Metric system – the preferred system of measurement throughout the world; it is based on the decimal system

Minim – the basic unit of volume in the apothecary system

Mixture – an incorporation of two or more substances, without chemical union, in which the physical characteristics of each component are retained

Modems – devices used to transfer information from one computer to another

Mortar – a cup-shaped vessel in which materials are ground or crushed

N

National Drug Code (NDC) – a unique and permanent product code assigned to each new drug as it becomes available in the marketplace; identifying the manufacturer or distributor, the drug formulation, and the size and type of its packaging

National Formulary (NF) – a database of officially recognized drug names

Nebulizer – a device used for inhalation that uses a small machine to convert a solution into a mist that a patient inhales through a facemask or a mouthpiece

Neurohormones – hormones produced and released by neurons

Neurohypophysis – posterior lobe of the pituitary gland

Neuromuscular blocking agents – drugs that block neuromuscular transmission at the neuromuscular junction; they cause paralysis of specific skeletal muscles

Neuron – the basic cell of the nervous system

Normal flora – the nonpathogenic microorganisms that exist externally and internally in humans

Nuclear pharmacy – a pharmacy that is specially licensed to work with radioactive materials; previously called radiopharmacy

Numerator – the number of the parts of the whole being considered

O

Ointment – a semisolid preparation that usually contains medicinal substances and is intended for external application

Opiates – narcotic alkaloids found in opium

Opioids – chemical substances that have morphine-like action in the body; commonly used for pain relief

Oral – pertaining to the mouth; medication given by mouth

Osteoporosis – a bone disease characterized by reduced bone mineral density, leading to an increased risk of fracture

Ounce – a unit of weight in the apothecary system; 1 oz = 8 drams

Overpayment – payment by the insurer or by the patient of more than the amount due

Over-the-counter (OTC) – a medication that may be purchased without a prescription directly from the pharmacy

P

Parasites – organisms that live in or on another organism and take their nourishment from the host organism

Parenteral – a dosage form usually intended to be administered intravenously, subcutaneously, or intramuscularly

Parenteral nutrition – a combination of amino acids, dextrose, fats, vitamins, minerals, electrolytes, and water administered intravenously that is capable of providing all the nutrients needed to sustain life

Parkinson's disease – a degenerative disorder of the central nervous system that usually impairs motor skills, speech, and other functions

Patient prescription system – a system of drug distribution in which a nurse supplies the pharmacy with a transcribed medication order for a particular patient and the pharmacy prepares a 3-day supply of the medication

Percent – a term referring to "hundredths"; a *percentage* is a fraction whose denominator is understood to be 100; for example, 25/100 is also expressed as 25 percent or 25%

Percentage markup system – a system of establishing price that assumes that total operating expenses are directly related to the acquisition cost

Peritonitis – inflammation of the peritoneum (the membrane lining parts of the abdominal cavity and visceral organs)

Perpetual inventory systems – inventory control systems that allow monthly drug use reviews

Personal digital assistants (PDAs) – handheld electronic devices that interface with computer systems to handle data such as patient charts, medical histories, and drug information

Personal protective equipment – gloves, gowns, face shields, goggles, laboratory coats, and masks used to protect against blood, bodily fluids, and microorganisms

Pestle – a solid device that is used to crush or grind materials in a mortar

Phagocytize – to engulf solid particles within a cell membrane to form an internal food vacuole (membrane-bound compartment)

Pharmaceutical care – the provision of drug therapy for the purpose of achieving the improvement of a patient's quality of life, which includes the prediction, detection, and resolution of drug therapy-related problems

Pharmacist – an individual who is educated and licensed to dispense drugs and to provide drug information to patients and other health-care providers

Pharmacodynamics – the study of the biochemical and physiological effects of drugs

Pharmacokinetics – the study of the absorption, distribution, metabolism, and excretion of drugs

Pharmacy – the art and science of dispensing and preparing medication and providing drug-related information to the public

Pharmacy compounding – the preparation, mixing, assembling, packaging, or labeling of a drug or device

Pharmacy technician – an individual who helps licensed pharmacists provide medications and other health-care products to patients

Pharmacy Technician Certification Board – a national organization that provides certification to pharmacy technicians based on a national examination and on continuing education

Physiology – the branch of science that deals with how body parts work and what they accomplish

Piggyback – a medication, many times an antibiotic, that is added into an IV bag of medication

Pill – a small, globular mass of soluble material containing a medicinal substance to be swallowed

Pipette – a long, thin, calibrated hollow tube, which is made of glass and used for measuring liquids

Placebo – an inactive substance or preparation used as a control in an experiment or test to determine the effectiveness of a medicinal drug

Placebo effect – a measurable improvement in a patient's health or condition after a placebo has been administered; it is thought to occur because of the patient's belief in the supposed drug administered

Plaster – a solid preparation that can be spread when heated and that becomes adhesive at body temperature

Point-of-sale (POS) master – an inventory control system that allows inventory to be tracked as it is used

Point-of-service (POS) – payment of services outside of an insurance plan at the time the service is rendered

Policies and procedures manual – a formal document specifying guidelines for operations of an institution; a set of standard procedural statements or documents that aid an organization in operating effectively and efficiently and support the overall goals of the organization

Policy limitation – policies that exclude certain types of coverage

Policy terms and financial obligations – policy that becomes effective only after the company offers the policy and the person accepts it and pays the initial premium

Potentiation – an effect that occurs when a drug increases or prolongs the action of another drug, the total effect being greater than the sum of the effects of each used alone

Powder – a dry mass of minute separate particles of any substance

Preauthorization – the requirement of notification and permission to receive additional types of services before one obtains those services

Preferred provider organization (PPO) – a managed care organization that contracts with a group of providers, who are called *preferred providers*, to offer services to the managed care organization's members

Prefix – a part of a word structure that occurs before or in front of the word and modifies the meaning of the root

Premium – the cost of the coverage that the insurance policy contains; this may vary greatly, depending on the individual's age and health and the type of insurance protection

PRN (as needed) medication order – an order for medication to be given in response to a specific defined parameter or condition

Professionalism – the conduct or qualities characterized by or conforming to the technical or ethical standards of a profession; exhibiting a courteous, conscientious, and generally businesslike manner in the workplace

Protected health information (PHI) – all of a patient's private information that is protected from unauthorized use

Proportion – the equality of two ratios

Purchase order – the document created when an order is placed

Q

Quotient – the answer to a division problem

R

Radiopharmaceutical – a drug that is or has been made radioactive to treat diseases (e.g., radioactive iodine) but most commonly used as diagnostic agents

Ratio – an expression that compares relative quantities

Receptor – the cell to which a drug has an affinity

Renal corpuscle – a filtration unit in the kidney that consists of a knot of capillaries (the glomerulus) surrounded by the Bowman's glomerular capsule

Renal tubule – the portion of the nephron in the kidney that contains the tubular fluid filtered through the glomerulus

Root – the main part of a word that gives the word its central meaning

S

Sanitization – a process of cleansing to remove undesirable debris

Scheduled intravenous (IV)/total parenteral nutrition (TPN) solution order – an order for medication given via an injection; these medications are to be prepared in a controlled (sterile) environment

Scheduled medication order – an order for medication that is to be given on a continuous schedule

Sebaceous – skin glands that secrete an oily substance called "sebum"

Sedation – the use of a sedative agent to reduce excitement, nervousness, or irritation; commonly prior to a medical procedure

Sedatives – substances that suppress the central nervous system and induce calmness, relaxation, drowsiness, or sleep

Seizure – a temporary, abnormal electrical brain condition that results in abnormal neuronal activity; it can affect mental ability and cause convulsions; recurrent, unprovoked seizures are called *epilepsy*

Side effect – an outcome other than that intended; most commonly used in the context of drug therapy in which a side effect is an unwanted consequence of the drug in use

Signa – a Latin term meaning "mark" or "label"; abbreviated as "Sig," the signa is the part of a prescription where the prescriber writes the directions for use

Software – a set of electronic instructions that tell the computer what to do

Solution – the incorporation of a solid, a liquid, or a gas into a liquid

Solvent – a liquid vehicle in which active ingredients are dissolved; a liquid drug that does not require shaking before use

Specific affinity – the attraction a drug has for particular cells

Spirits – an alcoholic or hydroalcoholic solution of volatile substances

Spores – forms that some bacteria assume to increase their chances of surviving heat, dehydration, and antiseptics or antibiotics

Squamous cell carcinoma – malignant tumor of the flat, scale-like cells of the most superficial layer of the skin, mouth, esophagus, bladder, prostate, lungs, and vagina

Standard precautions – a set of guidelines for infection control

Standards – established by authority, custom, or general consent as a model or example; something set up and established by authority as a rule for the measure of quantity, weight, extent, value, or quality

Starter kit – a group of medicines provided to a hospice patient to treat urgent problems that develop in the last days or weeks of life

State board of pharmacy (BOP) – the organization responsible for the registration of pharmacists, pharmacy interns, and pharmacy technicians

Sterile product – a substance that contains no living microorganisms

Sterilization – complete destruction of all forms of microbial life

Subcutaneous injection – the administration of a medication by means of a needle and syringe into the layer of fat and blood vessels beneath the skin

Sublingual – pertaining to the area under the tongue

Subscriber – the individual or organization protected in case of loss under the terms of an insurance policy

Subscription – the part of a prescription that includes directions for compounding; physicians seldom include it today, leaving product preparation to the pharmacist's discretion

Suffix – a word ending that modifies the meaning of the root

Superscription – the part of a prescription below the patient's name and address that begins the body of the actual prescription; it is usually designated by the symbol "Rx"

Suppository – a small, semisolid bullet-shaped dosage for ready insertion into a body orifice, other than the oral cavity (e.g., rectum, urethra, or vagina); made of a substance, usually medicated, that is semisolid at ordinary temperature but melts at body temperature

Surgical asepsis – the complete destruction of organisms before they enter the body

Suspension – a class of pharmacopeial preparations of finely divided, undissolved drugs dispersed in liquid vehicles for oral or parenteral use

Synergism – a combined action of two or more agents that produces an effect greater than would have been expected from the two agents acting separately

Syrup – a liquid preparation in a concentrated aqueous solution of a sugar used for medicinal purposes or to add flavor to a substance

T

Tablet – a solid dosage form containing medicinal substances with or without suitable diluents

Tablet triturate – solid, small, and usually cylindrically molded or compressed tablets

Tare – the weight of an empty capsule used to compare with the full capsule

Telepharmacy – the use of electronic communications to bring pharmacy services to patients who are not located close to a pharmacy

Third-party payer – the fee for services provided is paid by an insurance company and not by the patient

Time limit – the amount of time from the date of service to the date (deadline) the claim can be filed with the insurance company

Time purchase – the time that the purchase order was made but not paid at the time of purchase

Tincture – an alcoholic solution prepared from vegetable materials or from chemical substances

Tolerance – increasing resistance to the usual effects of an established dosage of a drug as a result of continued use

Topical – pertaining to a drug that is applied to the surface of the body

Total parenteral nutrition (TPN) – an intravenous feeding that supplies all the nutrients necessary to sustain life

Toxemia – the presence of toxins in the blood

Transdermal drug delivery (TDD) – pertaining to a passage through the skin; dosage forms that release minute amounts of a drug at a consistent rate

TRICARE – a federally funded comprehensive health benefits program for dependents of personnel serving in the uniformed services

Triturate – to reduce to a fine powder by friction

U

Unit-dose drug distribution system – a system for distributing medication in which the pharmacy prepares single doses of medications for a patient for a 24-hour period

Unit-of-use packaging – the packaging from bulk containers into patient-specific containers

Uremia – an illness accompanying renal failure involving urinary waste products contained in the blood

Urethritis – inflammation of the urethra caused by an infection such as chlamydia

U.S. Pharmacopeia (USP) – a database of drugs and their preparation that serves as the standard for drugs used in the United States

V

Venae cavae – the collective name for the superior and inferior *vena cava*, which are the veins that return deoxygenated blood from the body into the right atrium of the heart

Vial – a small glass or plastic bottle intended to hold medicine

Virus – the smallest of all microorganisms, it cannot grow or reproduce apart from a living cell

W

Waiting period – the period of time that an individual must wait to become eligible for insurance coverage (e.g., 30 days) before coverage commences or for a specific benefit

Want book – a list of drugs and devices that routinely need to be reordered

Water – a mixture of distilled water with an aromatic volatile oil

Wheal – a bump on the skin

Index